melodie cool'

Clinical and Diagnostic Procedures in Obstetrics and Gynecology

PART A: OBSTETRICS

REPRODUCTIVE MEDICINE

A Series of Textbooks and Monographs

Editors

Professor E. Malcolm Symonds, M.D.
Chairman
Department of Obstetrics and Gynecology
The University of Nottingham
Nottingham, England

Professor Frederick P. Zuspan, M.D.
Chairman
Department of Obstetrics and Gynecology
The Ohio State University
Columbus, Ohio

Volume 1 Practical Pediatric and Adolescent Gynecology, Sir John Dewhurst

Volume 2 Amniotic Fluid and Its Clinical Significance, edited by Merton Sandler

Volume 3 Clinical Sexuality, edited by Stephen F. Pariser, Stephen B. Levine, and Malcolm L. Gardner

Volume 4 Clinical and Diagnostic Procedures in Obstetrics and Gynecology. Part A: Obstetrics. Part B: Gynecology. Edited by E. Malcolm Symonds and Frederick P. Zuspan

Other volumes in preparation

Clinical and Diagnostic Procedures in Obstetrics and Gynecology

PART A: OBSTETRICS

Edited by

E. MALCOLM SYMONDS, M.D.
Department of Obstetrics and Gynecology
The University of Nottingham
Nottingham, England

FREDERICK P. ZUSPAN, M.D.
Department of Obstetrics and Gynecology
The Ohio State University
Columbus, Ohio

MARCEL DEKKER, INC.   New York and Basel

Library of Congress Cataloging in Publication Data

Main entry under title:

Clinical and diagnostic procedures in obstetrics and
gynecology.

(Reproductive medicine ; 4-)
Contents: pt. A. Obstetrics.
Includes bibliographical references and indexes.
1. Obstetrics—Addresses, essays, lectures.
2. Gynecology—Addresses, essays, lectures.
I. Symonds, E. M. (Edwin Malcolm) II. Zuspan,
Frederick P., [date]. III. Series. [DNLM:
A. Obstetrics—Methods. B. Gynecology—Methods.
W1 RE213P v. 4 / WQ 100 C6405]
RG101.067 1983   618   83-5341
ISBN 0-8247-1778-3 (pt. A)

MARCEL DEKKER, INC.

270 Madison Avenue, New York, New York 10016

Current printing (last digit):

10 9 8 7 6 5 4 3 2 1

PRINTED IN THE UNITED STATES OF AMERICA

About the Series

Some time ago, the publishers, Marcel Dekker, Inc., interested us in developing a new concept in editing a series of books on *Reproductive Medicine,* which would span the Atlantic Ocean by the editors' representation in Europe and in the United States. In general, many of the books destined for production in this series that relate specifically to obstetrics and gynecology will have an author or editor in Europe and one in the United States. This concept of bringing contributors from the two continents together permits an academic discussion of similar and dissimilar points of view in relation to any given topic.

Marcel Dekker is particularly well placed to introduce such a concept. Their previous experience has involved the development and merging of European publishing experience into the United States scene. At present, Dekker's main office is in New York, with supplementary offices in Europe. Hence, the amalgamation of authors, under joint editorship, and the established experience for distribution of books, have made this experiment one that is particularly well adapted to these publishers. This is a new venture in medical publishing and one which will grow and develop with time.

E. Malcolm Symonds, M.D.
Frederick P. Zuspan, M.D.

Preface

The editors believed that it was appropriate to develop a book that would be most helpful to those who care for the female patient, and especially for those who practice obstetrics and gynecology. A large number of very fine textbooks are devoted to obstetrics and gynecology, but none of them has exactly what we have aimed for in this book. Two volumes comprise *Clinical and Diagnostic Procedures in Obstetrics and Gynecology*: Part A addresses obstetrics, and Part B focuses on gynecology. The book is not designed to be a comprehensive, overall treatise, but is intended specifically to identify in depth clinical procedures that are performed for women who are either pregnant (Part A) or nonpregnant (Part B). We have deliberately excluded references to major operative procedures since it was not our intention to complete a compendium of obstetric or gynecologic surgery.

The editors have chosen gifted authors from Europe and the rest of the world, as well as the United States, to contribute in-depth chapters on specific procedures. We have intentionally not had authors from different parts of the world write on corresponding topics, but on related topics, and they tend to supplement and complement each other. We owe a considerable debt of gratitude to all of the contributors for agreeing to participate and for their prompt provision of manuscripts.

E. Malcolm Symonds, M.D.

Frederick P. Zuspan, M.D.

Contributors

RICHARD L. BERKOWITZ,* M.D., Associate Professor, Department of Obstetrics and Gynecology, Yale University School of Medicine, and Director, High Risk Obstetrical Service, Yale-New Haven Medical Center, New Haven, Connecticut

GEOFFREY CHAMBERLAIN, F.R.C.S., F.R.C.O.G., Consultant Gynecologist and Resident Medical Officer, Queen Charlotte's Hospital for Women, London, England

J. SELWYN CRAWFORD, F.F.A., R.C.S., F.R.C.O.G., Consultant Anesthestist, Department of Anesthesia, Birmingham Maternity Hospital, Birmingham, England

LACHLAN J. C. de CRESPIGNY, M.D., F.R.A.C.O.G., Obstetrician and Ultra-soundologist, Ultrasound Department, University of Melbourne, Royal Women's Hospital, Melbourne, Australia

MAURICE L. DRUZIN, M.D., Department of Obstetrics and Gynecology, New York Hospital-Cornell Medical Center, New York, New York

DENYS V.I. FAIRWEATHER, M.D., F.R.C.O.G., Professor and Director, Department of Obstetrics and Gynaecology, School of Medicine, University College London, England

*Present affiliation: Professor, Department of Obstetrics and Gynecology and Director, Division of Maternal-Fetal Medicine, Mt. Sinai School of Medicine, New York, New York.

EMILY A. FINE, M.D., Resident in Obstetrics and Gynecology, Yale-New Haven Hospital, New Haven, Connecticut

CHARLOTTE GIBBINGS, M.D., B.S., D.A., Resident Surgical Officer, Queen Charlotte's Hospital for Women, London, England

PAUL GRECH, M.D., F.R.C.R., Consultant Radiologist, X-ray Department, Northern General Hospital, Sheffield, England

ZEPH J. R. HOLLENBECK, M.D., Professor, Department of Obstetrics and Gynecology, The Ohio State University College of Medicine, Columbus, Ohio

JAY D. IAMS, M.D., Assistant Professor, Department of Obstetrics and Gynecology, The Ohio State University College of Medicine, Columbus, Ohio

IAN RICHARD JOHNSON, D.M., M.R.C.O.G., Department of Obstetrics and Gynecology, University Hospital, Queen's Medical Centre, Nottingham, England

JOSEPH J. KRYC, M.D., Assistant Professor, Department of Anesthesiology, Assistant Professor, Department of Obstetrics and Gynecology, and Director of Obstetrical Anesthesia, The Ohio State University, Columbus, Ohio

BRIAN A. LIEBERMAN, M.B., B.Ch., M.R.C.O.G., Consultant Obstetrician and Gynecologist, St. Mary's Hospital, Manchester, England

IAN MacGILLIVRAY, F.R.C.O.G., F.R.C.P., Regius Professor, University of Aberdeen, Aberdeen, Scotland

DAVID R. MILLAR, F.R.C.S., F.R.C.O.G., Consultant Obstetrician and Gynecologist, Jessop Hospital for Women, Sheffield, England

A. D. MILNER, M.D., F.R.C.P., D.C.H., Professor of Pediatric Respiratory Medicine, Department of Child Health, University Hospital, Nottingham, England

EBERHARD MUELLER-HEUBACH, M.D., Associate Professor, Department of Obstetrics and Gynecology, University of Pittsburgh School of Medicine, Magee-Women's Hospital, Pittsburgh, Pennsylvania

RICHARD H. PAUL, M.D., Professor, Department of Obstetrics and Gynecology, Los Angeles County/University of Southern California School of Medicine, Los Angeles, California

E. J. QUILLIGAN, M.D., Professor, Obstetrics and Gynecology, University of California at Irvine, Irvine, California

HUGH P. ROBINSON, M.R.C.O.G., F.R.A.C.O.G., Obstetrician-in-Charge, Ultrasound Department, University of Melbourne, Royal Women's Hospital, Melbourne, Australia

RUDY E. SABBAGHA, M.D., Associate Professor, Department of Obstetrics and Gynecology, Northwestern University Medical School, and Ultrasound Department, Northwestern University and Memorial Hospital, Prentice Maternity Center, Chicago, Illinois

PHILIP J. STEER, M.D., M.R.C.O.G., Senior Lecturer and Honorary Consultant, Department of Obstetrics and Gynecology, St. Mary's Hospital Medical School, London, England

HERMAN P. van GEIJN, M.D., Assistant Professor, Department of Obstetrics and Gynecology, Academisch Ziekenhuis der Vrije Univesiteit, Amsterdam, The Netherlands

H. VYAS, M.B., M.R.C.P., Research Fellow, Department of Neonatal Medicine and Surgery, City Hospital, Nottingham, England

B. ALAN WALDRON, M.B., B.S., F.F.A.R.C.S., Consultant Anesthetist, Department of Anesthesia, Nottingham City Hospital and University Hospital, Nottingham, England

R. H. T. WARD, M.A., F.R.C.O.G., Consultant Obstetrician and Gynecologist and Senior Lecturer, Department of Obstetrics and Gynecology, School of Medicine, University College London, England

FREDERICK P. ZUSPAN, M.D., Professor and Chairman, Department of Obstetrics and Gynecology, The Ohio State University, Columbus, Ohio

Contents

Clinical and Diagnostic Procedures in Obstetrics and Gynecology

PART A: OBSTETRICS

1

Diagnostic Ultrasound: Physics, Instrumentation, Early Pregnancy, and Placental Localization

HUGH P. ROBINSON and LACHLAN J. C. de CRESPIGNY / University of Melbourne, Royal Women's Hospital, Melbourne, Australia

A basic principle of current medical practice is that patient management and treatment should be based, where possible, on reliable information and accurate diagnosis. Until recently, this has been a difficult principle to follow in the field of obstetrics due to the relative inaccessibility of the uterus and its contents to established investigative techniques. As a result the management of patients with prenatal problems was often empirical at best, and at worst quite inappropriate. Among recent advances in obstetrical care, the introduction of diagnostic ultrasound has been a major contributor to improvements in prenatal diagnosis. The information this noninvasive technique provides when obtained by a skilled operator often influences patient management quite dramatically. Hence, the obstetrician may now have the option of adopting a more active approach to an individual problem which would otherwise have been untenable. In this context it is important to stress that the quality of the information provided is only as good as the experience of the operator and the care with which the scan is performed. We adhere to what we consider the ideal: all examinations are performed by medical personnel (almost all specialist obstetricians), who report their findings immediately on completion of the examination.

In this chapter a brief outline of the background physics of diagnostic ultrasound and current instrumentation will be given, followed by a description of the current role of this modality in early pregnancy problems and prepartum hemorrhage, together with our views on how the information gained in these areas is most appropriately integrated into patient management.

1

PHYSICS AND INSTRUMENTATION

Ultrasound may be simply defined as sound that lies above the range of human hearing, the upper level of which seldom exceeds 20,000 cycles/sec, that is, 20 kilohertz (KHz). In medical practice the sound frequencies used for diagnostic purposes are generally at least two orders of magnitude higher, in the region of 2-20 megahertz (MHz). However, despite this vast difference in frequency, ultrasound has most of the properties of audible sound. In an identical way to the echo produced by a person shouting towards a cliff face, an echo results when ultrasound reaches a plane within the body where tissues with different densities (acoustic impedances) are in apposition. It is these returning echoes, amplified and processed in various ways, on which the diagnostic modality of echography is based. Unlike audible sound, ultrasound can be produced such that it may be confined to a relatively narrow beam. This directional property allows the investigator to "point" an ultrasound beam down into the patient knowing that the echo information received will come only from along the path of the beam, with minimal extraneous information derived from adjacent areas. One other major difference between audible sound and ultrasound is that the latter will not penetrate a gas medium. As a result, diagnostic ultrasound has very limited application in the diagnosis of bowel and lung disorders and, unless a full-bladder technique is employed to push away gas-filled intestines, structures and organs within the pelvis are inaccessible to "visualization."

Very simply, ultrasound is produced by the excitation of an unusual type of crystal, known as a piezoelectric crystal, which, in response to an electrical "blow," vibrates at a predetermined frequency. By appropriate means the transmitting phase is made to last for only a very small fraction of a second. This mechanical "sound" energy, in the ultrasound range, then passes through the patient where it is progressively degraded by absorption, refraction, and reflection. Reflected echoes derived from structures in the path of the incident beam travel back to the piezoelectric crystal, which is now in its receiver phase. When reflected sound strikes the crystal, it resonates in sympathy and a potential difference is produced across its surface. The small voltages thus produced are amplified and processed in various ways and the information presented as a line of dots of varying intensity on suitable oscilloscope or television displays. Knowing the average speed of sound through living tissues (1540 m/sec) and the time delay between the ultrasound leaving the crystal and each of a series of echoes returning, it is a simple calculation for the equipment to determine the depth at which each echo originated and to plot the derived information on the display screen. In this way the single line of echo information is produced (Fig. 1).

At this point it is appropriate to consider the various types of ultrasound equipment in current use in obstetrical and gynecological practice. These may be conveniently divided into the *static* and the *real-time* scanners.

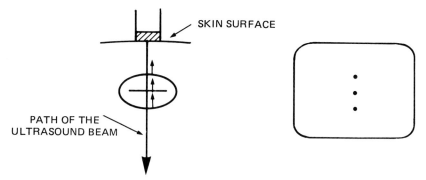

Figure 1. A single pulse of ultrasound is shown passing down through a fetal head. In this schematic diagram there are returning echoes from the anterior and posterior skull walls and from the midline structures. These echoes are represented by dots on the display screen.

With the static scanners, the ultrasound probe assembly is moved manually over the patient's skin. The position and orientation of the probe is recorded automatically by appropriate sensing devices. In this way each line of echoes received from within the patient can be recorded on the screen at a corresponding position and angle (Fig. 2). Most machines generate more than 1,000 of these lines each second. As the probe is moved over the patient the resulting lines on the screen merge, giving an integrated two-dimensional "slice" of information: the echogram or B-scan image. In contrast with real-time equipment, this system provides a constant frame of reference and, therefore, spatial orientation, of a single or a series of echograms. Again, because of the probe reference system, scanning and rescanning along a predetermined plane is greatly facilitated, which allows greater accuracy when measurements of the fetus are desired. Finally, static scanners allow viewing of interfaces from a number of different angles (compound scanning). Since echoes of maximal size are obtained when the incident ultrasound beam strikes tissue planes at right angles, the compounding facility provides the optimal method of outlining organs and structures under scrutiny.

There are three basic forms of real-time scanners; the linear-array, the mechanical, and the phased-array. The last mentioned is not yet in widespread use and will not be discussed. The scanning head of the linear array may house up to 100 or more individual transducer elements arranged sequentially along its long axis. In most currently available equipment the elements are activated in banks of four or five so that the ultrasound wavefront from each element will interact with those from its neighbors to produce a fairly narrow focused integral "beam." In its simplest form, elements 1-4 will be fired, and the returning echoes duly received; elements 2-5 will next be activated, and so on

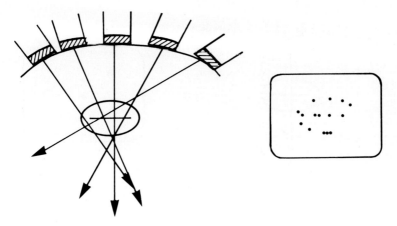

Figure 2. With movement of the transducer over the skin surface, individual pulses of ultrasound are directed from different positions and angles at the fetal skull, giving a two-dimensional slice of information.

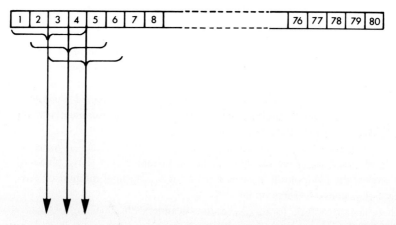

Figure 3. In the simple form of linear-array firing sequence as shown in this diagram, banks of four transducers are fired simultaneously such that each group produces a single "integral" beam of ultrasound energy.

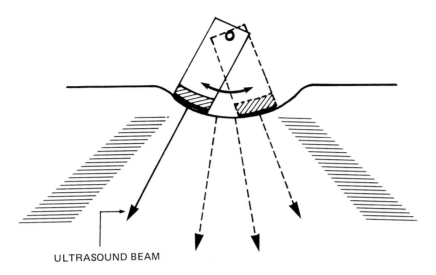

ULTRASOUND BEAM

Figure 4. In this form of mechanical real-time scanner, a single transducer is made to oscillate about its base. As the face of the transducer sweeps across the skin surface, pulses of ultrasound are generated and returning echoes received within each very small arc of movement. A wedge-shaped area of information is thus produced. In reality, a thin membrane separates the transducer and the skin.

(Fig. 3). This sequence is continued along the line of elements to complete one single frame comprising approximately the same number of lines of echo information as there are transducer elements in the array. The number of lines can be greatly increased by simple duplication and by sequencing the firing order in groups of four and five alternately. The sequence of firing then goes back to the beginning, the complete process being repeated about 25 times/sec, more quickly than the 15 frames/sec flicker rate of the human eye. Thus, the image becomes continuous or "real-time." Mechanical real-time scanners, on the other hand, have been designed with either a single oscillating transducer (Fig. 4), or a rotating wheel with three or more transducer crystals mounted on its periphery (Fig. 5). With both a wedge-shaped area of information is "viewed." Real-time scanners offer the advantages of ease of use, rapid survey of an organ or area of interest, and positive identification of moving or pulsating structures. However, since they produce only what is known as simple scans (in contrast with compound scans), the quality of the images produced is usually not as good as those achieved with

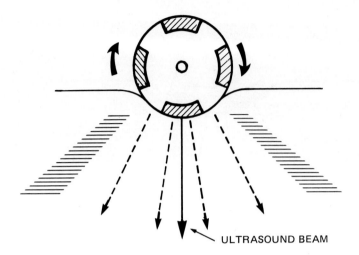

Figure 5. In this rotating system, there are four transducers in the assembly. Information is received from each as it comes in contact with and rotates across the skin surface. In a similar way to the oscillating transducer system, only a wedge-shaped area is examined.

the static scanners, although recent improvements in technology and design have improved picture quality greatly. In addition, since the frame of reference is that of the transducer, orientation may be difficult, especially when scanning an advanced pregnancy where only limited sections can be viewed at one time. Finally, due to the inherent limitations of their resolution capabilities and problems of orientating the transducer at a precise and predetermined angle and position, measurement, especially in obstetric practice, does not have precision equal to that obtainable with a static scanner (Adam et al., 1978, 1979).

EARLY PREGNANCY PROBLEMS

Before addressing the problem of the ultrasound assessment of an early pregnancy, it is relevant first to determine at what stage and how reliably the presence of a pregnancy may be confirmed. In a series of 49 patients with certain menstrual histories and periods of amenorrhea of between 35 and 42 days, an intrauterine sac was identified in 36 (Robinson, 1978). Thirty-four of these pregnancies continued normally, a diagnosis of a blighted ovum being made in the remaining two at a later examination. Of the 13 patients in whom no pregnancy was found, 10 "menstruated normally" within 2 weeks and three were later shown to have blighted ova which remained very small for date until abortion ensued. These results indicate that a careful ultra-sound examination will demonstrate the presence of a pregnancy provided that it is intrauterine, that at least 3 weeks have elapsed since conception, and that it is a normal pregnancy. These are important points when the role of ultrasound in the diagnosis or exclusion of ectopic pregnancy is considered.

Ectopic Pregnancy

With its associated potential for serious maternal morbidity and even mortality, ectopic pregnancy assumes an importance in the field of obstetrics and gynecology greatly exceeding its relative frequency. It is often difficult to diagnose on a clinical basis and, in view of its attendant risks, early surgical means of confirming or refuting the diagnosis have long been standard practice. It was not surprising, therefore, that great hope was held out for the use of diagnostic ultrasound as a means of allowing definitive diagnoses with a resulting decrease in the number of "unnecessary" laparoscopies and laparotomies. Unfortunately, while this technique has assumed an important role in this area, the results cannot be considered sufficiently reliable to be used as the sole arbiter in confirming or refuting the diagnosis.

From a practical standpoint, ultrasound should be regarded primarily as a means of determining the presence or absence of an intrauterine pregnancy. Given that there is no doubt that the structure visualized is a pregnancy and that it lies within the cavity of the uterus, then the diagnosis of an ectopic pregnancy can be virtually excluded, since the probability of a coexistent extrauterine pregnancy (approximately 1:30,000 pregnancies) is so rare as to be almost discounted. However, before diagnosing an intrauterine pregnancy, the ultrasonologist must be assured that the structure seen is not simply a blood clot or decidual cast and that the pregnancy is not outside the uterus, or lodged in the isthmus or cornual area. Should an intrauterine pregnancy be seen, the adnexa must still be examined to exclude a coincident problem that might account for the patient's symptoms, such as a twisted or ruptured cyst. However, the demonstration of an "empty" uterus by the clear visualiza-tion of a central cavity line is supportive, if circumstantial, evidence of an ectopic pregnancy in a patient whose clinical evidence suggests the diagnosis. In our own practice, when the clinical picture is not clear, we have found an elevated luteinizing hormone (LH) level (using a fast radioimmunoassay with a high cross-reactivity with human chorionic gonadotropin (HCG) (Hay et al., 1981) to be very useful when taken in conjunction with an empty uterus in deciding to undertake laparoscopy.

While the demonstration of the presence or absence of an intrauterine preg-nancy is the mainstay of the use of ultrasound in suspected ectopic pregnancies,

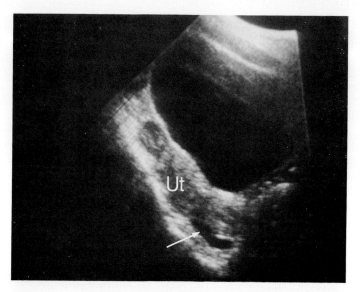

Figure 6. A patient with abdominal pain, a positive pregnancy test, and an empty uterus (Ut) on ultrasound examination. In the pouch of Douglas there was a small collection of free fluid (arrow), presumed to be blood.

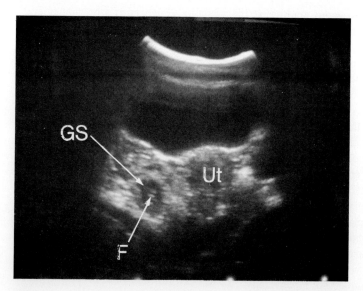

Figure 7. A transverse section showing an empty uterus (Ut) with a gestation sac (GS) containing a living fetus (F) in the adnexal area.

additional but inconstant features may lend support to the diagnosis. These include the presence of free fluid (presumptive blood) in the pelvis (Fig. 6), most readily seen in the pouch of Douglas, and the finding of an adnexal cystic mass. However, unless there is a demonstrably live fetus within such a "cyst" (a most uncommon circumstance) (Fig. 7), one must be cautious in interpreting this structure as an ectopic gestation sac. Such alternatives as a normal follicle, a corpus luteum cyst, hydrosalpinx, or an embryological or endometriotic cyst could give similar ultrasound appearances. Likewise, a chronic ectopic pregnancy is difficult to distinguish from pelvic inflammatory disease with abscess formation, or extensive endometriosis.

In a recent unpublished series from our own department, of 146 patients with clinical features suggestive of ectopic pregnancy the diagnosis was proven subsequently in 46. In 43 of these patients the uterus was demonstrated to be empty by ultrasound; the remaining three patients were initially thought to have small intrauterine blighted ova (empty sacs). However, at subsequent ultrasound examinations, the diagnoses were reversed. In 29 of the 46 patients (63%) there was clear evidence of free fluid (presumptive blood) in the pouch of Douglas and in 39 (85%) there was evidence of an adnexal mass. There were only two patients in whom an absolute diagnosis of ectopic pregnancy could be made by the unequivocal demonstration of a gestation sac containing a live fetus outside the uterus.

Bleeding in Early Pregnancy

For the purposes of this section it is assumed that the patient has an intra-uterine pregnancy and that the bleeding is from within the uterus.

Spontaneous abortion is very common, with most authors quoting rates in the order of 10% or greater. This figure, however, relates to the number of abortions occurring in patients in whom there had been good clinical and/or biochemical evidence of pregnancy. On the other hand, very much higher rates have been calculated for the *total* loss of conceptuses. Hertig and his co-workers (1959, 1967), in their classic series of studies, estimated that only 42% of pregnancies survive long enough to cause the patient to miss her expected menstrual period; of these, almost 30% abort with or without preceding clinical signs of pregnancy, giving an overall wastage rate of 60%. Similarly, Roberts and Lowe (1975), from some speculative calculations, concluded that at least 78% of conceptions are aborted. Clearly, therefore, the obstetrician in his or her management of the 10% or so of patients who have clinical evidence of spontaneous abortion is really only dealing with the "tip of the iceberg:" those pregnancies sufficiently "viable" to have grown large enough and for long enough to produce clinical signs and symptoms of pregnancy.

Almost without exception, spontaneous abortion is heralded by vaginal bleeding, a symptom which has thus come to be regarded as a very bad prognostic feature. Unfortunately, the equally large group of women who bleed in the early weeks of pregnancy but whose pregnancies continue normally is thereby subjected to considerable stress until it becomes obvious that the pregnancy is viable. Diagnostic ultrasound has assumed one of its major roles in obstetrics in this area through its ability to detect the presence or absence of fetal life.

Using Doppler equipment, where the ultrasonic beam is directed through the abdominal wall, fetal heart tones may be detected as early as 8 or 9 weeks of pregnancy and reliably from 12 weeks. With more sophisticated static B scanners it has been possible to determine the presence of fetal life from as early as 6-6½ weeks and with complete reliability from 7 weeks (Robinson, 1972). More recently, with the advent of good quality real-time scanners, the demonstration of fetal heart activity has also become feasible from around 8 weeks. These scanners also allow the visualization of fetal body and limb movements from the time of their inception between 8 and 9 weeks. Thus, ultrasound equipment in its various forms has become the most important diagnostic aid in patients who bleed in the early weeks of pregnancy. No other ancillary aid is as capable of providing the certainty of diagnosis of continuing fetal life in the first trimester and, indeed, as will be discussed below, of providing a definitive diagnosis in the event that the pregnancy is noncontinuing.

On an ultrasound basis, abortive pregnancies may be defined under the headings discussed below (Robinson, 1975).

Missed Abortions

This term includes those pregnancies in which a fetus can be clearly defined within the gestation sac but in which no fetal heart movements can be detected. In our experience, the fetus grows at a normal rate until its death, and the gestation sac continues to increase in volume thereafter, albeit at a reduced rate. Growth of the sac ceases on average some 2-3 weeks later, with spontaneous abortion ensuing within 1-2 weeks. In a series of 92 such cases (Robinson, 1978) in which the fetus was found at the time of abortion, 90% of the fetuses were estimated to have died before the 12th weeks, with the mean time of fetal death being 8½ weeks. Very few patients had a history of pain or bleeding at or around the estimated time of fetal death. The majority continued to feel pregnant and had positive results of urine pregnancy tests until shortly before the abortion occurred. For this group of noncontinuing pregnancies, a clear diagnosis using ultrasound is possible in every case given a careful and detailed examination. We are quite prepared to terminate such a pregnancy, at the parents' request, on the basis of a single examination.

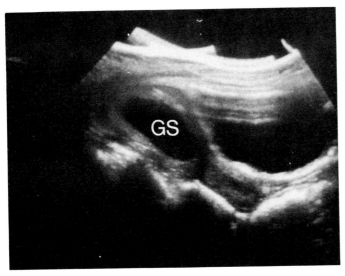

Figure 8. A patient with 12 weeks of amenorrhea but in whom the gestation sac (GS) is no more than 10 weeks' size. A careful search of the whole volume of the sac revealed no evidence of a fetus. In a sac of this size the absence of a fetus allowed a definite diagnosis of blighted ovum to be made.

Blighted Ovum

For the purposes of ultrasound diagnosis this term is used to designate a pregnancy in which no fetus can be found within the gestation sac. In all but a few of these pregnancies the gestation sac size is below the lower limit of normal for continuing pregnancies from a very early stage. However, we do not consider the finding of a "small-for-dates" gestation sac to be sufficient evidence to allow the diagnosis, since an error in "dates" could be an equally valid explanation. In view of this, a definitive diagnosis is only made at the first examination when there is absence of a fetus in a gestation sac of at least 7-8 weeks' size (Fig. 8). In a normal continuing pregnancy a fetus will be readily seen when the gestation sac has attained this size. In our view failure to meet these criteria demands a second and occasionally even a third examination, when an observed failure of normal growth of the gestation sac will allow the diagnosis. In a series of 100 blighted ova a clear diagnosis could be made in just under one-half at the time of the first examination, and in all but a few of the remainder a definitive diagnosis was possible at the second examination. We consider the diagnosis of blighted ovum to be one of the most difficult areas in early pregnancy and one which should only be made with extreme caution and acted upon only when reported by an experienced observer.

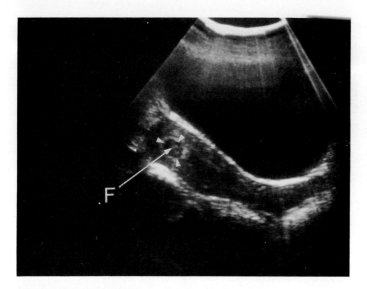

Figure 9. A pregnancy at 7 weeks by dates in which the fetus (F) is of normal size and is alive, but the gestation sac (arrowheads) is considerably smaller than expected for the period of amenorrhea. Spontaneous abortion occurred 3 days later.

Live Abortions

Included in this category are pregnancies which are clearly alive within 2 days of spontaneous abortion, or in which the fetus at the time of abortion shows no evidence of maceration. These abortions do not lend themselves to accurate prediction on the basis of data obtained at a prior ultrasound examination of heart rate, gestation sac size, or fetal length. However, for those who abort before the 12th week (early live abortions) a small gestation sac volume relative to the size of the fetus has been found to be a consistent feature (Fig. 9), although not one confined to such pregnancies (Robinson, 1975, 1978). Thus, this finding can only be considered as a worrying but not a diagnostic feature of impending abortion. For the "late live abortions" (>12 weeks), Reinold (1976) showed that sluggish fetal movements correlate well with subsequent abortion and that there is complete cessation of body and limb movements in the living fetus in the few days before spontaneous abortion.

Hydatidiform Mole

In the majority of cases, the diagnosis of hydatidiform mole leaves little room for doubt when it has the classic ultrasound appearances of a uterus filled with echoes (snowstorm appearance), and with no discernable gestation sac or fetus.

In some, however, the presence of hemorrhage within the molar tissue may engender some confusion, when one must consider the alternative diagnosis of a long-standing missed abortion with resorption of the amniotic fluid and perhaps hydropic degeneration of the trophoblast. In either event it is quite clear that the pregnancy is not a continuing one and is most appropriately managed by evacuation of the uterus.

If hydatidiform moles are excluded, the relative incidence of each of these groups in our experience is as follows: missed abortions, 40%; blighted ova, 45%; early live abortions, 3%; late live abortions, 12%. Chromosome studies performed on some of these pregnancies showed a 40% abnormality rate in the combined missed abortion/blighted ovum group, but an absence of abnormal karyotypes in the "live" abortion groups. Of further interest was that while there were cases of polyploidy and Down's syndrome in both the blighted ovum and missed abortion groups, trisomy 8 and 16s were confined to blighted ova and 45XO karyotypes to the missed abortions. While these data give some further insight into the etiology of the different groups, they must be used with caution in counseling patients.

Prognosis in Threatened Abortion

Having considered the efficacy of ultrasound, in careful hands, as a means of diagnosing and assessing the various forms of abortive pregnancies, it is relevant now to consider the prognosis for those patients who present with bleeding in early pregnancy. In a series of 367 patients who presented with bleeding in the first trimester of pregnancy and in whom the cervix was still closed, fetal heart movements were detected in 185 (50.4%) at the time of the first examination (Fig. 10). Of these pregnancies 160 (87%) continued beyond the 28th week; nine pregnancies in which fetal heart movements were detected initially, died subsequently, and the diagnosis was confirmed at a later examination. Of the 182 patients in whom no fetal heart movements were initially detected, five pregnancies continued; all five were less than 6½ weeks advanced in pregnancy at the time of the first examination. Since the sac sizes were well within the normal range for their ages, it was believed that the pregnancies were probably continuing. Later examinations confirmed fetal viability in this small group. Thus, the great majority of patients who present with a so-called "threat to abort" fall into two fairly well defined categories: those in whom an ultrasound examination shows definite or very suspicious evidence of a noncontinuing pregnancy and those in whom the pregnancy is clearly alive. The bleeding in the former group is then simply the initial stages of the spontaneous abortion process itself, while in the latter it would appear to have little prognostic significance, at least in the short term. For the long term, however, there is evidence for some increase in preterm delivery (Bennett and Kerr-Wilson, 1980) and perinatal mortality rates.

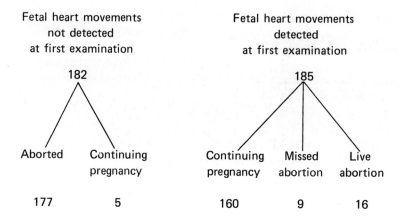

Figure 10. The outcome of 367 patients presenting with bleeding in the first trimester of pregnancy as related to the presence or absence of demonstrable fetal heart movements at the time of the first ultrasound examination.

The good prognosis for the pregnancies in which fetal heart movements were detected appeared not to be influenced by the gestational age at the onset of bleeding and the amount of blood loss; there were patients who required blood transfusions because of the volume lost and whose pregnancies continued.

Over the last few years, with improving resolution and grey-scale facilities, a proportion of patients have been identified with bleeding (approximately 5%) but whose pregnancies are ongoing in whom there is evidence of what can only be assumed to be intrauterine blood clot in association with the gestation sac (Fig. 1i). We recently reviewed the subsequent clinical course and outcome in a consecutive series of 41 such patients whose volume of the blood clot varied from 10 to 300% of the gestation sac volume. Two patients had their pregnancies terminated when their fear of fetal abnormalities could not be allayed. Of the remaining 39 pregnancies there were two spontaneous abortions, two early stillbirths (20 and 23 weeks), and a further pregnancy which was terminated on symptomatic grounds at 18 weeks because of recurrent episodes of very heavy vaginal bleeding. Prior to abortion in this last patient the uterus was demonstrated to be more than half filled with blood clot. This gives a pregnancy wastage rate of 5/39 (13%), identical to that found in our larger threatened abortion series. However, two other babies with fetal abnormalities died perinatally, one with an encephalocele and one with hydrocephaly and spina bifida cystica. Although a higher incidence of abnormality than one would expect in this small group, its significance remains doubtful. In many of our cases only 25-30% of the gestation sac was in direct contact with the

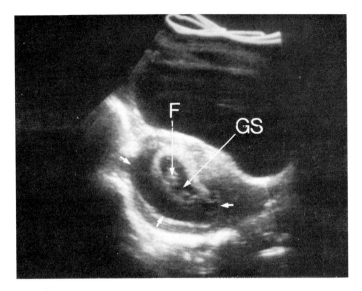

Figure 11. A patient at 8 weeks who presented with moderately heavy vaginal bleeding. The fetus (F) and gestation sac (GS) size were well within the normal limits and the fetus was demonstrated to be alive. Beneath the sac there is an echofree area (arrows) approximately twice the volume of the gestation sac which represents retained intrauterine blood clot. The pregnancy progressed normally following several weeks of intermittent vaginal staining.

uterine wall; despite this no baby was growth-retarded by weight. Finally, there were three preterm labors, giving an incidence of 9% (3/34). While the presence of intrauterine blood clot is a dramatic finding, the prognosis seems to be reasonably favorable.

PLACENTAL LOCALIZATION

Diagnostic ultrasound is the current technique of choice for placental localization in patients suspected of having a placenta previa. In experienced hands it has a high degree of accuracy (Morrison et al., 1972). Since the development of grey-scale systems, major errors in diagnosis should now be a rarity. Thus the management of patients presenting with prepartum hemorrhage can be more objective, in contrast with the previous empirical conservative approach when no or less reliable methods of placental localization were used. However, problems can and do arise in defining accurately the lowermost edge of the placenta in some patients, especially when it is sited posteriorly.

A prerequisite to accurate placental localization is a moderately full bladder. This helps to elevate the lower segment up out of the pelvis and provides a clear "window" through which to view the area. Care must be taken, on the other hand, to avoid overfilling since a grossly distended bladder may compress the anterior and posterior walls of the lower uterus thus giving a false impression of where the internal os lies. Thus, the lower edge of the placenta may appear to be much lower than in reality. Generally the entire outline of the anterior placenta is easy to define and, providing that a thick lower uterine wall is not mistaken for placental tissue, a confident diagnosis of its extent should be readily made. As mentioned above, the posterior placenta may pose difficulties especially if there is a degree of oligohydramnios and/or if the head has entered the pelvis. While there are means of overcoming these problems in most cases, given a detailed and careful examination, there remains a group of patients in whom the presence or absence of a placenta previa cannot be definitely determined. In such patients we consider it imperative that such doubt be reported and that a "best guess" not be made. Our philosophy is very much one of being prepared to accept the opprobrium of a colleague for the false-positive reports and the inconvenience thus engendered, rather than lull him or her into a false sense of security with the risk of an inappropriate and perhaps disastrous action being taken on the basis of an erroneously negative report.

"Placental Migration"

Since the placenta can be visualized just as readily in the second and early third trimesters of pregnancy as in the latter weeks, it has become possible for the first time to follow sequentially the alterations in placental site from these earlier stages. It has become evident that in a disproportionately large number of patients (±30%) the placenta appears to be previa or at least "low-lying" early in the second trimester, but only a very small number have a placenta previa at term (King, 1973; Badria and Young, 1976; Young, 1978). In an attempt to explain this phenomenon, the concept of "placental migration" has been introduced (King, 1973). While the placenta occupies one-half to one-third of the area of the uterine wall at 16 weeks, this proportion falls to no more than one-quarter at term (Young, 1978). There is, therefore, asynchrony of the growth rate of the uterus and the placenta with an overall but relative reduction in the area of placental attachment. It is proposed that the dynamic changes involved are made possible by the separation and subsequent reattachment of anchoring villi to the uterine wall. However, these dynamic processes provide no explanation for the ultrasound observation that the placenta always "migrates" in an upward direction and rarely, if ever, moves from a site in the upper segment down to or over the cervix.

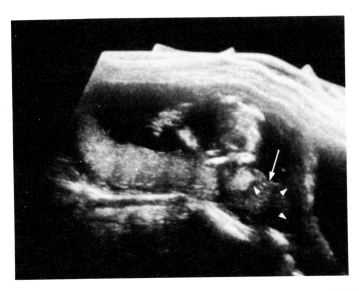

Figure 12. A posterior placenta in a pregnancy at 19 weeks. The lower edge of the placenta extends to the point marked by the arrow. The arrowheads define a localized myometrial contraction.

There must therefore be some stimulus for preferential upward growth or, alternatively and more likely, the low position of the inferior placental edge must be more apparent than real. In support of the latter is the observation that while a low-lying placenta is commonly seen with ultrasound in the middle of pregnancy, it is unusual to have major intrapartum bleeding problems when therapeutic abortion is performed at this stage. How to reconcile these conflicting observations?

Firstly, the observations of Buttery and Davison (1978) of the occurrence of localized myometrial contractions serve to explain how, in some cases, a false diagnosis of a low-lying placenta might be made. Since these contractions, which produce a localized "heaping up" of the myometrium, frequently occur near the internal os, their similar ultrasound appearance to placental tissue will lead to errors in diagnosis by the unwary (Fig. 12). With high-quality grey-scale equipment such errors should be avoidable. In a similar way, a blood clot which has formed in the lower pole of the uterus often appears in continuity with the placenta, making its lower edge difficult and at times impossible to define precisely (Williams et al., 1976). Secondly, during the formation of the lower segment from the isthmus of the uterus, the edge of a placenta which earlier appeared to reach to the cervix is in fact carried upwards away from the internal os. In conclusion, the evidence suggests that

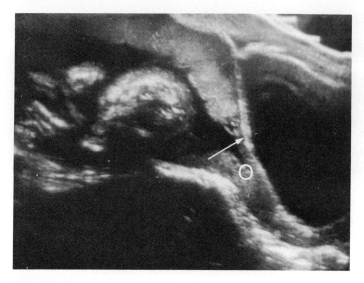

Figure 13. A pregnancy at 22 weeks in which the lower edge of the anterior placenta (arrow) terminates 1 cm short of the internal os (O).

many of the so-called low-lying placentas of the earlier weeks are more apparent than real but that there might still be come mechanism for preferential growth of the upper part of the placenta rather than at its lower edge.

Implications for Clinical Management

Before 20 Weeks
Unless the placenta is seen to cover completely the area of the internal os in these early weeks, no action need be taken on what appears to be a low-lying placenta. Indeed, we believe that a written diagnosis of placenta previa is rarely justified at this stage because of the unnecessary concerns it might cause to both the patient and her physician. Furthermore, a repeat ultrasound placental localization need only be performed if there is a subsequent clinical indication or if the initial examination showed a central placenta previa. Since we have never seen growth of a placenta downwards towards the cervix, the clear finding of a placenta at this stage with its lower edge more than 1 cm away from the internal os virtually excludes the possibility of a placenta previa for the remainder of the pregnancy (Fig. 13).

After 20 Weeks
A formal description of how low the placenta extends should be part of any examination report after the 20th week. The subsequent management of

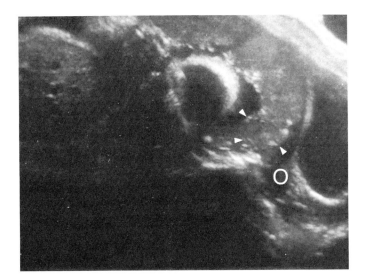

Figure 14. A patient at 32 weeks with a major degree of placenta previa. The placenta is mainly anterior but extends across the area of the internal os (O) onto the posterior wall (arrowheads).

patients with a low-lying placenta then depends on the presence or absence of vaginal bleeding, the age of the pregnancy, and the extent of the presumed placenta previa. When noted as an incidental finding, and in the absence of vaginal bleeding, it is reasonable to continue outpatient management until at least 30-32 weeks when at least those patients with a major degree of previa should be admitted. Those with recurrent bleeding and an ultrasound finding of a low-lying placenta are more safely managed in hospital irrespective of gestational age.

Delivery

A repeat examination is recommended in the last few weeks of pregnancy to allow the obstetrician to plan the timing and mode of delivery. We believe it to be unnecessary and potentially dangerous to perform an examination under anesthesia in patients shown by ultrasound to have a definite major degree of placenta previa (Fig. 14). In such patients an elective cesarean section is more appropriate. For those in whom there is any doubt, or if only a minor degree of previa is suspected, an examination in the operating room must be performed (with or without general anesthesia) with preparations made for immediate cesarean section. A clinical decision can then be made as to the mode of delivery. Patients who have had an prepartum hemorrhage but in whom the

placenta has been shown by an experienced observer to be located entirely
and without question in the upper segment, need not, in our view, undergo a
formal examination in the operating room.

Accidental Hemorrhage

Ultrasound does not have a major part to play in either the diagnosis or
management of this condition. A minor degree of accidental hemorrhage
is basically a diagnosis of exclusion. Notwithstanding, attempts are often made
to search for a small retroplacental clot. While sonolucent areas beneath the
placenta are often found, they are difficult to distinguish from large venous
sinuses and "blood lakes" (Callen and Filley, 1980), and even from the artefactual echofree areas not infrequently seen in the normal uterine wall.
Patients with a major abruption are seldom referred to the sonar department,
and rightly so, since their management is most unlikely to be influenced by
what is found.

REFERENCES

Adam, A. H., Robinson, H. P., Fleming, J. E. E., and Hall, A. J. (1978). A
    comparison of biparietal measurements using a real-time scanner and a con-
    ventional scanner equipped with a coded cephalometry system. *Br. J.
    Obstet. Gynaecol. 85*:487-491.
Adam, A. H., Robinson, H. P., and Dunlop, C. (1979). A comparison of
    crown-rump length measurements using a real-time scanner in an antenatal
    clinic and a conventional B-scanner. *Br. J. Obstet. Gynaecol. 86*:521-524.
Badria, L., and Young, G. B. (1976). Correlation of ultrasonic and soft tissue
    X-ray placentography in 300 cases. *J. Clin. Ultrasound 4*:403-406.
Bennett, M. J., and Kerr-Wilson, R. H. J. (1980). Evaluation of threatened
    abortion by ultrasound. *Int. J. Gynaecol. Obstet. 17*:382-384.
Buttery, B., and Davison, G. D. (1978). The dynamic uterus revealed by time-
    lapse echography. *J. Clin. Ultrasound 6*:19-22.
Callen, P. W., and Filley, R. A. (1980). The placental-subplacental complex:
    A specific indicator of placental position on ultrasound. *J. Clin. Ultra-
    sound 8*:21-26.
Hay, D., Tasker, P., Horacek, I., and Johnston, I. (1981). Two hour lutropin
    assay during ovulation. *Clin. Chem.* (in press).
Hertig, A. T. (1967). The overall problem in man. In *Comparative Aspects
    of Reproductive Failure.* K. Benirschke (Ed.). Springer-Verlag, Berlin,
    Heidelberg, and New York, pp. 11-41.
Hertig, A. T., Rock, J., Adams, E. C., and Menkin, M. C. (1959). Thirty-four
    fertilized human ova, good, bad and indifferent, recovered from 210
    women of known fertility. *Pediatrics 23*:202-211.

King, D. L. (1973). Placental migration demonstrated by ultrasonography. *Radiology 109*:167-170.

Morrison, J., Lachelin, G. C., and Blackwell, R. J. (1972). The accuracy of diagnosing placenta praevia with compound ultrasonic scanning. *Aust. N.Z. J. Obstet. Gynaecol. 12*:220-224.

Reinold, E. (1976). *Ultrasonics in Early Pregnancy: Diagnostic Scanning and Fetal Motor Activity.* S. Karger, Basel.

Roberts, C. J., and Lowe, C. R. (1975). Where have all the conceptions gone? *Lancet 1*:498-499.

Robinson, H. P. (1972). Detection of fetal heart movement in first trimester of pregnancy using pulsed ultrasound. *Br. Med. J. 4*:466-468.

Robinson, H. P. (1975). The diagnosis of early pregnancy failure by sonar. *Br. J. Obstet. Gynaecol. 82*:849-857.

Robinson, H. P. (1978). The evaluation of early pregnancy and its complications by diagnostic ultrasound. M.D. Thesis, University of Glasgow, Glasgow.

Williams, C. H., Van Bergen, W. S., and Prentice, R. L. (1976). Extra-amniotic blood clot simulating placenta praevia on ultrasound scan. *J. Clin. Ultrasound 5*:45-47.

Young, G. B. (1978). The peripatetic placenta. *Radiology 128*:183-188.

2

Cervical Encirclage

GEOFFREY CHAMBERLAIN and CHARLOTTE GIBBINGS / Queen Charlotte's Hospital for Women, London, England

Most spontaneous abortions that occur in the first trimester of pregnancy are associated with an embryonic abnormality incompatible with life. From the 13th week onward, however, the capacity of the mother's genital tract to hold a pregnancy often becomes the deciding factor. One of the causes of such midtrimester abortions is an incompetent cervix; this is most commonly treated in the Western world by cervical encirclage.

BACKGROUND

The concept of an incompetent cervix is not new. Gream, in 1865, first described it in the *Lancet*. Lash and Lash (1948) quoted Sproat Heaney who, discussing cervical incompetence, said that "the greatest contributing factor to this condition is tearing of the cervix by labour or by instrumental dilatation and incomplete healing after vaginal Caesarean section or vaginal hysterotomy." In the same paper Lash and Lash illustrated the concept well (see Fig. 1) and made the important point that the incompetence is nearly always anterior.

The incidence of an incompetent cervix has been reported in a wide range of between 0.1% (Lipshitz, 1975) and 1% of all deliveries (Duda and Lighezan, 1963), while up to 20% of midtrimester abortions have been associated with an incompetent cervix (Mann et al., 1961). The surgical treatment of this condition is therefore attractive. Several authors published reports just after the Second World War on the repair of the isthmus and upper cervical canal in the nonpregnant woman. Usually a plastic operation was done, excising some

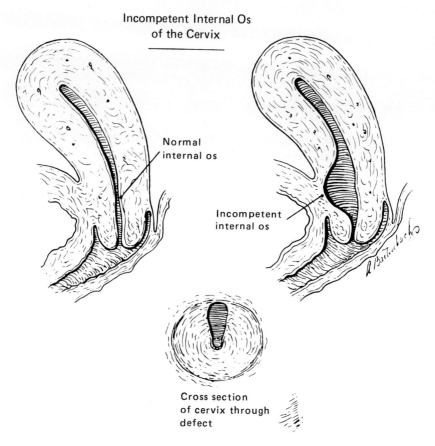

Incompetent Internal Os
of the Cervix

Normal
internal os

Incompetent
internal os

Cross section
of cervix through
defect

Figure 1. Cervical incompetence shown diagramatically. (From Lash and Lash, 1950.)

of the tissues in the area and reuniting the connective tissue and muscle fibers in an attempt to make a smaller internal os (Palmer, 1950; Lash and Lash, 1950). The operation described by the latter is shown in Figure 2. This would be a very sanguinous operation if performed in pregnancy and so a less traumatic cervical encirclage was developed; a band of inabsorbable suture material encircles the cervix as near to the internal os as possible.

The first time this operation was performed has often been in debate. Professor Shirodkar of Bombay published an account in 1955 of an operation he had done encircling the cervix with chromic catgut. MacDonald in Melbourne, publishing in 1957, reported a series of cases the first being a woman on whom

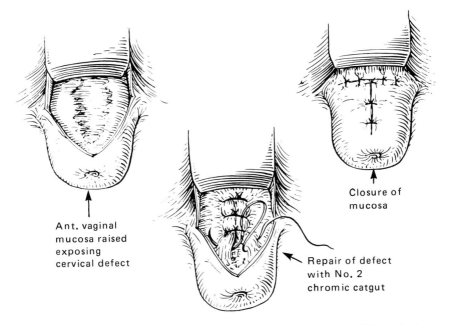

Figure 2. Repair of cervical canal in the nonpregnant woman. (From Lash and Lash, 1950.)

he had operated in February, 1952. However, Shirodkar had shown a film of such an operation in 1951 so that, although he had not published, he had showed details of the operation on the film. MacDonald, with typical generosity, has acknowledged Shirodkar's precedence in the operation consisting of the dissection of the anterior fornix, pushing up of the bladder base, and the insertion of an encircling tape buried under the epithelium of the cervix which was closed at the end of the operation. Thus it involved a moderate amount of dissection and anaesthesia to remove the suture. This operation, which should strictly be known as a Shirodkar stitch, is now rarely performed. As described later, there is a simpler procedure also called encirclage, correctly termed MacDonald's operation, involving multiple bites of the cervix. This is now more commonly performed in the Western world.

Aspects of cervical encirclage are considered in this chapter. As well as the work quoted from other centers, in order to provide up-to-date information, we have reviewed 136 women who in 1977-1978 had the procedure performed while pregnant, at Queen Charlotte's Hospital for Women (QCH). In that time 7938 women were delivered but incidence rates should not be derived since this is a selected hospital population. Some women with sutures inserted might not have delivered at QCH. Others may have had sutures inserted elsewhere and joined our clinic later. So for these and other reasons, no background population analyses can be performed of this group.

ETIOLOGY

A deficiency of the internal cervical os is due to an inadequacy of the circular muscle at this level. Care should be taken not to seek too firm an anatomical site for the internal sphincter of the cervix. There is a latticework of muscle fibers at the isthmocervical junction; in early pregnancy these rearrange themselves and become predominantly circular. There is probably not an anatomical sphincter in the sense of the pylorus but probably more a condensation of muscle as in the cardia of the stomach. Cervical incompetence may be congenital in origin, but it is more likely to be acquired, following overstretch of the internal sphincter. In either case, there is a slight gape of the cervical internal os and, in consequence, the growing gestation sac bulges down into the isthmus. The resistance to cervical opening in the normal uterus is deficient and so the upper end of the cervical canal opens further allowing this bulge of membranes to protrude into the canal. This will have the double effect of acting as a conical wedge pushing down to open up the rest of the canal and providing a place of added weakness in the membranes due to local overstretch and possible low-grade inflammation. Hence, the cervix may be dilated more or the membranes may rupture at this point. Both these events lead on to midtrimester abortion or early premature labor.

Congenital Cervical Incompetence

This is less common. For example, in the QCH series, only 4% of the women with cervical incompetence had not been pregnant before. It is postulated that a congenital weakness of the muscle at the level of the internal os had always been present. It is difficult to imagine this as an isolated structural alteration of the Müllerian duct system; one would expect it to be associated with other congenital defects. Goldstein (1978), following up 284 women with a history of stilbestrol exposure in utero while seeking adenosis of the vagina, found that five out of the nine in the series who had never conceived had a congenital deficiency of the cervix. Stilbestrol exposure may have impaired the development of the entire duct system to some degree and the cervix may have been the area to show first.

Acquired Cervical Incompetence

Most women with an incompetent cervix have had some dilatation of the cervix previously. In the QCH group, 60% had had at least one spontaneous abortion, and 49% at least one vaginal termination of pregnancy, almost half being over 10 weeks' gestation, while a quarter had had more than one vaginal termination. MacDonald (1980) found 68.8% of patients in his personal series of 269 women with incompetent cervix had had a previous history of dilatation and curettage while 7.8% had had a conization and 3% an amputation; thus about 80% had some surgery to the cervix. There may be a tear in one or other fornix after an obstetrical procedure, particularly after a difficult forceps rotation or when forceps are wrongly applied before the cervix is fully dilated.

INDICATIONS

Cervical encirclage is done for a woman who is either pregnant or considering becoming pregnant and who is judged to have cervical incompetence. This is exemplified by:

1. A history of a previous midtrimester abortion
2. A history of an early premature labor with rupture of the membranes before or at the onset of labor
3. Examination during pregnancy showing an abnormal degree of effacement or dilatation of the cervix

All these groups would include mostly women who have had some past history of gynecological or obstetrical problems.

In addition to the groups thought to have cervical incompetence encirclage has been used more recently in an effort to:

1. *Maintain a multiple pregnancy.* It has been suggested that sewing up the cervix will result in its not effacing as early. Thus, premature labor in women with an overdistended uterus containing twins would not occur as readily. Such reports as that of Zakut et al. (1977) are often quoted, but these are not well-controlled studies and have a bias in patient selection. A study from Liverpool (Weekes et al., 1977) compared the effects in these groups of women with twins of bed rest alone, bed rest and cervical suture, and no active treatment. There were no differences between the three groups in the gestational age, birth weight, or rate of perinatal deaths of the babies. They therefore concluded that there is no justification for indiscriminate cervical suture in the management of uncomplicated twin pregnancies. To take this problem further would undoubtedly demand a prospective randomized trial but there is sufficient doubt about the effectiveness of cervical encirclage in twin pregnancies to justify this being done.

2. *Prevent further bleeding in woman with a placenta previa.* By sewing up the cervix it was hoped that the lower segment would not be pulled up as soon

in pregnancy and not as much of the placenta would shear off. Hence pregnancy could be carried further and the fetus be more mature when the eventual cesarean section were performed. There is no substantial evidence that this is true and putting an encircling suture high into the cervix of a woman with the increased blood supply of placenta previa is sanguinous.

Cervical encirclage in nonpregnant women is usually performed only on those who have had enough damage to the cervix at a previous delivery or operation to be detected on clinical examination. A very badly lacerated cervix after obstetrical trauma should be repaired formally by colporrhaphy and not left to encirclage. However, some gynecologists insert a suture before pregnancy on the grounds that in their experience of encirclage in pregnancy, the sutures all have either been put in too late or disturbed the pregnancy so much that it aborted. Others think it unwise to perform interval encirclage because the presence of a suture may alter cervical function and impair fertility. Further, if the fetus is grossly abnormal a spontaneous abortion in the first trimester may be wholly or partially prevented; and subsequent evacuation of any retained products would be made difficult by a buried suture placed before pregnancy.

DIAGNOSIS

Cervical encirclage is performed when the cervix is judged to be incompetent, but the diagnosis of this condition can rarely be absolute.

History

Many physicians diagnose the presence of cervical incompetence only by its probability after the history of a previous midtrimester abortion or an early premature labor. Others include precipitating events such as a vaginal termination of pregnancy in the first trimester or a dilatation and curettage, particularly if this caused wide dilatation of the cervix as used to be done for dysmenorrhea. Occasionally, previous operative vaginal deliveries are associated with incompetence, particularly a forceps delivery of a large child, or a rotation forceps extraction. The precise percentage of those who have such a previous history varies from one reported study to another and obviously depends on the criteria of the investigator, the background obstetrical practice, and the social habits of the population. For example, MacDonald in 1957, reporting from North London, found that 54 of his 70 cases had had previous surgery of the cervix. Twenty years later in the QCH study of 136 women in West London who had a cervical encirclage in 1978 and 1979, 49% had had previous vaginal termination of pregnancy.

The number and proportions of those with any etiological factor will vary according to the population served and those selected to enter any study of cervical encirclage. Generally, however, they are multiparous (96% of the QCH study), have had a previous midtrimester abortion or premature labor (60%), may have had a previous vaginal procedure (54%), and have often had cervical encirclage in a previous pregnancy (32%).

Examination

Examination of the cervix between pregnancies is often unrewarding. It may be helpful to see if the cervix will accept a dilator: it is commonly considered that if a Hegar's cervical no. 8 dilator (8 mm diameter) enters the cervix easily, some incompetence is present.

Johnstone et al. (1972) refined this procedure by assessing the diameter of the internal os with a variably dilating device that measured the retaining capacity of the cervix with more precision. Alternatively, some wait to examine the cervix by serial vaginal examinations in pregnancy, to see how it responds to the enlarging gestational sac. Careful examination in the early weeks of pregnancy can detect a cervix which is effacing and starting to dilate. However, such prenatal surveillance is intermittent, usually at 1- or 2-week intervals and the cervix might dilate between these visits. Unfortunately, cervical incompetence is too often diagnosed only when the patient presents in the emergency room with uterine contractions, the cervix already 2-4 cm dilated, and a bulging bag of membranes at the os. Although encirclage can be done when the cervix is partly effaced and up to 5 cm dilated, the most successful operations are those performed before any dilatation or effacement occurs.

Investigations

The major investigations which may be performed are radiological. Funnelling of the internal os can be shown (see Figs. 3 and 4) but the functional significance of such anatomical findings is not clear. Some estimate of cervical function may be attained by using a Foley catheter (Soihet, 1974). When the blown-up balloon is pulled down onto the internal os it can mimic the effect of a bulging bag of membranes. However, even this is not a very physiological test, since the influence of the high progresterone levels of pregnancy are not seen in the nonpregnant internal os of the cervix.

Hysteroscopy in skilled hands may give some indication of cervical incompetence. As the hysteroscope is passed up the cervical canal, flushing the dilating fluid ahead of it, the distance travelled may appear rather short and the canal shelves away from the scope too soon.

In pregnancy, a carefully performed ultrasound examination can show the bulging bag of membranes funnelling the internal os, but this is very late

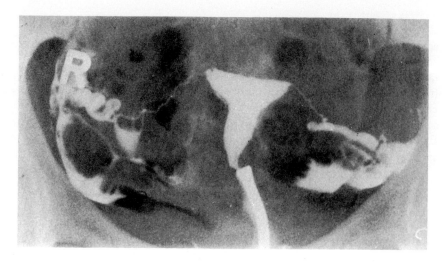

Figure 3. Hysterogram showing normal internal os of cervix.

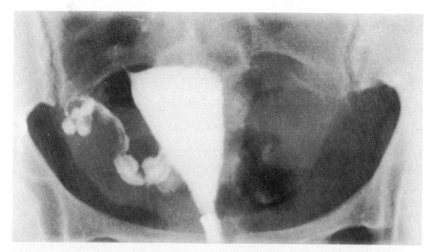

Figure 4. Hysterogram showing funnelling of the incompetent cervix.

in the process. Before this stage, ultrasound is less useful because the acoustical density of all the solid tissues in this region is similar.

The diagnosis of cervical incompetence is most commonly arrived at by considering the obstetrical history of midtrimester abortions or early premature labors. Next to this the physical appearances of the pregnant cervix examined serially in midgestation are the most useful at present. In the QCH series, 33% of the women had an encirclarge based on past obstetrical history grounds alone, 51% on examination in pregnancy, and 16% on a combination of both of these.

OPERATIVE PROCEDURES

Most cervical encirclage is done in pregnancy and, for the reasons already mentioned, after the 12th week, often with a preoperative ultrasound examination to confirm a live fetus and the gestational age. Procedures may be divided into those done electively and those done as emergency procedures. Figure 5 shows the distribution of weeks of pregnancy at which this procedure was performed in the QCH study.

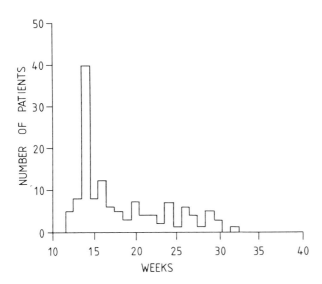

Figure 5. Distribution of weeks of gestation at which an encirclage was performed in the QCH series.

Elective Encirclage in Pregnancy

Preoperative Preparation

Since the procedure is elective and the woman is not in labor, she should be admitted to hospital for some hours before the operation and fully prepared for a general anesthesia. The pudenda should be shaved and a bath with a mild antiseptic may be given. No douching or cleaning of the vagina should be performed before the operation.

Anesthesia

Encirclage is a painful procedure involving pulling on the uterus and its ligaments; hence a general or epidural anesthetic is recommended although some have performed this procedure under paracervical block without ill effect.

Technique

Two groups of operation may effect cervical encirclage.

The Shirodkar operation. The cervix is gripped anteriorly with a vulsellum forceps and pulled down. An incision, about 1 inch long is made transversely at the apex of the anterior fornix, the bladder is pushed up by blunt dissection, and hemostasis is achieved (Fig. 6). The cervix is then lifted up and a small incision made in the midline of the posterior fornix. An aneurysm, or Reverdin, needle is then passed up from the posterior incision anteriorly and a nonabsorbable tape is pulled down around the cervix (Fig. 7). The tape is pulled out posteriorly and another needle then carries the tape up anteriorly again around the other side of the cervix into the region of the anterior incision (Fig. 8). The tape is then tied anteriorly and the knot cut short (Fig. 9). Both anterior and posterior incisions in the cervical epithelium are closed with catgut.

Knowing exactly how tightly to tie the tape is always a problem. There is no precision in this and probably it is not critical since the cervix has such a good blood supply in pregnancy that it is unlikely that any tissues will become ischemic. However, too loose a suture would be ineffective and a waste of time. Most aim to tie, with sufficient compression, to close off the canal. The disadvantage of the true Shirodkar stitch is that it is buried and cannot be removed without an anesthetic. This is a bloody procedure which may be performed just before labor starts. Many surgeons who employ this technique will deliver the child by cesarean section, leaving the stitch in place for a subsequent pregnancy.

The MacDonald-type stitch. This is a lesser surgical procedure and consists of a series of bites taken around the cervix. MacDonald's own technique uses an atraumatic needle with Mersilene tape inserted around the cervix as high as it will go, roughly level with the internal os. It is inserted in four or five

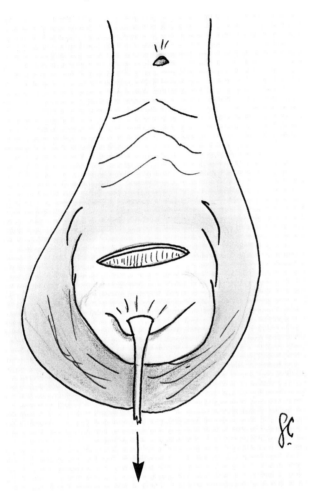

Figure 6. The Shirodkar type of encirclage: the anterior incision.

bites (Fig. 10) and the knot is tied anteriorly on the surface of the ectocervix, the ends being left long enough to make it easy to remove. Again, it is a problem to know how much pressure to use on the knot; MacDonald says that it should be enough to close the internal os completely, but this is often difficult. How can the surgeon know, from external pressure, what he or she is doing internally in the canal?

Most Western surgeons now use a 5-mm-wide Mersilene tape prepared on a double-ended traumatic needle (see Fig. 11). This allows the suture to be

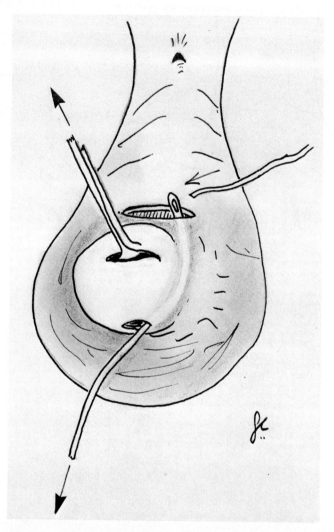

Figure 7. The Shirodkar type of encirclage: the posterior incision and passage of an aneurysm needle from behind forwards.

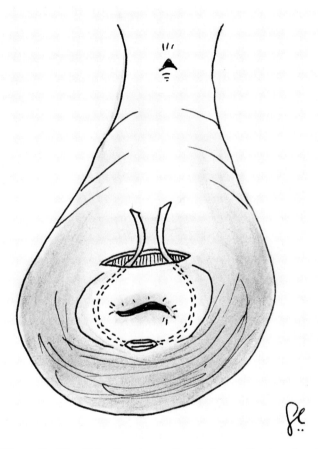

Figure 8. The Shirodkar type of encirclage: the tape has been drawn back and then passed forwards on the other side of the cervix.

started in the midline posteriorly so that less tape is dragged through the substance of the cervix on each side but the knot is still tied anteriorly..

The authors' technique uses two bites only, instead of the four to five MacDonald describes (see Fig. 12). The posterior lip of the cervix is grasped with a vulsellum and elevated. Each needle is introduced in turn at the midline as near to the internal os as possible and then swung in a complete semicircle through the substance of the cervix to leave anteriorly in the midline. With care, each of the needles can be introduced through the same hole

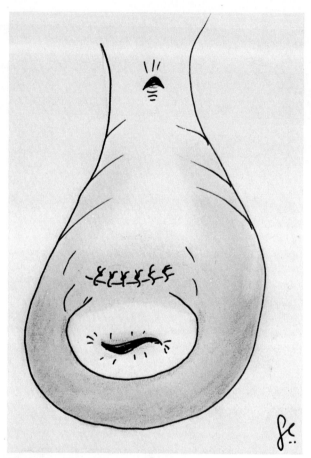

Figure 9. The Shirodkar type of encirclage: the knot is tied, cut short, and buried anteriorly.

posteriorly so that no tape is exposed to the vagina except the knot anteriorly (see Fig. 13). This seems a good compromise between the two techniques, avoiding on the one hand the more extensive dissection under the bladder base which Shirodkar used to do and on the other the multiple bites of MacDonald which leave more tape in contact with the vagina, providing a more irritating foreign body for the rest of pregnancy.

Emergency Encirclage in Pregnancy

The operative technique must be modified if the woman is in labor when the suture is inserted. If the cervix is up to 4 cm dilated with the membranes

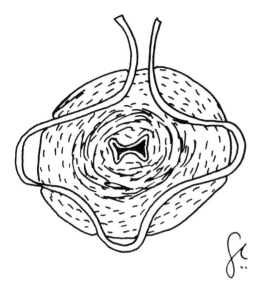

Figure 10. The MacDonald type of encirclage.

intact, they are usually bulging through the cervix and present a formidable risk of being pricked by the needle entering and leaving the cervical substance. It is wise to replace them with a gauze swab damped in saline on a pair of sponge-holding forceps, pushed up through the cervix. This takes the membranes out of the operative field. Then a MacDonald-type suture can be done, still using only two bites as described before if the surgeon wishes. As the ends are being tied, the assistant slowly removes the forceps and swab.

A slightly more elaborate but equally effective method has been described by Orr (1973). A Foley catheter with a 30-ml balloon is used instead of a swab on a stick. The end of the catheter beyond the balloon is amputated and the deflated balloon is passed up through the cervix against the membranes. The balloon is then slowly blown up and if the catheter stays in the right place, it carries the membranes up. The suture is inserted and, as the knot is tied, the fluid is released from the balloon so that the catheter can be withdrawn easily as the stitch is tied gently. We have not found this method to have any great advantage, but those who use it consider it to be less traumatic than the use of a saline-damped swab.

Basically, the MacDonald type of stitch is probably the best primary measure for all pregnant women irrespective of the number of bites used. It is certainly the method to use if the cervix has started dilating since it is much simpler and less traumatic. The Shirodkar type of suture is best used

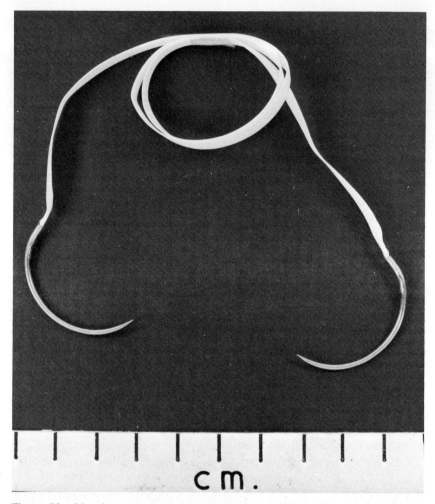

Figure 11. Mersilene tape with an atraumatic needle in each end used for MacDonald encirclage.

if there is obvious damage to the cervix such as a lateral laceration. Some also consider that the Shirodkar stitch should be used if the simpler stitch has failed in earlier pregnancy.

Encirclage Between Pregnancies

When no pregnancy is present, more extensive procedures may be performed safely, bearing in mind the reservations made already. The Shirodkar procedure

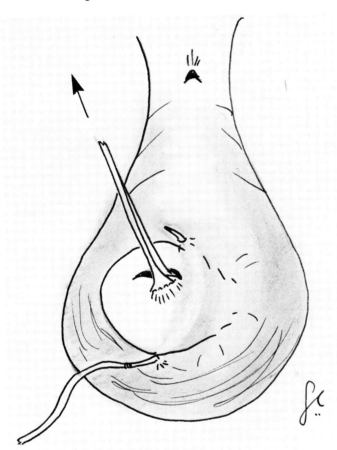

Figure 12. Buried encirclage with two bites only: insertion of needle from behind, bringing it out in the anterior fornix.

is used by some but MacDonald (1980) has described an elegant technique. He circumcizes the cervix and uses a ligature of portex tubing. This is inserted above the level of the uterosacral ligaments, the bladder having been pushed up first. He passes a Hegar's dilator in the cervix so that he can tie the polyvinyl tubing firmly onto this and still leave a reasonable canal for subsequent menstruation and the passage of sperm. He sews down the cut ends with silk so that they do not bulge onto the epithelium. The cervical epithelium is then closed by a series of sutures leaving the nonabsorbable suture in place. He considers this encirclage permanent so that all subsequent deliveries should be made by cesarean section.

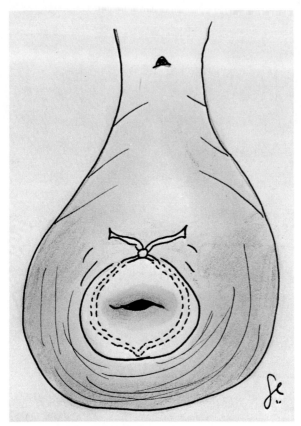

Figure 13. Buried encirclage with two bites only: the other needle passes along the other side of the cervix and, when the suture is tied, only the knot is in the vagina.

Occasionally, the cervix has been so damaged that a vaginal approach to insert a suture would be extremely difficult because of the dense fibrosis. This may follow a cervical amputation during a Manchester repair or an extensive cone biopsy, particularly if infection followed either. The lower segment of the uterus and upper cervix are then best approached abdominally. A transverse incision is made in the vesicocervical fold and the bladder is pushed down carefully by blunt and sharp dissection. A pair of curved forceps is passed around the barrel of the cervix through the uterosacral ligaments but keeping close to the cervical wall. A tape or portex flexible rod is passed circumferentially from the front of the cervix and tied anterior to the cervical substance at the level of the internal os. The peritoneum is repaired and the abdomen closed. Such an encirclage would require a cesarean section in any subsequent pregnancy since the stitch cannot be removed without an abdominal operation. This procedure is rarely needed and in the last 7 years we have done all extensive cervical repairs vaginally.

A newer technique of what may loosely be called cervical encirclage has recently been described in Europe. Bayer (1977) has used a Mayer ring pessary inserted around the cervix in outpatients. No anesthetic is required and the procedure is obviously simple. This appliance has been used in Eastern Europe and Bayer claims a consistent reduction in perinatal mortality from prematurity. It is quick and simple and it is said that the pessary can still be used at 3 cm dilatation of the cervix. It would obviously cause much less damage to the cervix than suturing and is less likely to start contractions of the myometrium. Since the paper in 1977 no other studies have been published in the Western literature and attempts to obtain such pessaries to perform a clinical trial in the United Kingdom have been unsuccessful.

Complications

The most immediate complication is failure of the operation and myometrial contractions. This is more likely if the encirclage is performed after cervical dilatation has started. Most reports say that the failure rate of an elective procedure in pregnancy was low (e.g., Lipshitz in 1975 reports four cases in 71 women).

Sepsis is another serious complication; the incidence seems to vary from one series to another. Kuhn and Pepperall (1977) found an 18.6% sepsis rate in a series of 242 pregnancies, the common organisms being *Escherichia coli,* and *Clostridium perfringens.* Two women died of endotoxic shock. If cervical encirclage is performed after membrane rupture, infection has a higher incidence. In the QCH series, 30 out of 136 women showed evidence of local infection (judged by a purulent vaginal discharge). Figure 14 shows that only 10 of these occurred within 3 weeks of insertion of this stitch, the rest occurring after that.

Hemorrhage can be a problem if the stitch is pulled on by the dilating cervix and the woman does not report immediately for medical help. However, the other causes of prepartum suture hemorrhage must be excluded. Thirty-one women in the QCH series reported this and the distribution of their bleeding in relation to insertion of the stitch is shown in Figure 15.

A less likely problem is malfunction of the cervix in labor after the suture has been removed, possibly necessitating abdominal delivery because of cervical stenosis. Commonly there is a mild degree of fibrosis which may be associated with some delay in the earlier stages of labor. However, once the cervix has started to dilate, this proceeds at a normal pace. Cervical

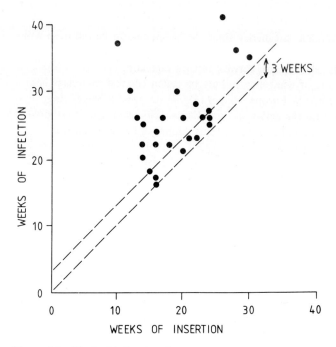

Figure 14. Vaginal infection first noted in relation to gestation at encirclage in the QCH series. Mostly it occurred more than 3 weeks after the operation.

lacerations or even a rupture of the uterus may occur if there are strong contractions before the suture is removed.

Most of these complications are preventable by careful prenatal surveillance and a proper explanation to the patient, warning her to report to the hospital if bleeding, uterine contractions, or loss of liquor occurs. These are all treatable risks and should be weighed against the patient's desire to have a mature baby after a series of obstetrical complications.

Immediate Postoperative Care

The patient should be prepared to stay in hospital for several days because myometrial contractions are most likely within the first 3 days after the operation. Initially she should rest in bed and only get up to use the toilet. Mobilization is started gradually and, if there are no complications, the patient is allowed home between the 3rd and 5th postoperative day. Analgesics should be given according to need. The usefulness of a prophylactic antibiotic is doubtful. Should there be a spike of temperature, broad-spectrum antibiotics should be given after a high vaginal swab is taken.

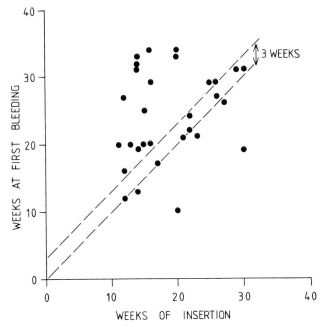

Figure 15. Bleeding first noted in relation to gestation at encirclage in the QCH series. Few cases occurred close to the procedure; some occurred before and the majority more than 3 weeks later.

Uterine muscle relaxants are of dubious use. Jennings (1972) used isoxuprine hydrochloride with no great improvement in results, while Lauersen and Fuchs (1973) showed no increased success rate when alcohol was given after the operation. More recently, salbutamol has been given and there is no evidence that this improves the success rate. It us unlikely to be a major adjunct since, in the earlier stages of pregnancy when the stitch is usually put in, salbutamol would have little effect on uterine musculature.

Later Postoperative Care

The patient should be seen frequently for the rest of the prenatal period. Weekly, or at the most fortnightly, visits should take place and at each of these a gentle vaginal examination should be performed. The lower uterine segment soon pulls up on the stitch and after this there should be a reasonable length of cervix left below the suture.

If all goes well, the patient will carry into the last weeks of pregnancy without the stitch cutting out. If this does occur, it usually happens posteriorly with the knot remaining in place anteriorly.

Removal of the Stitch

If there are no symptoms of earlier cervical activity, the suture is left until the fetus is well mature at 38 weeks. With the MacDonald procedure, the knot is in the anterior cervical fornix where it can be felt easily and seen using a Cusco's speculum. The running end is grasped with a pair of artery forceps and gently pulled down; the encircling tape in the cervix is then exposed and cut close to the knot. Removal is usually easy and of minimum inconvenience to the patient. Sometimes, however, fibrosis occurs so that the suture is buried and more traction is required to move it.

The Shirodkar-type suture is buried and removal requires an anesthetic and a formal opening of the epithelium of the anterior cervix. Such buried sutures are often difficult to remove even when exposed and many obstetricians would consider their presence an indication for a cesarean section, leaving the suture undisturbed for a future pregnancy.

Whoever inserts an encircling cervical suture must note in the patient's records, and tell the patient, whether the knot is tied anteriorly or posteriorly. In the vast majority it is an anterior knot but occasionally, with variations of technique, the knot is posterior. This can present problems to another obstetrician who may have to remove the knot in an emergency.

Method of Delivery

Many women delivery by spontaneous vaginal delivery soon after the stitch is removed. Figure 16 shows the time from removal of the stitch to delivery in the QCH series. About half the patients went into immediate labor on the same day as the stitch was removed and in the rest, labor was delayed for an increasing interval. Thirty-two percent of these women had to be induced with Syntocinon for postmaturity. Fifty-four percent delivered vaginally spontaneously, 30% required forceps, and 16% were delivered by cesarean section. Of these last group, failure to progress was the commonest indication, and a prepartum hemorrhage the next.

The cesarean section rate of those who have the simplest circlage may be much lower than the Shirodkar method (MacDonald, 1980). These data are based on series done in different centers and there is no randomized comparative trial of both techniques on the same population by the same surgeons.

If a cesarean section has to be performed in the prenatal period before suture removal, it may be wise to leave the suture there to help another pregnancy. If the knot is on the surface of the fornix, its tails should be trimmed short at the end of the operation since the foreign body will remain in the vagina for several years. A high Shirodkar-type suture or an abdominally placed one may cause fibrosis and distortion of the lower segment causing difficulty in pushing down the bladder in the early stages of cesarean section. Care should be taken, because bladder damage occurs easily.

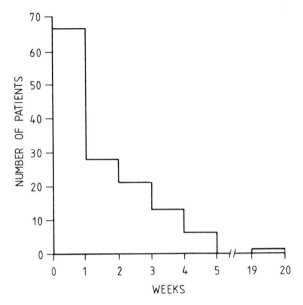

Figure 16. Interval from removal of suture to delivery in the QCH series (weeks).

Results

In medicine generally, intervention procedures are favored: both the doctor and patient feel that they are doing more good by doing something than by awaiting events. Often this is right, but it is difficult to prove. Cervical encirclage is widely used in the Western world and one must presume that the surgeons are all convinced that it improves fetal salvage. It is difficult to be certain what would have happened if the uterus had been left alone. Objective evidence of the value of the procedure is difficult to obtain. MacDonald's original report in 1957 showed a 47% fetal salvage rate in 70 patients. Late reports improve on this. From Melbourne, Kuhn and Pepperall (1977) have an 80.6% success rate in 242 patients while Lauersen and Fuchs (1973) in New York found a 83% salvage rate in 159 patients. But how can we be certain that we are doing good?

The salvage rates are impressive, particularly when, as in the Melbourne series, the rate among the same women in a previous pregnancy had been 28%. This would seem, superficially, to be a threefold improvement. Some would say that a change of this order should not need any statistical assessment to show what a good technique it must be. However, it is not good enough to compare patients with their own obstetrical history.

Patients in different pregnancies obviously differ in their age and parity while obstetrical techniques vary between centers and at different times. Similarly, one cannot compare one hospital with another since populations vary, obstetrical staff perform different procedures (as well as just the encirclage stitch), and data-recording methods differ. While these results seem good, some obstetricians are still sceptical and demand more objective evidence of the value of cervical encirclage.

Seppala and Lavera in 1971 devised a ratio based upon population studies; to do this would require total data collection for the population in a compact, well-organized, national obstetrical system. They expressed the total number of en-circlage operations in relation to the total deliveries in the population. The success rate of these operations was then derived along with the previous fetal salvage rate for the same patients. The current and previous success rates were calculated and a ratio of these two fetal salvage rates compared with a similar ratio calculated from the experience of multiparous normal women of a similar parity who did not have encirclage. From these two ratios a minimum benefit rate was obtained. Though these groups might not include exactly similar populations, some of the effects of variation could be diminished if careful parity matching was performed.

Ideally, a trial providing an acceptable control is required. A sequential cross-over trial using the same women in different pregnancies would not answer this because the cervix would be in a different state in each pregnancy. A random-ized controlled trial would take a population of women for whom cervical encirclage was indicated and then randomly allocate them into one group where the suture was performed prophylactically or to a second group in which this was not done. This might be difficult to organize: some surgeons would ask if it was ethical to do a randomized trial on such a well-established treatment. This might be answered by posing the counter question: is it ethical to submit women to an operation with a known complication rate and an unknown cure rate? Some gynecologists believe that they have the answer already and therefore would not consider randomization. They might suggest that another way would be to perform a randomized trial in a part of the world where the operation has not yet been routinely performed and is not yet universally available. Unfortunately, in areas where this would hap-pen, data collecting methods are so poor that the trial would have great difficulty in proving the question.

At present the Medical Research Council and the Royal College of Obstetricians and Gynaecologists in the United Kingdom are performing a multi-center randomized trial of cervical encirclage which will answer some of the criticisms raised.

As well as the fetal salvage rate, one should perhaps consider the quality of the babies born. Figure 17 shows the birth weights of the babies who were

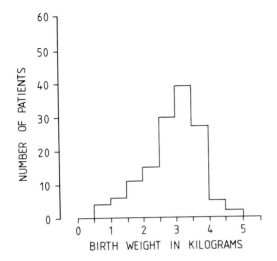

Figure 17. Distribution of birth weight in the encirclage group (QCH series).

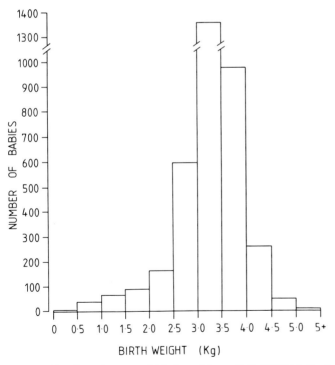

Figure 18. Distribution of birth weights of all QCH births in 1978.

born to the 136 women in the QCH series. They may be compared with the birth weights of all the babies born at QCH in the same year (Fig. 18). There is a skew to the left towards the lighter weights in the babies of the sutured patients. Perhaps a better comparison would be of what happened to those women with cervical incompetence of similar parities who delivered babies without a suture, but this is at present unknown because most are treated. This skew in distribution towards light birth weight might be expected in a condition that leads to premature babies anyway, and the fact that the bulk of children weighed more than 2.5 kg is a point in favor of the procedure.

CONCLUSIONS

Cervical suture is a commonly performed procedure simple to do, and appears to be helpful. Complication rates are low but its real value is still in doubt. In order to assuage those doubts, before extending the indications for this operation, its value and effectiveness should be proved by one of the methods mentioned in this chapter.

REFERENCES

Bayer, H. (1977). Einige neue Gesichtspunkte bei der Prophylaxe und Therapie der drohenden Frühgeburt. Sbl Gynah *99*:547-551.

Goldstein, D. P. (1978). Incompetent cervix in offspring exposed to diethylstilbestrol in utero. *Obstet. Gynecol. 52* (Suppl.):735-755.

Gream, G. T. (1865). Dilatation of the cervix uteri. *Lancet i*:381.

Jennings, C. L. (1972). Temporary submucosal circlage for cervical incompetence. *Am. J. Obstet. Gynecol. 113*:1097-1102.

Johnstone, F. D., Boyd, I. E., and McClure-Browne, J. C. (1972). Instrument for measuring the available diameter of the internal cervical os. *Lancet ii*:1294.

Kuhn, R., and Pepperall, R. (1977). Cervical ligation. *Aust. N. Z. J. Obstet. Gynaecol. 17*:79-83.

Lash, A. F., and Lash, S. R. (1950). Habitual abortion: The incompetent maternal os of the cervix. *Am. J. Obstet. Gynecol. 59*:68-76.

Lauerson, N. A., and Fuchs, F. (1973). Experience with Shirodkar's operation and preoperative alcohol treatment. *Acta Obstet. Gynaecol. Scand. 52*:77-81.

Lipshitz, J. (1975). Circlage in the treatment of incompetent cervix. *S. Afr. Med. J. 49*:2013-2015.

MacDonald, I. (1957). Suture of the cervix for inevitable miscarriage. *J. Obstet. Gynaecol. Br. Emp. 63*:346-352.

MacDonald, I. (1980). Cervical circlage. *Clin. Obstet. Gynaecol.* 7:461-479.

Mann, E. C., McLaren, W. D., and Hoyt, D. B. (1961). The physiology and clinical significance of the uterine isthmus. *J. Obstet. Gynaecol. 81*:209-213.

Orr, C. (1973). An aid to cervical circlage. *Aust. N.Z. J. Obstet. Gynaecol.* *13*:114.

Palmer, R. (1950). Le rôle de la beme de l'isthme utérin dans l'avortement habituée. *Res. Gynecol. Obstet. 47*:905-909.

Sappala, M., and Vara, P. (1971). Standardization of the results of Shirodkar's operation. *Acta Obstet. Gynaecol. Scand. 50*:66

Shirodkar, V. N. (1955). A new method of operative treatment for habitual abortion. *Antiseptic 52*:229-235.

Soihet, S. (1974). Surgical treatment in the incompetent cervix. In *Recent Advances in Human Reproduction.* Excerpta Medica, Amsterdam.

Weekes, A. R. L., Menzies, D. N., and de Boer, C. H. (1977). The relative efficacy of bed rest, cervical suture and no treatment in the management of twin pregnancy. *Br. J. Obstet. Cynaecol. 84*:161-164.

Zakut, H., Inster, V., and Serr, D. M. (1977). Elective cervical suture in preventing premature delivery in multiple pregnancies. *Isr. J. Med. Sci. 13*: 488-492.

3

Fetoscopy

DENYS V. I. FAIRWEATHER and R. H. T. WARD / School of Medicine,
University College London, England

DEVELOPMENT OF METHODS AND INSTRUMENTATION

The term *fetoscopy* was introduced first in 1969 by Scrimgeour of Edinburgh
to describe the technique of intrauterine visualization of the fetus. However,
the first report and description of a technique allowing direct viewing of the
fetus in utero was in October 1954. Westin, in a letter to *The Lancet* titled
"Hysteroscopy in Early Pregnancy," reported that, under general anesthesia in
two cases, and local anesthetic in a third, a 10 mm McCarthy's panendoscope
had been introduced through the cervix into the amniotic cavity prior to therapeutic termination of pregnancies between 14 and 18 weeks' gestation. He
succeeded in observing and photographing the fetus and, in the case where local
anesthesia was used, fetal movements and fetal swallowing were seen. Full de-
tailes of those and an additional six cases were not published until 1957 when
Westin suggested that this hysteroscopic technique opened new possibilities for
obtaining information on the physiology of the fetus.

The next approach was described in 1967 by Mandelbaum and his colleagues
who used an amnioscope passed per abdomen through a 14-gauge needle into
the uterus as for amniocentesis, together with a second needle (16-gauge) for
insertion of a lighting system and the transfusion catheter as a method of
visualizing the fetus to aid intrauterine transfusion of the fetus in Rhesus disease. Neither the stage of gestation nor the success of the procedure was
recorded, although it was suggested that *amnioscopy* might open new research
avenues related to intrauterine existence, hematologic testing of the fetus, and

photographic recording of prenatal events. In 1969 Wade and colleagues, using a modified pediatric fiberoptic cystoscope, reported intrauterine fetal transfusion in two patients using transabdominal amnioscopy to insert the transfusion needle into the fetal peritoneal cavity. Only one case was successful and the authors believed that the 5-mm diameter of the cannula was potentially too traumatic. In the unsuccessful case, amniotic fluid leakage and premature labor supervened.

The next report came from Valenti in 1972, again using a modified pediatric cystoscope inserted under epidural anesthesia through an abdominal and uterine incision in six patients who were to undergo hysterotomy for termination of pregnancy between 14 and 18 weeks of gestation. He described a technique for fetal tissue (skin and muscle) biopsy. In the following year (Valenti, 1973), he extended the application of the technique (again in patients about to undergo termination of pregnancy). He inserted a 27-gauge needle into the umbilical cord 1 in. from its insertion into the fetal abdominal wall to take fetal blood samples in an attempt to diagnose hemoglobinopathies prenatally. At about the same time Scrimgeour (1973a,b), using a fiberoptic telescope with outside diameter of 2.2 mm and length of 20 cm, introduced through an appropriately sized trocar and cannula, reported his experience of fetoscopy in 28 patients in midtrimester where termination of pregnancy was already planned. The procedure was carried out under general anesthesia through a small suprapubic incision to display the uterus, the wall of which was then incised to expose the amniotic membrane in an area free of placenta (the placenta having been previously localized by ultrasound). The trochar was inserted into the amniotic sac, and then removed, leaving the cannula down which the telescope was passed. Escape of amniotic fluid was kept to a minimum by tension on two mattress sutures inserted at the ends of the small uterine incision. On completion of the procedure, the trochar wound was closed, and the pregnancy was then terminated by hysterotomy. This series verified that it was possible to carry out visual inspection and photography of the fetus in the midtrimester and that around 18 weeks' gestation was the optimal time for the procedure. Scrimgeour then went on to carry out fetoscopy in six patients at high risk of having a fetus with a neural tube defect and was the first to apply the technique to pregnancies which were intended to continue if no fetal abnormality was detected. In three no problems were encountered and the fetuses proved to be normal on delivery around term. The other three presented problems; one thought normal went into premature labor at 34 weeks and the baby had spina bifida and hydrocephaly; one failed entry may have caused fetal damage and the pregnancy was terminated, showing spina bifida; in the third, good visualization was obtained but abortion occurred after 48 hr and the placenta was found damaged close to cord insertion. These caused Scrimgeour to conclude that at that time fetoscopy could not be considered as a practical technique where continuation of the pregnancy was desired.

In April and May 1974, Hobbins and his colleagues at Yale, still working in patients scheduled for midtrimester termination of pregnancy, reported the use under local anesthesia of fetoscopy with a 1.7-mm diameter Dyonics needle-scope through a 2.7 X 2.2 mm diameter oval cannula for fetal skin biopsies (26 cases) and fetal blood sampling (eight cases). This instrument was originally designed for orthopedic purposes (arthoscopy) and has subsequently, with minor modifications, been used by the majority of fetoscopists. The abdominal approach was as for amniocentesis.

The next report with a pregnancy continuing after fetoscopy came from Laurence and his associates from Wales in 1975. Visualization of the fetus at 18 weeks' gestation was obtained through a Richard Wolf 9-mm rigid end-view laparoscope inserted under general anesthesia using a technique similar to that reported by Scrimgeour. Digital abnormalities were excluded and the pregnancy continued despite liquor leakage from 26 weeks until 35 weeks' gestation when delivery was achieved by cesarean section. In 1976, Benzie et al. reported another case going to term after fetoscopy at 16 weeks' to exclude arthrogryposis multiplex congenita. Alter and her associates (1976) reported four cases where fetoscopy (carried out twice in two of the four) for fetal blood sampling between 19 and 25 weeks' gestation for antenatal diagnosis of β-thalassemia major showed nonaffected fetuses. The infants were subsequently delivered healthy at or near term. Both these groups used the Dyonics needle-scope (details of which are given below) with local anesthesia for the procedure.

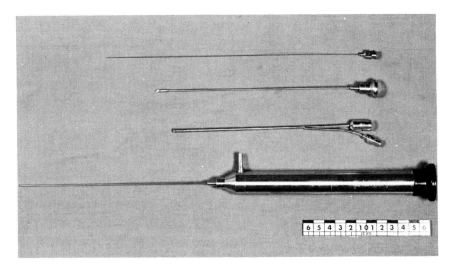

Figure 1. Dyonics needlescope with Hobbins cannula and sharp trochar for insertion and 25 G needle for fetal blood sampling.

In 1976, Gustavii and Cordesius described a transvaginal approach for fetoscopy. Under local anaesthetic in six patients undergoing termination of pregnancy, they inserted the needlescope through the anterior fornix into the uterus and amniotic cavity and were able to visualize fetal vessels on the chorionic plate of the placenta from which blood samples were obtained. No further reports of this approach which, it was suggested, was particularly applicable when the placenta was anteriorly situated, have appeared.

Since 1977 experience with the abdominal approach for fetoscopy under local anesthesia used for a variety of indications has increased rapidly, as has the literature on the subject.

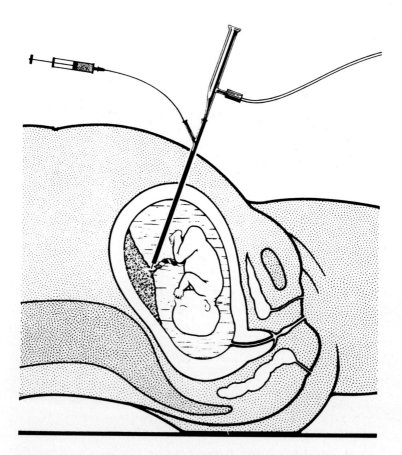

Figure 2. Needlescope in use for blood sampling from vessel close to cord insertion.

Fetoscopes

A variety of fetoscopes produced by different manufacturers are currently available and have a range of diameters from 1.7 mm upwards. The require cannulas of diameters from around 2 mm upwards for their insertion. The cannula may be provided with a side-arm to give access for a sampling needle or to allow attachment of a flushing system. The available angle of vision varies from 55 to 105°, depending on the optical system, and the diameter of the visual field, magnification, and focus varies with the distance from the fetoscope tip to the object in view. The length of the instrument is normally 15 cm. To date, only rigid instruments have been commercially produced, although preliminary trials with a flexible-ended instrument have been undertaken (Fairweather, 1980). Illumination is provided by a fiberoptic guide from a high-power light source.

The Dyonics needlescope shown in Figure 1 is a 1.7-mm diameter by 15 cm long rigid-rod endoscope, the image being carried by a solid self-focusing lens surrounded by fibers along which light is transmitted. For insertion into the uterus it is passed through a 2.7×2.2 mm oval cannula. Its focal length is about 2 cm with a 70° angle of visualization and magnification of 2-5 times. Figure 2 illustrates diagramatically the fetoscope in use for fetal blood sampling.

FETOSCOPY TECHNIQUE

Preparation

Timing
If visualization of the fetus is the main indication for fetoscopy, this is best timed between 15 and 17 weeks'. For fetal blood sampling or fetal tissue biopsy, fetoscopy is best delayed until the 18th-20th week when the fetal blood volume (18.5 ml at 16 weeks' increasing to 32 ml at 18 weeks' and 45 ml at 20 weeks' [Ward and Modell, 1981]) has increased sufficiently to improve the margin of safety. Later than the 20th week the vision may be impaired by clumps of desquamated squamous cells, which give a clouded appearance to the amniotic fluid.

Assessment of the Pregnancy before Fetoscopy
Ideally, a B-scan ultrasound is performed some weeks beforehand to confirm the presence of a single, viable fetus, or twins, and allow accurate calculation of the gestational age. This examination is also valuable when confirming subsequent fetal growth, particularly in patients who have threatened to abort and yet still wish to have prenatal diagnosis.

Expert counseling is mandatory for all couples before prenatal diagnosis, but particularly when fetoscopy is required, since it carries greater risks than

amniocentesis. The couple at risk of a condition for which fetoscopy is indicated should have a full explanation of the nature, limitations, and hazards
of the procedure. Furthermore, the problems associated with midtrimester
therapeutic abortion should be raised. Prenatal diagnosis in the presence of
twins raises special problems. The possibility of failure to make a diagnosis at
all, or of succeeding in only one fetus, should be discussed, as well as the
ethical dilemma when considering abortion of an unaffected with an affected
fetus (Camba et al., 1981).

Equipment
The following sterile equipment is needed:

Drapes and four towel clips.
Sponges and antiseptic solution in gallipot.
Packet of 4 X 4 in. swabs.
Sponge-holding forceps.
Kidney dish, filled with sterile water.
Various syringes: for local anesthetic (1 X 5 ml), collection of amniotic fluid
    (1 X 20 ml), and fetal blood sampling (4 X 1 ml), flushed with heparin.
Two 21-gauge 1½- or 2-in. hypodermic needles.
One 25-gauge hypodermic needle.
No. 11 scalpel blade.
In a gallipot: heparin 100,000 U freeze-dried mixed with 5 ml 0.9% sodium
    chloride (for prenatal diagnosis of hemophilia, sodium citrate is used as the
    anticoagulant).
Needlescope (Dyonics Inc.) and light cable.
Hobbins cannula and both sharp and blunt trochars. The operating channel of
    amniotic fluid and also helps to control the sampling needle. (A hole is made
    in the diaphragm with a No. 1 needle).
Two 23-cm-long 25-, 26-, or 27-gauge needles for fetal blood sampling, flushed
    with heparin).
Nonsterile equipment: light source, Coulter cell channelyser, real-time
    ultrasound.

Care of the Needlescope Equipment
The needlescope and light cable are sterilized by being placed in a metal tank
containing Cidex (glutaraldehyde) for 20-30 min. Before the procedure they
are removed from the tank, rinsed with sterile water in the kidney dish, and
dried. Particular attention should be given to the lens and eye-piece of the
needlescope. Between cases, the needlescope and light cable are washed and
reimmersed in Cidex for sterilization. When not in use, the needlescope should
be kept in its box to minimize damage, particularly to the lens.

The other equipment can be conveniently prepared and packed in a C.S.S.D. pack. However, the sharpness of the trochar may be better safeguarded if the cannula and trochar are kept and sterilized on site.

General Fetoscopy Procedure

The procedure is performed in an operating room under strict aseptic conditions. Premedication with diazepam 10 mg orally is given to the patient and she is made comfortable in the dorsal position with one pillow under her head. An operating table that allows both lateral and vertical tilt is ideal, but a delivery bed with a firm mattress can be used. In particularly apprehensive patients, and when fetal examination is indicated, a "butterfly" needle is inserted into a vein in the dorsum of the patient's hand so that diazepam may be injected as necessary. Before fetal blood sampling is undertaken, a maternal blood sample is taken to demonstrate the maternal cell size peak on the Coulter channelyser and for estimation of serum alpha-fetoprotein and the patient's Rh group, if this is not already known. At this stage, prior to scrubbing up, the surgeon should palpate the abdomen to determine the height and size of the uterus, and note any abdominal scars or excess obesity that may complicate the procedure. Real-time ultrasound immediately before the procedure is the key to success, and identification of the various intrauterine structures may take as long as the fetoscopy procedure itself.

Selection of the site for cannula insertion depends on the position of the placenta, site of the cord insertion, position of the fetus, and the availability of a satisfactory pool of amniotic fluid (see Fig. 3).

When the placenta is posterior, care is necessary because it is easy to "overshoot." It is helpful to measure the distance to the chorionic plate. In the majority of patients in whom the placenta is predominantly anterior, it is possible to find a placenta-free window. Although a site directly over the fetal body is best avoided, it is wisest to choose an approach where there is a pool of amniotic fluid, suitably splinted to some extent by fetal limbs. Because of the comparative shortness of the cannula (particularly in the obese patient), undue angulation to the uterine entry site may lead to failure to enter the amniotic cavity, or stripping of the membranes, or the cannula being dislodged from the amniotic cavity. The whereabouts of the cord insertion must be taken into account in planning the optimum insertion site. Blood samples can be safely taken from a vessel near the cord insertion (Rodeck and Campbell, 1979) and this site may be preferred. However, if samples need not be 100% fetal, smaller vessels elsewhere on the chorionic plate can be used. When the main indication for fetoscopy is visualization, the exact site of insertion of the fetoscope must be determined by the way the fetus is lying. To alter the fetal position, the patient may be asked to

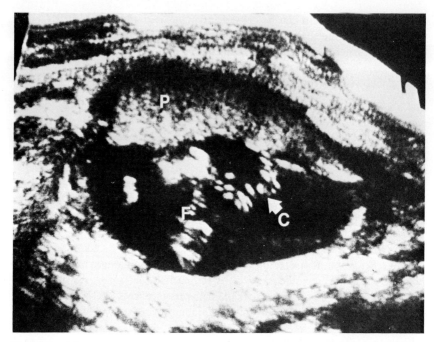

Figure 3. Ultrasound display showing placental site (P), fetal parts (F), and umbilical cord (C) of 16-week pregnancy.

empty her bladder at this stage. However, a full or half-full bladder may be helpful when the placenta is predominantly anterior. Relative contraindications will be apparent at this stage in a few cases. These are discussed later (see Technical Difficulties).

The cord insertion and the proposed site for insertion of the cannula are marked on the patient's abdominal skin (a small coin, pressed firmly, is ideal for this purpose). The surgeon and assistant don hats and masks and, after a surgical scrub, put on gowns and gloves. It is our practice then to assemble the needlescope in the cannula and confirm patency of the 27-gauge needles by flushing with heparin. The light cable is attached to the needlescope and the optical system checked. The patient's abdominal skin is cleaned with antiseptic and draped, leaving a wide area to allow access for real-time ultrasound scanning. The 5MHz transducer and lead of the real-time scanner are cleaned with chlorhexidine in spirit, and the surface covered with sterile KY jelly. The whole transducer is placed in a size 8 sterile glove and sterile KY jelly applied over the gloved transducer head. (Alternatively, the transducer can be placed in a sterile polythene bag and sterile liquid paraffin used for acoustic coupling) (Rodeck, 1980).

Rescan under sterile conditions is now performed and, while the intrauterine anatomy is visualized, the patient should be instructed to remain still, breathe normally, and refrain from coughing.

Once the site of entry and the depth of insertion necessary are determined, local anesthetic (1% lignocaine) is infiltrated down to the rectus sheath. A small skin incision is then made with a No. 11 scalpel blade. The cannula with the sharp trochar in situ is inserted first through the abdominal wall, and then with a deliberate thrust into the uterine cavity. For the surgeon who is experienced in amniocentesis, a similar feeling of sudden lack of resistance is evident when the amniotic cavity is entered. The trochar is removed and amniotic fluid usually flows back up the cannula. To take a specimen for alpha-fetoprotein examination and, if indicated, cell culture, it is necessary to block the side-arm of the cannula. Great care must be taken not to dislodge the cannula from the amniotic sac. If blood is aspirated at this stage, the real-time scanner will usually resolve the difficulty. The tip of the cannula can be readily identified, enabling the surgeon to advance, withdraw, or angle it as necessary. Any blood-stained specimen of amniotic fluid should be tested for fetal cells. The needlescope is now passed down the cannula and preliminary visualization undertaken. Occasionally the cannula may "overshoot" into a posterior placenta, or bleeding from the uterus itself may lead to blood-staining of the amniotic fluid.

Success or failure of the procedure will then depend on the amount of bleeding and the speed with which visualization or a sample of fetal blood can be safely obtained. A modest amount of blood in the amniotic fluid will clear within a week, but it has been our experience that heavy blood contamination makes subsequent fetoscopy with visualization impossible.

After successful fetoscopy, the needlescope is withdrawn from the cannula and replaced by the blunt trochar. The insertion of the trochar before withdrawal of the cannula is important to prevent any evagination of the membranes. The cannula, along with the trochar, is withdrawn quickly, the puncture site compressed with the finger for 30 sec, and then covered with a plastic dressing and bandage.

Further Management

Medication

Some centers favor prophylactic antibiotics either given to the patient before fetoscopy or injected intra-amniotically. Tocolytic agents given before and/or after the procedure to damp down uterine activity have also been used but the value of those measures has not been established and opinion is divided. Anti-D 100 μg is given intramuscularly to all Rh-negative patients who do not already have antibodies.

Records

An accurate record of the procedure should be made immediately, describing any technical problems. The site of the cannula entry and cord insertion are noted, as well as the placental position and whether the amniotic fluid was clear at the end of the procedure. This latter point is important for the rare occasions that a repeat procedure is necessary.

General

We make a practice of demonstrating the fetal heartbeat immediately after fetoscopy since bradycardia has been noted in some cases, although this does not necessarily mean that there has been fetal or placental trauma. In addition, it provides some comfort to the patient to see that her fetus is unharmed by the procedure. The patient remains recumbent for 10 min and is then transferred to a bed to rest for the remainder of the day. Although we have kept patients overnight in the past, we have recently reverted to allowing them to return home the same day with instructions to avoid all but light activity and to abstain from coitus for a week. After a technically difficult procedure, or when the amniotic fluid is left heavily blood-stained, we consider stricter bed rest advisable in an attempt to reduce subsequent complications. The patient is told to report any fever, pain, contractions, vaginal bleeding, or amniotic fluid leakage.

Technique for Fetal Examination and Skin Biopsy

Depending on the area of the fetal anatomy to be visualized or biopsied, the fetoscope approach may have to be delayed until the fetus is in a favorable position. When necessary, the fetus can be effectively sedated by suitable medication to the mother via the butterfly needle. Specific parts of the fetus can readily be identified by fetoscopy, although there may be difficulties in orientation and a total examination of fetal surface anatomy is rarely achieved. Indeed, even total visualization of the back or entire length of the fetal spine may be difficult. The earlier in gestation the more body parts are visible but, of course, they are then less well differentiated. Skin biopsy specimens are usually taken from the fetal scalp or trunk. For the information and guidance of the surgeon, the synchronous use of real-time ultrasound is essential. When a suitable area has been located, the endoscope is removed, the biopsy forceps are inserted, real-time ultrasound checks approximated to the fetus, and the biopsy is performed. It is essential to use the ultrasound to check that fetal movement has not occurred between removing the endoscope and taking the biopsy specimen.

Technique for Fetal Blood Sampling

Fetoscopy

Under direct vision via the fetoscope either the cord insertion or a suitable fetal vessel on the chorionic plate is identified. We have not had a preference

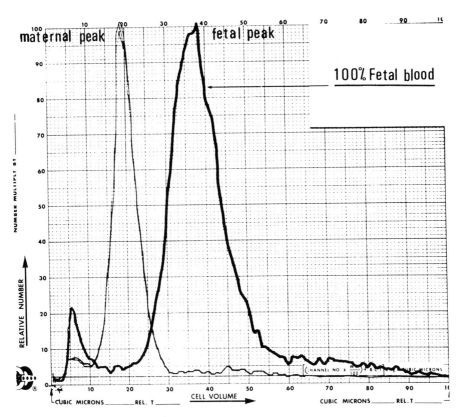

Figure 4. Maternal and fetal cell size distribution curves.

for a vein or artery although the latter bleeds for a few seconds longer than the
vein when sampling is completed. The 27 gauge needle is threaded through the
side arm of the cannula and a 1 ml syringe attached. The needle point is visualized by the surgeon and inserted with a deliberate thrust into the chosen
vessel. Aspiration usually produces fetal blood if the tip of the needle is within
the vessel, but if there is no flow the needle is very slowly withdrawn until
blood is obtained. It is rarely necessary to collect more than 0.5 ml but 1-2 ml
can be safely taken. Each sample of blood is immediately examined for fetal
cells with a cell-size analyser such as the Coulter channelyser. Fetal blood is
readily distinguished from maternal by the larger size of the fetal cells (see
Fig. 4). If pure fetal blood is not necessary for diagnosis, it is possible to
aspirate amniotic fluid in the immediate vicinity of the puncture site, which
is invariably rich in fetal cells. The bleeding from the fetal blood vessel stops

within 15-20 sec. As stated, fetal blood samples may be obtained from vessels on the chorionic plate, or from the cord, usually at the placental insertion. The latter has the advantages that pure fetal blood is consistently obtained, there is little risk of fetomaternal haemorrhage, and hemostasis is rapid (Rodeck and Campbell, 1979).

When an effort is made to sample from a vessel, either arterial or venous on the chorion plate, the amnion may slide in front of the sampling needle. Furthermore, the vessel may be transfixed so that initially maternal blood is sampled from the intervillous space, a situation which leads to fetomaternal hemorrhage. Withdrawing the needle into the lumen of the fetal vessel, if done carefully, still allows satisfactory fetal samples to be collected. In either case, we always aspirate a sample of amniotic fluid after withdrawing the needle, as often this contains 100% fetal blood.

If inadvertent blood-staining occurs after insertion of the cannula, a 20-ml syringe can be used to remove some of the blood-stained amniotic fluid. However, when heavy bleeding occurs, we have occasionally used a flushing system with Hartman's solution. This manoeuver allows a flow of clear fluid to emerge gently ahead of the fetoscope and continue while blood sampling is done. The solution is delivered via a system consisting of a drip set and plain extension tubing attached to a "T" connection with the operating arm of the cannula. The rate of flow should be enough to allow adequate visualization. When a satisfactory sample has been obtained (or the procedure abandoned) the amount of solution infused is estimated (usually about 50 ml) and excess amniotic fluid removed to avoid overdistention of the uterus.

The role of the assistant. When fetal blood samples are being taken, an assistant should be responsible for inserting the 27-gauge sampling needle (previously introduced through the diaphragm of the rubber stopper) into the side-arm of the cannula, attaching a 1 ml heparinized syringe, and gently moving the plunger when instructed. When blood is obtained (or if either amniotic fluid or no blood appears in the syringe) the assistant should tell the surgeon. When the syringe is being changed, suction on the plunger should be discontinued (to release the vacuum).

Placentacentesis, Placental Aspiration, Blind Needling
These synonymous terms describe the second method of midtrimester fetal blood sampling which was developed as a direct result of experience with amniocentesis, to obtain samples of fetal red cells, especially from patients in whom initially it was believed that fetoscopy was not possible because the placenta was anteriorly situated. As indicated above, fetoscopy is now generally found to be possible, regardless of the situation of the placenta.

The technique was first described by Kan's group in 1974 in 19 patients who were undergoing termination of pregnancy between 18 and 22 weeks' gestation. They were successful in obtaining samples containing 2-95% of fetal cells in 11. Later that year, the group (Chang et al., 1974), still working on patients undergoing termination of pregnancy, confirmed the feasibility of using the mixed samples obtained by this technique for in utero diagnosis of hemoglobinopathies and in, May, 1975 (Kan et al., 1975) they described the first successful application of prenatal diagnosis in a pregnancy at risk for homozygous β-thalassemia, using this technique. The fetus was reported non-affected and the pregnancy continued until 39 weeks' when a normal infant was delivered. Since then, a number of workers, particularly our own group in London (Fairweather et al., 1980), have continued to report successful use of the technique in selected cases.

Technique. The selection and preparation of patients are similar to that for fetoscopy. The placenta is localized and under local anesthesia and real-time ultrasound control, similarly to amniocentesis, a 19-21-gauge spinal needle is directed to where the tip is just inside the chorionic plate of the placenta. This should allow the entering or traversing of a fetal vessel in the plate and aspiration of small amounts of blood or blood-stained amniotic fluid into a heparinized syringe. The presence of fetal cells in the sample is checked (as for fetoscopy cases) using the Coulter channelyser. The samples often contain mixtures of fetal and maternal red cells and their value for diagnostic purposes depends both upon the percentage of fetal cells present and the type of disorder for which prenatal diagnosis is being employed. For this reason the technique may be useful, for example, for diagnosis of β-thalassemia (where as little as 2-5% of fetal cells may be adequate) but is less satisfactory where 100% fetal sample is necessary (e.g., for hemophilia) for diagnostic purposes. Where fetoscopy has failed, and the amniotic fluid is subsequently too blood-stained or turbid to allow visualization, placentacentesis may be the only alternative method of obtaining a sample suitable for diagnostic purposes. For this reason we still believe that this technique has a place, albeit limited, for use in centers where midtrimester fetal blood sampling is carried out regularly.

TECHNICAL DIFFICULTIES

Maternal Obesity

Because of the relatively short effective length of the cannula, fetoscopy may not be possible in the very obese patient.

The Anterior Placenta

Initially, only patients with posterior placentas were considered as suitable candidates but, with experience, successful fetoscopy is possible in the majority of patients with an anterior placenta. A careful search will usually identify a "window" since the placenta rarely completely covers the anterior uterine wall. Tilting the patient laterally to encourage uterine rotation in the long axis, or waiting until her bladder fills, may be helpful. If the situation remains hopeless, it is worth delaying the procedure for a week or more. If at that time no placentafree area is found, the surgeon has a choice of selecting a site where the placenta is thinnest, or performing placentacentesis. The former has the disadvantage that maternal bleeding may occur not only into the amniotic fluid, obscuring a satisfactory view, but also retroplacentally. The latter is inappropriate when pure fetal blood is essential for diagnosis.

The Posterior Placenta

"Overshooting" and puncturing the placenta can occur with consequent heavy blood-staining of the amniotic fluid. Ironically, this is more likely to occur in the very thin patient, particularly if the placenta bulges into the amniotic cavity. Careful assessment of the depth of the chorionic plate beforehand, and selection of a site where there is a good pool of amniotic fluid, preferably splinted by fetal parts, should minimize this problem. Occasionally the fetus intervenes between the surgeon and the best source of blood. Access may be obtained by careful manipulation of the needlescope or by tilting the patient.

Oligohydramnios

A reduced amount of amniotic fluid is a major problem. Delaying the procedure for as long as possible gives the surgeon the opportunity to confirm that normal fetal growth is occurring and the best hope for successful fetoscopy.

Failure to Penetrate the Membranes

This is nearly always due to a blunted trochar. If a substitute sharp trochar is not available, the procedure is best delayed. Alternatively, substitution of the trochar with a very long 22-gauge needle, passed through the membranes may allow the cannula to be introduced through the hole (Mahoney, 1980). The trochar needs to be sharpened at regular intervals.

Visualization

This can be due to blood or turbidity of the amniotic fluid, both of which reduce the chance of successful fetoscopy. Blood-staining may be the result of earlier amniocentesis or threatened abortion, while fresh bleeding can be induced at fetoscopy. Flushing the contaminated field with Hartman's solution is occasionally successful (See Fetoscopy).

Abdominal Scars

Previous gut surgery or peritonitis may lead to adhesions beneath the scars, so that in such patients great care should be taken in choosing a suitable site for the cannula insertion. A too lateral approach is also to be avoided because of the risk to the uterine vessels, which may be particularly vulnerable in the presence of uterine rotation.

Twin Pregnancy

Successful sampling from both fetuses depends very much on the position of the placentas and access to both sacs. It has been our practice, to enter each sac separately through two different skin incisions (Camba et al., 1981), but Rodeck and Wass (1981) have described blood sampling in twin pregnancies using a single approach. The injection of methylene blue into one sac after successfully sampling both fetal circulations confirms that both sacs were indeed separately entered. In addition, the risks of premature delivery after prenatal fetal blood sampling in a twin pregnancy are considerable (see below).

SAFETY AND COMPLICATIONS

Fetoscopy

The obstetric risks of fetoscopy are not yet fully known and individual series are too small to define the problems. Certain risks have been identified from the world experience of fetoscopy (Prenatal Diagnosis, 1980).

Maternal Risks
Local pain at the site of insertion may be due to a hematoma, in either the abdominal wall or uterine muscle. Other risks include local infection at the insertion site and, rarely, septicemia following amnionitis. Maternal sensitisation may occur in the Rh-negative mother with an Rh-positive fetus. A double dose of anti-D may be more appropriate when a mixed blood sample is obtained at fetoscopy or after blind needling.

Fetal Risks
The incidence of fetal loss decreases as individual obstetricians acquire experience in the technique of fetoscopy. Unfortunately the data from many of the series could not be readily compared because both diagnostic cases and procedures before therapeutic abortion were reported and results sometimes did not take account of undelivered pregnancies. A group of fetoscopists

Table 1. Collected Data on Pregnancy Outcome after Fetoscopy for Visualization or Fetal Blood Sampling, and after Placentacentesis

	Total fetoscopies	Fetoscopy for visualization only	Fetoscopy for fetal blood sampling	Placentacentesis only	Placentacentesis following fetoscopy
Total cases	331	54	277	153	29
Total fetal and perinatal[a] loss (%)	10.2	11.4	9.9	12.7	26.1
Fetal loss within 7 days of procedure (%)	3.0	3.7	2.9	9.8	20.7
Fetal loss after 7 days of procedure and perinatal loss (%)	5.1	6.1	4.9	0	0
Premature delivery (%)	11.2	15.2	10.2	5.6	23.5

[a]Including neonatal deaths in first 7 days.
Summary from Prenatal Diagnosis, 1980.

Table 2. Fetal Loss Before 26 Weeks Following 205 Diagnostic Fetoscopies[a] in 198 Pregnancies

Method used and number of pregnancies	Therapeutic abortions for thalassemia major	Pregnancies intended to continue	Number of IUFD[b] (%)	Number of spontaneous abortions (%)	Pregnancies continuing beyond 26 weeks
Fetoscopy only 147 (154 fetoscopies)	33	114	3 (2.6)	6 (5.3)	105
Both fetoscopy and placentacentesis 51	11	40	7 (17.5)	4 (10)	29

[a]All for midtrimester fetal blood sampling.
[b]IUFD = intrauterine fetal deaths.

(Prenatal Diagnosis, 1980) first met in November 1979 in an attempt to clarify the true nature of the fetal risks. Their findings are summarized in Table 1.

Early fetal loss. Fetal loss within a week of the procedure includes intra-uterine fetal death (IUFD) and spontaneous abortion. When IUFD occurs, it is usually noted immediately after the procedure and can be caused by direct fetal or placental trauma, fetal exsanguination, and occasionally amnionitis, which may be secondary to spontaneous amniotic fluid leakage. However, spontaneous abortion may be delayed for several weeks and in our experience has a strong association with amniotic fluid leakage. The initial experience at Yale in a series of 102 fetoscopies (Mahoney, 1980) gave a 6% loss due to abortion or amnionitis. In a later report (DeVore et al., 1980) the risk of spontaneous abortion was less than 5% and Rodeck (1980) had an early loss of 3.7% of continuing pregnancies. Our own experience (Ward et al., 1981) of 154 diagnostic fetoscopies for fetal blood sampling in 147 pregnancies (Table 2) gave an incidence of 7.9% for early IUFD and spontaneous abortion. If fetoscopy had to be followed by placentacentesis to obtain a suitable sample (51 pregnancies), the early fetal loss rate rose to 27.5%.

Amniotic Fluid Leakage

This may occur soon after the procedure or be delayed for many weeks. Such a delay may follow failure of the hole in the membranes to heal after fetoscopy (Rocker and Laurence; 1978). The reported incidence of amniotic fluid leakage varies between series: 2.7% (Mahoney, 1980) to 8% (Rodeck, 1980). In our series (Ward et al., 1981) (Table 3), following successful fetoscopy the incidence was 6.8% but rose to 21.6% when placentacentesis was also required. One in three of the pregnancies complicated by amniotic fluid leakage ended in spontaneous abortion.

Prematurity

The fetoscopy group's (Prenatal Diagnosis, 1980) combined data gave a pre-maturity rate of 11.2%. Individual series have shown rates of 11% (Mahoney, 1980) and 12.7% (Rodeck, 1980). (Eight patients of the 63 delivered pregnancies.) In our series (Ward et al., 1981) the rate was 14.3% following success-ful fetoscopy but rose to 37.9% when placentacentesis was also required, giving an overall rate of 19.4% (Table 4). However, many of these deliveries occurred in the 35th and 36th weeks and the two twin pregnancies that were delivered at 27½ and 30 weeks have been included. Furthermore, the in-cidence of previous terminations of pregnancy was high in this population (Modell et al., 1980) before prenatal diagnosis became available, predisposing to cervical incompetence with subsequent higher rates of both spontaneous abortion and premature rupture of membranes.

Table 3. Outcome of 21 Pregnancies in which Amniotic Fluid Leakage Occurred after Fetoscopy[a]

Method used and number of pregnancies	Therapeutic abortions for thalassemia major	Spontaneous abortions	Premature delivery	Mature delivery	Total number (%)
Fetoscopy only 147 (154 fetoscopies)	1	4	4	1	10 (6.8)
Both fetoscopy and placentacentesis 51	1	3	4	3	11 (21.6)
Total 198	2	7	8	4	21 (10.6)

[a]All cases for midtrimester fetal blood sampling.

Table 4. Time of Delivery (after 26 weeks) in 134 Continuing Pregnancies after Fetoscopy[a]

Method used and number of pregnancies	34 weeks or less (%)	35 and 36 weeks (%)	Total up to 36 weeks (%)	37 weeks and over	Incomplete data on maturity
Fetoscopy only 105	7[b] (6.7)	8 (7.6)	15[b] (14.3)	83	7
Both fetoscopy and placentacentesis 29	8[b] (27.6)	3 (10.3)	11[b] (37.9)	17	1
Percentage of total pregnancies	11.2	8.2	19.4	—	—

[a]All cases for midtrimester fetal blood sampling.
[b]Includes one twin pregnancy.

Total Fetal and Neonatal Loss

The fetoscopy group (Prenatal Diagnosis, 1980) gave an overall loss of 10.2%. However, when corrected for those fetuses lost which were subsequently found to have thalassemia, or which had lethal anomalies unrelated to the procedure, the figure was 8.8%. In Rodeck's series (1980) four losses were attributed to the procedure in 108 pregnancies. (There were, however, two other late fetal deaths in this series and 41 patients still undelivered.) Our own experience (Ward et al., 1981) shows an overall fetal loss of 22 fetuses in 198 pregnancies (11.1%), 20 of which were early losses and two were neonatal deaths, one at 30 weeks and a twin at 27½ weeks. The corrected figure (excluding the one fetus with thalassemia major) was 10.6%.

The risks to any pregnancy of failed fetoscopy must be considered carefully since occasional failure is inevitable even when considerable experience has been obtained.

Placentacentesis

Although the technique is disarmingly simple, the risk of damage (with subsequent fetal exsanguination) to a large fetal vessel is much greater than with the 25- or 27-gauge needle used for fetal blood sampling under direct vision by fetoscopy. Early fetal loss from abortion or intrauterine death is, therefore, more likely with this technique. Because the 19-21-gauge needle is much smaller than the 2.2 X 2.7 mm fetoscope cannula, consequently making a smaller rent in the membranes, the risk of amniotic fluid leakage and premature labor is, however, less than with fetoscopy. There is an overall fetal loss rate of 12.7% (Prenatal Diagnosis, 1980). Our own experience (Ward et al., 1981) in 137 pregnancies where placentacentesis (181 procedures) was performed, showed an early fetal loss rate of 15% corrected to 11%) for the 97 pregnancies remaining after therapeutic abortions had been excluded, but the immediate fetal loss can be as low as 3.5% (Angioni, personal communication).

The incidence of amniotic fluid leakage and premature delivery was 4 and 10%, respectively.

Present Status

The international fetoscopy group met again in Edinburgh in July, 1980, and reported (Fairweather, 1980) (Table 5) their conclusion that for experienced operators, while fetoscopy carried a lower overall fetal loss (3-5%) than placentacentesis (6-9%), the prematurity rate was greater after fetoscopy. When both procedures were used, the risks of both fetal loss and prematurity were greatly increased.

Table 5. Current Results of Experienced Operators (%)

Procedure	Fetoscopy and fetal blood sampling	Placentacentesis alone	Both fetoscopy and placentacentesis
Success with first procedure	80-95	80-90	
Fetal and perinatal loss	3-5	6-9	30-40
Premature labor	16	4	33

[a]Data collected by Fetoscopy Group (Fairweather, 1980).

APPLICATIONS OF FETOSCOPY

The applications of fetoscopy can be considered under four main headings.

Visualization of Fetal Anatomy

Fetoscopy for prenatal diagnosis of genetic abnormalities which are detectable or able to be excluded by inspection of the exterior of the fetus for a marker feature is usually combined with ultrasound examination.

Recent technical advances with ultrasound have so increased the definition, dimensions, and quality of pictures produced (see Fig. 5) that ultrasound may displace fetoscopy in this role; it has the added advantage that it is a noninvasive technique. In cases where there are other conflicting or indeterminate data (e.g., high alphafetoprotein levels although ultrasound fails to demonstrate a neural tube defect) fetoscopy may continue to be useful.

To date, abnormalities that have been reported diagnosed or excluded by the use of fetoscopy include:

Limb or digit deformities:
   Polydactyly and syndactyly
   Ectrodactyly (lobster-claw hands)
   Abnormal thumbs
   Split-hand syndrome
   Hypoplastic limbs, diastrophic dwarfism
   Single-limb amelia
   Popliteal pterygia

Neural tube deformities:
   Meningomyelocele
   Spina bifida

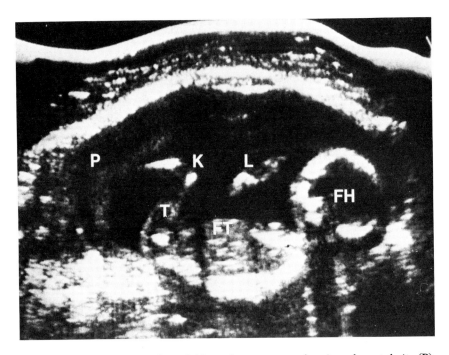

Figure 5. Ultrasound display of 13-week pregnancy showing placental site (P) and knee (K), thigh (T), trunk (FT), upper limb (L), and head (FH) of fetus.

Facial Clefts:
   Cleft lip, cleft palate

Combination deformities or syndromes:
   Ellis-van Creveld syndrome (chondrodystrophy, polydactyly, dysplasia of
       nails
   Arthrogryposis multiplex congenita (abnormal limbs)
   Meckel's syndrome (microcephaly, encephalocele, cleft palate, polydactyly)
   Smith-Lemli-Opitz syndrome (microcephaly, typical facies, genital ab-
       normalities in male syndactyly)
   EEC syndrome (ectrodactyly, ectodermal dysplasia, cleft lip and palate)
   Teacher-Collins syndrome (typical facies, ocular abnormalities, external ear
       abnormalities)
   Laurence-Moon-Biedl syndrome (retinitis pigmentosa, hypogenitalism and
       postaxial polydactyly)
   Cornelia de Lange's syndrome (skeletal abnormalities)
   Holt-Oram syndrome (congenital heart disease, upper limb phocomelia, or
       thumb abnormalities)

Clearly other possible conditions may be amenable to diagnosis by fetoscopy; Mahoney and Hobbins (1979) recently listed more than 50 of these.

Fetal Tissue Biopsy

Up to now fetal skin has been the only tissue biopsied in pregnancies which were destined to continue if no abnormality was detected. The disorders studied were congenital bullous ichthyosiform erythroderma (Golbus et al., 1980), lamellar ichthyosis congenita (nonbullous congenital ichthyosiform erythroderma) Elias et al., 1979). The former is an autosomal dominant and the latter a recessive disorder, often referred to as harlequin syndrome.

Midtrimester Fetal Blood Sampling

Theoretically, access to pure fetal blood samples could allow prenatal diagnosis of a whole range of congenital disorders that manifest an abnormality of any of the fetal blood elements (red blood cells, white blood cells, platelets, or plasma), and lists of such disorders have already been constructed (DeVore et al., 1980). In practice, however, the application has been limited to the following, where specific hematological or biochemical microtechniques have been developed for sample analysis.

1. *Hemoglobinopathies (Which Represent the Main Indications at Present)*
   β-thalassemia major (analysis of globin chain synthesis for β to γ ratio).
   Other thalassemias (globin chain analysis) including:
   $\delta\beta/\beta$-thalassemia, hemoglobin E-thalassaemia
   Hemoglobin Lepore/β-thalassemia, Homozygous α_1 thalassemia
   Hemoglobin S-thalassemia
   Sickle-cell anemia (analysis of globin chain synthesis for presence of γB^s and absence of B^A)

2. *Hemophilia*
   Hemophilia A(classic) (Factor VIII analysis)
   Hemophilia B (Christmas disease) (Factor IX analysis)
   Homozygous van Willebrand's disease (Factor-VIII-related antigen analysis)

3. *Chronic Granulomatous Disease (Enzyme Nadp Activity)*

4. *When Patients Presented Too Late for Amniotic Cell Culture or When Culture was Unsuccessful*
   a. Galactosemia (enzyme galactose 1-phosphate uridyl transferase activity)
   b. Chromosomal analysis to exclude Down's syndrome (Technique allowing chromosome analysis within 72 hr).

5. *Rhesus Isoimmunization.*
   Where the husband is heterozygous and because of previous history of Rh-affected infants, the couple were unwilling to accept another pregnancy in which the fetus is liable to be affected (Rh-positive).

6. *Other Applications Reported Which Must Still be Considered Research*
   Rather than Clinical Practice
   a. *Duchenne's Muscular Dystrophy (DMD).* There have been a number of
      reports of attempts to use fetal blood samples for assay of creatinine
      phosphokinase (CPK) activity to detect this disorder. Several wrong
      predictions have now been documented and it is concluded that mid-
      trimester determination of fetal CPK activity is not an accurate marker
      of this disorder. Other markers are currently being investigated including
      studies of red-cell and white-cell membranes and plasma myoglobin con-
      centrations, but at present accurate in utero diagnosis or exclusion of
      DMD is not possible.
   b. *In utero Fetal Infection.* A few attempts have been made using mid-
      trimester fetal blood samples to detect in utero infection with rubella
      or toxoplasmosis but at present results have failed to show that this
      application is useful or reliable.
   c. *In utero Manipulations.* As indicated in the introduction to this chapter,
      one of the earliest applications suggested for fetoscopy was for placement
      of catheters for in utero intraperitoneal transfusion of the fetus in severe
      Rh disease. While this might be a valuable technique between 18 and 22
      weeks' gestation, few workers resort to intrauterine transfusion as early as
      this stage of gestation. As gestation advances, the practicability of
      fetoscopy diminishes because of the increasing size of the fetus, turbidity
      of the amniotic fluid, and general reduction in available space. Combined
      radiological and ultrasound control for the relatively few cases that now
      require intrauterine transfusion offers a much more satisfactory approach
      than does fetoscopy.

There is no doubt, however, that fetoscopy allows the placement of fine
needles or catheters into the lumena of fetal vessels. Clearly, in the future this
might permit direct infusions of substances for therapeutic purposes. At the
present, however, this is still at the research stage. In the same manner it would
be possible to utilize fetoscopy for transplantation of tissue (e.g., bone marrow)
into the fetus in utero and this approach has already been used in research involving animals.

CONCLUSIONS

Fetoscopy requires the skills of highly trained personnel who are able to use the
technique regularly and are familiar with the difficulties and complications associated with the procedure. It is not a technique for the occasional operator.
Because of the invasive nature of fetoscopy, with its resultant dangers to a
continuing pregnancy, together with the documented increased risks should
fetoscopy fail and a second procedure be required, the indications for employ-

ing the technique must be carefully considered against the severity of the condition suspected and the risk of its occurrence. It should not be used if an alternative, less invasive (e.g., amniocentesis) or noninvasive (e.g., ultrasound) technique can provide the required information. Because of the increased risk of premature labor following fetoscopy, access to skilled neonatal care as well as obstetric expertise, is a necessary consideration when setting up a fetoscopy service.

Although fetoscopy used to provide pure fetal blood samples has enabled prenatal diagnosis of inherited diseases that were previously undetectable through amniocentesis (e.g., β-thalassemia), advances in molecular biological techniques for DNA analysis of amniotic fluid fibroblasts using restriction enzymes to examine specific gene sequences are rapidly changing the scene. These techniques have recently been used on cells obtained by midtrimester amniocentesis to diagnose at least two hemoglobinopathies and the way now seems open to the development of further diagnostic methods which may detect diseases resulting from deletions of gene sequences.

If fetoscopes of smaller diameter become available, the applications of fetoscopy may expand but at present there seems to be a relatively limited field for use of this technique, and even present indications must be kept under review in the light of developments in other technology.

ACKNOWLEDGMENTS

The authors wish to acknowledge the help of Dr. Bernadette Modell and support of their many other colleagues at UCH who have cooperated to make these studies possible. We wish to thank Mr. V. Asta for the art work in Figure 2 and Dr. I. Shirley for providing Figures 3 and 5.

REFERENCES

Alter, B. P., Modell, B., Fairweather, D., Hobbins, J. C., Mahoney, M. J., Frigoletto, F. D., Sherman, A. S., and Nathan, D. G. (1976). Prenatal diagnosis of hemoglobinopathies. A review of 15 cases. *N. Engl. J. Med.* *295:*1437-1443.

Benzie, R. J., Malone, R. M., Miskin, M., Rudd, N. L., and Schofield, P. A. (1976). Prenatal diagnosis by fetoscopy with subsequent normal delivery. Report of a case. *Am. J. Obstet. Gynecol. 126:*287-288.

Camba, L., Ward, R. H. T., Shirley, I., Matsakis, M., Mouzouras, M., and Modell, B. Antenatal diagnosis for thalassemia in twin pregnancies. (In preparation 1981).

Chang, H., Hobbins, J. C., Cividalli, G., Frigoletto, F. D., Mahoney, M. J., Kan, Y. W., Nathan, D. G. (1974). In utero diagnosis of hemoglobinopathies: Hemoglobin synthesis in fetal red cells. *N. Engl. J. Med. 290*:1067-1068.

DeVore, G. R., Mahoney, M. J., and Hobbins, J. C. (1980). Fetoscopy: An update. *Clin. Obstet. Gynecol. 23*:481-498.

Elias, S., Mazur, M., and Simpson, J. L. (1979). Prenatal diagnosis of ichthyosis congenita. *Am. J. Hum. Genet. 31*:70A.

Fairweather, D. V. I. (1980). Personal communication.

Fairweather, D. V. I. (1980). Fetal Blood Sampling in Early Pregnancy. Communication to Plenary Session of 22nd British Congress of Obstetrics and Gynaecology, Edinburgh, July.

Fairweather, D. V. I., Ward, R. H. T., and Modell, B. (1980). Obstetric aspects of midtrimester fetal blood sampling by needling or fetoscopy. *Br. J. Obstet. Gynaecol. 87*:87-99.

Golbus, M. S., Sagebiel, R. W., Filly, R. A., Gindhart, T. D., and Hall, J. G. (1980). Prenatal diagnosis of congenital bullous ichthyosiform erythroderma (epidermolytic hyperkeratosis) by fetal skin biopsy. *N. Engl. J. Med. 302*: 93.

Gustavii, B. and Cordesius, E. (1976). Transvaginal approach for sampling of fetal blood. *Lancet 2*:375.

Hobbins, J. C. and Mahoney, M. J. (1974). In utero diagnosis of hemoglobinopathies: Technic for obtaining fetal blood. *N. Engl. J. Med. 290*:1065-1067.

Hobbins, J. C., Mahoney, M. J., and Goldstein, L. A. (1974). New Method of intrauterine evaluation by the combined use of fetoscopy and ultrasound. *Am. J. Obstet. Gynecol. 118*:1069-1072.

Kan, Y. W., Valenti, C., Carnazza, V., Guidotti, R., and Rieder, R. F. (1974). Fetal blood sampling in utero. *Lancet 1*:79-90.

Kan, Y. W., Golbus, M. S., Klein, P., and Dozy, A. M. (1975). Successful application of prenatal diagnosis in pregnancy at risk for homozygous β-thalassaemia. *N. Engl. J. Med. 292*:1096-1099.

Laurence, K. M., Prosser, R., Rocker, I., Pearson, J. F., and Richards, C. (1975). Hirschsprung's disease associated with congenital heart malformation, broad big toes and ulnar polydactyly in siblings—A case for fetoscopy. *J. Med. Genet. 12*:334-338.

Mahoney, M. J. (1980). *Prenatal Approaches to the Diagnosis of Fetal Hemoglobinopathies*. Y. W. Kan and C. D. Reid (Eds.), N.I.H. Publication no. 1529, pp. 5-8.

Rodeck, C. H. and Wass, D. Sampling pure fetal blood in twin pregnancies by fetoscopy using a single uterine puncture. *Prenatal Diagnosis 1*:43-49.

Mahoney, M. J. and Hobbins, J. C. (1979). Fetoscopy and fetal blood sampling. In *Genetic Disorders and the Fetus-Diagnosis, Presentation and Treatment.* A. Milunsky (Ed.), Plenum, New York and London, pp. 501-526.

Mandelbaum, B., Pontarelli, D. A., and Brushenko, A. (1967). Amnioscopy for prenatal transfusion. *Am. J. Obstet. Gynecol. 98*:1140-1143.

Modell, B., Ward, R. H. T., and Fairweather, D. V. I. (1980). Effect of introducing antenatal diagnosis on reproductive behaviour of families at risk of thalassaemia major. *Br. Med. J. 1*:1347-1350.

Prenatal Diagnosis. (1980). Past, present and future. Report of an International Workshop. *Prenatal Diagnosis.* Special Issue Dec. 1980. 29-33. John Wiley and Sons, Chichester and New York.

Rocker, I. and Laurence, K. M. (1978). Defect in fetal membranes after fetoscopy. *Lancet 1*:716.

Rodeck, C. H. (1980). Fetoscopy guided by real-time ultrasound for pure fetal blood samples, fetal skin samples and examination of the fetus in utero. *Br. J. Obstet. Gynaecol. 87*:449-456.

Rodeck, C. H. and Campbell, S. (1979). Umbilical cord insertion as source of pure fetal blood for prenatal diagnosis. *Lancet 1*: 1244-1245.

Scrimgeour, J. B. (1973). Other techniques for antenatal diagnosis. In *Antenatal Diagnosis of Genetic Disease.* A. E. R. Emery, Ed., Churchill Livingstone, Edinburgh and London, pp. 40-57.

Scrimgeour, J. B. (1973b). Fetoscopy. In *Birth Defects,* Proceedings of the International Conference, Vienna, 1973. A. G. Motulsky and W. Lentz (Ed.), Excerpta Medica, Amsterdam, International Congress Series no. 310, pp. 234-239.

Valenti, C. (1972). Endo-amnioscopy and fetal biopsy—A new technique. *Am. J. Obstet. Gynecol. 114*:561-564.

Valenti, C. (1973). Antenatal detection of hemoglobinopathies—a preliminary report. *Am. J. Obstet. Gynecol. 115*:851-853.

Wade, M. E., Ogden, J. A., Anderson, G. G., and Davis, V. D. (1969). Intrauterine fetal transfusions. *Am. J. Obstet. Gynecol. 105*:962-971.

Ward, R. H. T. and Modell, B. Physiology of midtrimester. In *Fetoscopy.* K. M. Laurence and I. Rocker, (Eds.). Elsevier/North Holland Biomedical Press, B.V., pp. 3-31.

Ward, R. H. T., Modell, B., Fairweather, D. V. I., Shirley, I., Richards, B. A., and Hetherington, C. P. The obstetric outcome and problems of mid-trimester fetal blood sampling for antenatal diagnosis. *Br. J. Obstet. Gynaecol. 88*:1073-1080.

Westin, B. (1954). Hysteroscopy in early pregnancy. *Lancet 2*:872.

Westin, B. (1957). Technique and estimation of oxygenation of the human fetus in utero by means of hystero-photography. *Acta Paediatr. 46*:117-124.

4
Amniocentesis

JAY D. IAMS / The Ohio State University, Columbus, Ohio

The current widespread use of amniocentesis for multiple indications has its origins in the reports of Schatz who in 1882 performed the procedure to relieve polyhydramnios, and of Menees et al. who in 1930 performed amniographic placental localization. The reports by Bevis (1950, 1952, 1956) in the 1950s of the correlation between amniotic fluid optical density and the severity of Rh hemolytic disease in the fetus, and the subsequent positive experience with the procedure in the management of Rh-sensitized gravidas, revealed the procedure to be less hazardous than formerly believed. The modern era of amniotic fluid analysis in prenatal diagnosis of congenital disorders and assessment of fetal maturity and well-being was initiated by the publication in 1966 by Steele and Breg of successful fetal cell cultivation from amniotic fluid, and by Gluck et al. in 1971 of the utility of the lecithin-sphingomyelin ratio in assessing fetal lung m turity. It is now a common procedure, with an estimated 15,000 procedures performed annually in the second trimester alone. Frequency of amniocentesis in the third trimester is more difficult to estimate, but it is clearly a commonly performed procedure.

INDICATIONS

Therapeutic

Relief of Hydramnios
Schatz' initial indication for amniocentesis in decompression of hydramnios remains valid today. Amniocentesis should be limited in cases of hydramnios

to those women who experience respiratory embarrassment because of limitation of diaphragmatic excursion by the overdistended uterus. Most of these patients will have acute hydramnios in the second trimester, and require multiple procedures to drain the fluid which can reaccumulate rapidly (Pitkin, 1976; Queenan and Gadow, 1970). Slow drainage over several hours using an indwelling catheter is recommended to avoid sudden decompression with consequent placental abruption. The more chronic forms of hydramnios seen in the third trimester rarely produce sufficient maternal symptoms to warrant intervention.

Therapeutic Abortion

Midtrimester therapeutic abortion may be accomplished using intra-amniotic instillation of hypertonic saline, urea, and/or prostaglandin. It is often expedient to withdraw a portion of the amniotic fluid before instillation, but care must be taken to ensure the continuing intra-amniotic placement of the needle before injection to avoid m ternal side effects. A recent case of selective intrauterine fetal cardiac puncture and exsanguination in a twin pregnancy discordant for genetic disease has been reported with successful continuation of the remaining gestation (Kerenyi and Chitkara, 1981).

Intrauterine Fetal Transfusion

First reported by Liley in 1963, this procedure offers some chance of survival to fetuses severely compromised by fetal-maternal isoimmunization. Although some centers continue to report success with fluoroscopy and amniography, ultrasonography is now the method of choice to identify successful placement of the transfusion catheter within the fetal peritoneal cavity (Berkowitz, 1980).

Other

Intra-amniotic instillation of various nutrients, hormones, and drugs has been attempted as intrauterine fetal therapy for various disorders, but none of these approaches has become an established technique.

Diagnostic

Implicit in the use of amniocentesis as a diagnostic procedure is a careful assessment of the risks and benefits and, most importantly, the limitations of the information to be gained from amniotic fluid analysis. Clinical decision-making based on amniotic fluid emphasizes the positive laboratory result, for example, the lecithin-sphingomyelin (L-S) ratio indicating lung maturity, or the amniocyte karyotype showing trisomy 21. These two examples are typical of most amniotic fluid analysis: a negative result does not necessarily means that the fetus has immature lungs if the L-S is 1:1 or that the fetus is free of birth defects if the karyotype is normal. Unless clinicians consciously remind themselves of the limitations of a "negative" result from amniotic fluid, the value of the data obtained may be overestimated and the risks of the procedure underestimated. A detailed discussion of the clinical uses of amniotic fluid is beyond the scope of this chapter, but it is important to remember the risks of the procedure for mother and fetus outlined here.

Second Trimester Amniocentesis
Amniotic fluid analysis in the second trimester is only one step in the prenatal detection of birth defects, albeit the most dramatic and risky. The most important and least emphasized step in prenatal diagnosis is, of course, a careful screening history to identify women who might choose further studies. In order to ask the right questions for all but the most obvious indication (advanced maternal age), the physician must develop a genetic "consciousness." Incomplete or inaccurate inform tion from the patient's history can lead to unnecessary testing, erroneous counseling, and, most tragically, unnecessary termination of a normal pregnancy or continuation of an unwanted abnormal gestation. An obstetrical history of repeated losses or congenital anomalies is especially important. Frequently the history will suggest the possibility of a defect whose etiology is obscure and not familiar to the physician. This requires a careful search of the literature and, occasionally, telephone consultation with a perinatal center before further counseling or testing is carried out. Sixteen weeks' gestation (14 weeks after conception) is the best time to perform the procedure. The volume of fluid nearly doubles between 14 and 16 weeks, and the likelihood of recovering viable fetal fibroblasts is highest at 16 weeks. Taps done beyond 18 weeks have a lower recovery rate of viable cells and may not yield a diagnosis in time to effect termination, if that is the patient's choice. Taps attempted at 14 weeks are less likely to obtain fluid, and if successful have fewer viable cells.

Once identified, the gravida who might benefit from amniotic fluid analysis usually is defined by one of four categories.

Chromosomal disorders. Amniotic fluid karyotype analysis should be offered to women of advanced age, to women who have previously borne a child with a chromosomal aberration or undiagnosed multiple anomalies, or where one parent is known to be a balanced translocation carrier. Hook (1981) has recently published a useful tabulation of the rate of chromosomal abnormalities according to maternal age.

X-linked disorders. A personal or family history of an x-linked disorder such as Duchenne's muscular dystrophy is an indication for offering fetal karyotype analysis to determine fetal sex. The knowledge that an x-linked recessive disorder will affect half of male offspring and none of female offspring may be useful to the family, although the disease itself cannot yet be detected directly.

Table 1. Inborn Errors of Metabolism Detectable in Utero by Antenatal
Diagnosis by Assessment for Presence or Absence of an Enzyme in Amniotic
Fluid

Mucopolysaccharidoses	
Disorder	Inheritance
Hurler's syndrome	AR
Scheie's syndrome	AR
Hurler-Scheie compound	AR
Hunter's syndrome (severe)	XLR
Sanfilippo's syndrome A	AR
Sanfilippo's syndrome B	AR
Morquio's syndrome	AR
Maroteaux-Lamy syndrome (2 types)	AR
Beta-glucuronidase deficiency	AR
Carbohydrate metabolism	
Glycogen storage disease type II (Pompe's disease)	AR
Glycogen storage disease type III	AR
Glycogen storage disease type IV	AR
Glycogen storage disease type VIII	XLR
Galactosemia	AR
Glucose 6-phosphate dehydrogenase deficiency	XLR
Fucosidosis	AR
Mannosidosis	AR
Phosphohexose isomerase deficiency	AD
Pyruvate decarboxylase deficiency	AR
Pyruvate dehydrogenase deficiency	AR
Lipidoses and sphingolipidoses	
Generalized gangliosidosis (GM_1 gangliosidosis type 1)	AR
Juvenile GM_1 gangliosidosis type 2)	AR
Tay-Sachs disease (GM_2 gangliosidosis type 1)	AR
Sandhoff's disease (GM_2 gangliosidosis type 2)	AR
Juvenile GM_2 gangliosidosis (GM_2 gangliosidosis type 3)	AR
GM_3 sphingolipodystrophy	AR
Gaucher's disease (three types)	AR
Neimann-Pick disease type A	AR
Neimann-Pick disease type B	AR
Krabbe's disease (globoid cell leukodystrophy)	AR
Lactosyl ceramidosis	AR
Metachromatic leukodystrophy	AR

Table 1 (continued). Inborn Errors of Metabolism Detectable in Utero by Antenatal Diagnosis by Assessment for Presence or Absence of an Enzyme in Amniotic Fluid

Mucopolysaccharidoses	
Disorder	Inheritance
Fabry's disease	XLR
Farber disease	AR
Refsum's disease	AR
Wolman's disease	AR
Cholesterol ester storage disease	AR

Amnio acid metabolism	
Argininosuccinicaciduria	AR
Aspartyglucosaminuria	AR
Citrullinemia	AR
Cystathioninuria	AR
Cystinosis	AR
Cystinuria	AR
Hartnup disease	AR
Histidinemia	AR
Homocystinuria due to cystathionine synthetase deficiency	AR
Homocystinuria due to methylene-tetrahydrofolate reductase deficiency	AR
Hyperammonemia I	AR
Hyperammonemia II	AR
Hyperargininemia	AR
Hyperlysinemia	AR
Hypervalinemia	AR
Iminoglycinuria	AR
Isoleucine catabolism disorder	AR
Isovalericacidemia (infantile and intermittent forms)	AR
Methylmalonicaciduria I (vitamin B_{12}-unresponsive)	AR
Methylmalonicaciduria II (vitamin B_{12}-responsive)	AR
Methylmalonicaciduria III	AR
Methyltetrahydrofolate methyltransferase deficiency	AR
Ornithinemia	AR
Phenylketonuria	AR
Propionicacidemia	AR
Vitamin B_{12} metabolic defect	AR

Porphyrias	
Acute intermittent prophyria	AD
Congenital erythropoietic porphyria	AR

Table 1 (continued). Inborn Errors of Metabolism Detectable in Utero by Antenatal Diagnosis by Assessment for Presence or Absence of an Enzyme in Amniotic Fluid

Mucopolysaccharidoses	
Disorder	Inheritance
Other disorders	
Acatalasemia	AR
Adenosine deaminase deficiency (severe combined immunodeficiency)	AR
Ehlers-Danlos syndrome VI	AR
Familial hyperlipoproteinemia	AD
Leigh encephalopathy	AR
Lesch-Nyhan syndrome	XLR
Lyosomal acid phosphate deficiency	AR
Mucolipidosis III	AR
Oroticaciduria (two types)	AF
Xylosidase deficiency	AR

AD = Autosomal dominant.
AR = Autosomal recessive.
XLR = X-linked recessive.

Source: Iams, J. D. (1982). Prenatal diagnosis of congenital defects. In *Practical Manual of Obstetric Care*. F. P. Zuspan and E. J. Quilligan (Eds.), C. V. Mosby, St. Louis. Modified from Refs. 45, 55, and 60.

Metabolic disorders.   There are currently more than 100 metabolic disorders, usually autosomal recessive in inheritance, which can be diagnosed from studies on amniocytes or amniotic fluid. The time required for such studies is usually longer than the 3-5 weeks for karyotype analysis, and special transportation of samples to distant laboratories may be required. Disorders currently detectable are listed in Table 1, but the list is likely to grow steadily and this sample should not be viewed as current.

Amniotic fluid alpha-fetoprotein (AFAFP) determination.   AFAFP is useful in detecting the presence of open neural tube defects and abdominal wall defects. Defects covered by skin may not be associated with elevated AFAFP and may therefore be missed by this assay alone. Ultrasound is therefore a necessary adjunct. The risk of bearing a child with a neural tube defect is 2-5% for a couple with one affected first degree relative (child, parent, or sibling), and rises to 10% with two affected first degree relatives. Similar risk estimates apply to other defects of multifactorial causation.

THIRD TRIMESTER INDICATIONS

Amniocentesis in the third trimester is used to assess fetal well-being and to estimate fetal maturity.

Assessment of Fetal Well-being

Fetomaternal Isoimmunization
Amniotic fluid analysis of the difference in optical density at 450 nm between the expected and tested values (ΔOD 450) is the cornerstone of management of the pregnancy complicated by fetomaternal isoimmunization. The majority of cases will be caused by Rh incompatibility, but other irregular antibodies such as Kell or JKA may cause similar fetal disease. Amniocentesis in affected pregnancies is usually begun at 24 weeks' gestation and repeated at intervals depending upon the values obtained.

Meconium
The presence of meconium-stained amniotic fluid has traditionally been regarded as evidence of fetal stress or distress in high-risk pregnancies. The value of meconium-stained fluid in predicting an adverse outcome is in doubt, however, because it is at once a sign of and, in the meconium aspiration syndrome, a cause of fetal morbidity (NICHD, 1979).

Fetal Maturity Studies

Phospholipid Studies
The most useful index of fetal maturity is obtained from amniotic fluid phospholipid analysis. The ratio of lecithin to sphingomyelin is at present the standard indicator of fetal pulmonary maturity. An L-S ratio of 2:1 or greater using Gluck's techniques correlates very well with the absence of the neonatal respiratory distress syndrome (RDS) (Gluck et al., 1971). It is again important to note that not all infants born following an amniocentesis showing a ratio less than 2:1 will develop RDS (Harvey et al., 1975). Kulovich et al., (1979; Kulovich and Gluck, 1979) have recently championed the use of an amniotic fluid phospholipid profile. The most useful of the individual phospholipids is the presence of phosphatidylglycerol, especially in the pregnancies of diabetic women (Bustos et al., 1979)..

Optical Density
There have been several reports of the value of the optical density of amniotic fluid at 650 nm in predicting fetal pulmonary maturity (Copeland et al., 1978; Sbarra et al., 1978). The basis of this association between the OD 650 and neonatal pulmonary outcome is uncertain. This test is rapid and simple enough to be performed in a hospital laboratory without special equipment or personnel. Doubt remains, however, of its reliability because of other less optimistic reports (Planche et al., 1981).

Cytology
Desquamated fetal cells in amniotic fluid show an increased fat content with
advancing gestational age, demonstrated with the Nile blue sulfate stain.
Brosens (1966) demonstrated that the percentage of nile-blue-positive cells increased from less than 1% before 34 weeks' gestation to 10-50% at 38-40 weeks'
gestation. This test is also simple and rapid but, like the absorbance at 650 nm,
does not directly assess the fetal lung maturation.

Creatinine
Amniotic fluid creatinine concentration increases with gestation as a result of
the increasing fetal muscle mass and m turity of the fetal kidneys. A value of
2 mg% will be noted in 94% of fetuses by 37 weeks' gestation (Pitkin and
Zwirek, 1967). Research from Dr. Brian Andresen's laboratory at Ohio State
University has recently (Andresen et al., in press) demonstrated an increase in
hippuric acid with advancing gestation thought also to be due to increasing
maturity of the fetal kidney.

Other
Amniotic fluid osmolarity and, in the absence of fetomaternal isoimmunization,
the Δ OD 450, have been used as well to estimate fetal maturity.

TECHNIQUE OF AMNIOCENTESIS

The technique of needle insertion does not differ substantially in the second
and third trimesters, and is summarized in Table 2.

Since the ratio of risk to benefit is more difficult to quantify numerically
in the second trimester, more attention is generally paid to counseling before
amniocentesis. Nevertheless, proper consent should be the first step in
amniocentesis regardless of gestational age. Ascertainment of blood type and
antibody status is the next step. Unsensitized Rh-negative women syould be
given Rhogam after the procedure (ACOG, 1981).

The use of ultrasound before amniocentesis has somewhat surprisingly
continued to be a subject of considerable controversy in the literature. In
part, this may be explained by differences in study design. Some report
results when compound scanning was performed within 24-48 hr of the tap
(Miskin et al.), others report data from patients scanned in one location, and
then immediately transported to another location for the tap (Karp et al., 1977),
and still others utilize real-time scanning performed by the same individual who
then immediately or simultaneously does the amniocentesis (Bartsch et al., 1980;
Golbus et al., 1979). Of these various approaches, only the last, when the
tap is done at the same time as the scan without first emptying the bladder,
has utility (Kerenyi and Walker, 1977). The position of the placenta and fetus
relative to the abdominal wall may vary depending on the size of the bladder.

Table 2. Technique of Amniocentesis

1. Obtain all necessary data: past history, obstetric history, blood type and Rh, antibody screen
2. Counsel patient regarding risks and benefits, problems, etc
3. Perform ultrasound with full bladder: locate placenta, rule out multiple gestation, estimate amniotic fluid volume, look for anomalies, fibroids, establish gestational age
4. Identify safest access to amniotic fluid sac: if necessary, have patient empty bladder, repeat scan, or have patient return at a later date
5. Prepare abdomen: povidone-iodine scrub; infiltrate skin with locan anesthetic, verbal anesthesia
6. 22-gauge needle inserted
7. First 3 cc fluid discarded
8. 15-20 cc fluid in sterile container to lab for karyotype
9. 5 cc fluid for alpha-fetoprotein determination

It is therefore important to perform the tap immediately following the ultrasonographic exam without changing the patient's position or having her empty the bladder. Occasionally, an overdistended bladder may be fully or partially emptied, revealing safe access to the amniotic sac where none existed before. No consensus exists regarding a beneficial effect of ultrasound in diminishing the number of bloody taps. However, there is little argument that ultrasound is of value for several other reasons (Chandra et al., 1979). Avoidance of the placenta, or at least of the likely area of cord insertion, is possible with ultrasongography, as is avoidance of needle insertion into a fluid pocket containing multiple loops of cord. Diagnosis of fetal death and multiple pregnancy may be made, and accurate gestational dating for second trimester taps is imperative. Just as important is avoiding even an attempt at amniocentesis when the fluid volume is not sufficient to expect success. In second trimester prenatal diagnosis, the patient may be asked to return in 7-10 days when the fluid volume is larger. In the third trimester, severe oligohydramnios evident on scan may indicate that prospects for success are minimal while risk of cord or fetal puncture is increased. Uterine fibroids may be noted also on the sonogram and should be avoided.

The three most commonly selected sites for amniocentesis in the third trimester are behind the fetal neck, beneath the fetal head, and in the area of the fetral small parts. Teramo and Sipinen (1978) reported variable rates of success and spontaneous membrane rupture following third trimester amniocentesis in 200 patients. Their results, summarized in Table 3, reveal the enhanced success and diminished risk when taps are done beneath the elevated fetal head or in the area of the small parts compared with attempts behind the fetal neck.

Table 3. Success and Spontaneous Rupture of Membrane (SROM) by Site of Amniocentesis

Site selected	% Successful	Mean % attempts	Risk of SROM within 5 days (%)
Suprapubic	98	1.2	8.6
Small parts	93	1.3	4.9
Behind fetal neck	89	1.7	24.0

[a]$p < 0.05$

Source: Teramo and Sipinen (1978).

Selection of the needle insertion site should include maternal as well as fetal considerations. Taps through the lateral third of the rectus muscle may puncture the epigastric vessels and result in hematoma formation. Indeed, a patient recently cared for at Ohio State University Hospital developed such a complication after a tap through the middle of the rectus muscle, and required multiple transfusions and abdominal exploration to control the bleeding. A midline insertion is always preferable whenever possible. Despite the complication noted above, other sites are acceptable if they offer the only safe access to fluid, and the benefit of amniotic fluid analysis outweighs the risk.

The diameter of the needle also affects the incidence of complications, as indicated in the NICHD amniocentesis survey (1976). We prefer a 22-gauge Whitacre needle for two reasons: first, its small diameter minimizes risk; second, the relatively blunt tip gives a good "tissue feel" not found with a standard hypodermic needle, and affords less likelihood of fetal or cord laceration should the fetus move during the procedure (Fig. 1).

The site selected should be carefully scanned in longitudinal and transverse fashion to be sure that the apparent pocket of fluid adequate in one diameter is not insufficient in the other. The angle of needle insertion should be perpendicular to the skin whenever possible to minimize errors in the angle of entry. The entry site should be marked, either by indenting the skin with the tip of a ballpoint pen or by an indelible marker.

Careful skin cleansing is mandatory. Infection is a rare but definite risk and should always be avoidable with proper attention to antiseptic technique.

Following site selection it is important to remember the beneficial effects of "verbal anesthesia." It may be reassuring to divert the patient's attention through small talk, or to explain each subsequent step in detail, depending on her anxiety level. The use of local anesthesia is optional. Some favor its use while others believe that the needle insertion itself is no more uncomfortable than administering a local anesthestic. The author's preference is a local

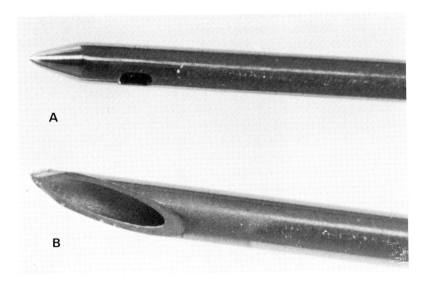

Figure 1. A: Tip of 22-gauge Whitacre needle; B: Tip of 20-gauge spinal needle, oblique view.

injection of xylocaine in the skin and parietal peritoneum. Observing the response to injection of local anesthetic is helpful in anticipating patient co-operation during the actual procedure. In addition, when a Whitacre needle is used, it is frequently necessary to puncture the skin with a hypodermic needle first since the Whitacre needle tip may not be sharp enough to pierce the skin. A local anesthetic facilitates this step as well.

The actual needle insertion should be done with a firm thrust to the depth anticipated by the ultrasound examination, noting the gentle "pop" as the needle passes through the amniotic sac. Use of a sharp hypodermic tip may make this change in resistance imperceptible. Although ultrasonographic depth measurements are useful, these should be combined with a tactile appreciation of proper intra-amniotic location. This tactile sense of uterine anatomy can be appreciated after relatively few amniocenteses.

The stylet should always be in place during needle insertion to avoid occlusion of the lumen with maternal tissue. In the case of amniocentesis to determine fetal karyotype, this maternal tissue may grow in cell culture and yield spurious results (one hopes, normal female). Once inserted, the needle stylet is withdrawn and the hub observed for appearance of amniotic fluid.

The 22-gauge needle does not allow spontaneous egress of fluid as rapidly as a larger-bore needle, so patience is necessary. If no fluid is forthcoming, aspiration and rotation of the needle to displace the side hole may be attempted. If blood is returned spontaneously or with aspiration, the needle may be advanced until fluid is returned. Clear fluid should be sent whenever possible, but even bloody fluid can be sent for study. In the case of maturity studies, blood may alter the L-S ratio, but will not affect the determination of phosphatidylglycerol (Strassner et al., 1980). Even alpha-fetoprotein measurement need not be abandoned when bloody fluid is obtained: although maternal blood will elevate the AFAFP, this increase will not ordinarily exceed three standard deviations above the mean, which is the customary upper limit of normal. Even small amounts of fetal blood may significantly elevate the AFAFP, however. Identification of fetal cells with the Kleihauer-Betke technique (Doran et al., 1977) and measurement of amniotic fluid acetylcholinesterase may be helpful in such instances (Seller et al., 1981).

If the first needle insertion produces no fluid, it may be useful to repeat the ultrasound examination to be sure the site originally selected is satisfactory. The likelihood of success diminishes, and the risk of complication increases, after two unsuccessful attempts (NICHD, 1976). The patient should therefore be asked to return at a later date if fluid is not obtained after two attempts.

Taps done in the vicinity of the maternal bladder always raise the question of whether maternal urine was obtained. Urine and amniotic fluid may be distinguished by the ferning reaction and protein content (Elias et al., 1979). For genetic taps, the first 3 cc of fluid should be discarded to avoid contamination with maternal cells. Proper handling of fluid samples requires that they be kept sterile for cell culture or bacteriologic studies, and that they be protected from light to avoid alteration of the Δ OD 450. Prompt transport of the fluid to the appropriate laboratory is also necessary. Schwartz et al. (1981) found that amniotic fluid phospholipids remained stable for up to 24 hr at room temperature, but must be frozen or refrigerated if analysis cannot be performed within that time. These authors as always emphasize the importance of strict adherence to protocol if results are to be valid.

Mailing specimens to referral laboratories for cytogenetic analysis may result in an unacceptably high rate of culture failures and should be avoided (Golbus et al., 1979). It is occasionally necessary to send fluid samples to distant laboratories for specialized testing (e.g., sphingomyelinase assay for Niemann-Pick disease). In such cases prior arrangement of prompt transport is essential.

Postamniocentesis fetal surveillance is indicated whenever there is a possibility of extrauterine fetal survival, beginning at 26-28 weeks gestation. The duration of monitoring should be at least 20-30 min, with longer observation whenever multiple attempts or bloody fluid complicate the procedure (Klein et al., 1981).

RISKS OF AMNIOCENTESIS

Maternal

Significant maternal hemorrhage is uncommon but has been reported (DiFrancesco, 1972; McBride et al., 1978). Avoiding the lateral third of the rectus muscle can minimize this risk. Although not serious, maternal syncope is not uncommon. In late pregnancy, aortocaval compression with supine hypotension may be expected in 20% of gravidas, and a vagal response with syncope may be seen at any time in pregnancy. Women should therefore not be unattended as they arise after the procedure.

Maternofetal

Maternofetal bleeding may initiate maternal antibody formation in the unsensitized mother, and may stimulate additional antibody production in the sensitized patient (Queenan and Adams, 1964). Mennuti et al. (1980) have demonstrated fetomaternal bleeding following genetic amniocentesis, using pre- and post-tap maternal serum alpha-fetoprotein (MSAFP) assays. They found post-tap elevations of MSAFP in 28 of 333 consecutive patients (8.4%). Four of these 28 patients (14.3%) experienced spontaneous abortion, compared with 3 of 305 (0.98%) whose pre- and post-tap MSAFP values did not differ. In a small study, Hill et al. (1980) documented Rh-sensitization during pregnancy in three (5.4%) of 56 unsensitized Rh-negative gravidas who underwent amniocentesis. Harrison et al. (1975) found that ultrasound diminished the likelihood of significant fetomaternal transfusion from 9.0 to 4.5% in mid-pregnancy taps, and from 10 to 4% in late-pregnancy taps. Ultrasonographic placental localization and use of Rhogam in unsensitized Rh-negative patients are indicated on this basis.

Amniotic fluid leakage was found in 1.2% of the NICHD (1976) study patients, and could theoretically lead to premature labor or intrauterine infection. We have observed this event twice in 400 patients undergoing second trimester amniocentesis; both patients stopped leaking after 2-4 days and experienced no adverse sequelae. Teramo and Sipinen (1978) reported a 13.5% incidence of spontaneously ruptured membranes within 5 days of third trimester amniocentesis (see Table 3). The likelihood of premature labor following amniocentesis increases with advancing gestation. Premature labor following amniocentesis without amniorrhexis is a question of uncertain magnitude. Uterine contractions occur frequently following needle insertions, but rarely lead to labor in a patient not otherwise at risk of premature delivery. The British amniocentesis study (Report to the MRC, 1978) reported an increased incidence of subsequent preterm delivery in women who had second trimester genetic amniocentesis, but the study design was flawed by a large number of women with elevated MSAFP in the amniocentesis group, increasing the proportion of twin gestations and infants with anomalies in the study group. The NICHD amniocentesis survey (1976) found no increase in the incidence of preterm delivery, and the large study of Crandall et al. also found no increase in low-birth-weight delivery (Crandall et al., 1980).

Fetal

Abortion

Abortion was reported in 3.5% of women undergoing second trimester genetic amniocentesis compared with 3.2% of age-matched controls in the NICHD amniocentesis registry (1976). Although this difference is not statistically significant, there is certainly some risk of abortion associated with genetic amniocentesis. Golbus et al. reported that 1.5% of 3000 women who underwent genetic amniocentesis delivered earlier than 28 weeks' gestation, and 1.2% of women registering for amniocentesis and counselling miscarried during the week before the appointment. Crandall et al. (1980) reported a total fetal loss of 2.7% (1.3% spontaneous abortion before 28 weeks', 1.4% stillbirth and neonatal death) in 2000 women who had second trimester taps, compared with 2.2% in a control population. Verjaal et al. (1981) reported 23 losses (1.5%) within 3 weeks of the procedure among 1500 midtrimester amniocenteses. There was a marked relationship in this series of fetal loss to operator experience. The risk of loss within 3 weeks of the tap was 3.7% with operators who had performed fewer than 10 punctures, and only 0.3% if the operator had performed more than 50.

There are numerous case reports of fetal injury following amniocentesis, but little prospectively collected data is available. The NICHD registry study (1976) found no evidence of physical injury resulting from amniocentesis. The British study (1978) identified 4 cases of needle injury in 1379 infants born to women who had amniocentesis, but found similar injury in 3 of 1395 control infants whose mothers had not had amniocentesis. Karp and Hayden (1977) studied 190 women who had 234 midtrimester amniocenteses between 1971 and 1975. Four needle punctures were found, but none of these had been noted on routine newborn examination. Two of the four infants were born to women who required multiple needle insertions. They concluded that this risk was diminished with increasing operator experience. Epley et al. (1979) examined 107 infants born after second trimester amniocentesis performed between 1970 and 1977, and found that 10 of these (9%) had unusual cutaneous scars, one of which was serious. There were no injuries among 64 study infants who had had only one needle insertion. Six of 27 women (22%) who required two punctures delivered infants with unusual scars, and four of seven infants delivered after four punctures had scars. The procedures were performed with a 20-gauge spinal needle and were preceded by compound ultrasound examination, although not necessarily performed immediately before the procedure.

At the Ohio State University Prenatal Diagnostic Clinic, no needle marks have been identified at routine newborn examination among 230 infants born to women who had genetic amniocentesis from 1979 to 1981. These infants have not, however, been subjected to a specific examination aimed at identifying needle injury.

There are case reports of fetal exsanguination (Kirshen and Benirsche, 1973), splenic injury (Egley, 1973), cardiac tamponade (Berner et al., 1972), pneumothorax (Leake et al., 1974), skin punctures (Broome et al., 1976), loss of an eye (Cross and Naumenee, 1972), and arteriovenous (Gottdiener et al., 1975), and ileocutaneous (Rickwood, 1974) fistulae following taps at various times in gestation. The risk of such serious injuries appears small, probably less than 1 in 300, but should not be omitted from discussion with the patient, for this sort of injury is frequently uppermost in her mind. Howard and Crandall administered the Gesell Developmental Evaluation to 150 children between 8 and 37 months of age born to women who had midtrimester amniocentesis and to 64 control infants, and found no difference in development (Howard and Crandell, 1979).

AMNIOCENTESIS IN MULTIPLE PREGANCY

The possibility of multifetal gestation is another indication for ultrasound examination before amniocentesis at any gestational age. Analysis of fluid from one sac may or may not be applicable to the other fetus(es), depending on the indication for the procedure. Spellacy et al. (1977) have reported no significant difference in the lecithin-sphingomyelin ratios obtained from both sacs in 14 diamniotic gestations, but caution that this finding may not be applicable in cases of discordant growth. In such cases it would be wisest to tap the sac of the larger fetus who is less likely to show pulmonary maturity than the small and presumably stressed twin. Again the role of ultrasonic fetal evaluation is obvious. If the indication for amniocentesis is for genetic studies or evaluation of Rh-sensitization, however, fluid from one twin is not necessarily applicable to both. Twins may be of different Rh types, and even if both are Rh-positive, may have different degrees of hemolysis (Beischer et al., 1969). Cytogenetic analysis may, of course, differ in dizygotic twin gestation. The presence of one normal twin and one with trisomy 21 raises an obvious ethical dilemma which must be discussed fully with the parents (Kerenyi and Chitkara, 1981).

The technique of successfully sampling all sacs in multiamniotic gestation relies heavily on careful ultrasound evaluation to evaluate the position of each fetus and, if possible, identify a dividing membrane. After successfully obtaining fluid from the first sac, a small amount (approximately 0.5 cc) of either indigo carmine or Evans blue dye should be introduced, and the needle withdrawn. Methylene blue dye has been reported to cause methemoglobinemia and should be avoided (Cowett et al., 1976). A red dye may be confused with blood and is therefore also best avoided. Repeat scanning after the first sac has been tapped is recommended to identify the safest site for the second insertion. If clear fluid is obtained, the second sac has been successfully entered; if blue-tinged fluid is obtained, the same sac has been entered again.

SUMMARY

Amniotic fluid has been shown to be a valuable source of inform tion about the fetus. Our immediate challenge is proper patient selection, rational interpretation of the data obtained, and diminution of known risks. The future challenge is finding alternate noninvasive means of determining fetal status without subjecting the mother and fetus to the risks of amniocentesis.

REFERENCES

American College of Obstetricians and Gynecologist (1981). Technical Bulletin, No. 61. The selective use of Rho(D) immune globulin(RhIG).

Andresen, B. D., Ng, K., and Iams, J. D. Variations in amniotic fluid hippuric acid levels with gestational age. *Am. J. Obstet. Gynaecol.* (In Press).

Bartsch, F. K., Lundberg, J., and Wahlstrom, J. (1980). One thousand consecutive midtrimester amniocenteses. *Obstet. Gynecol. 55*:305.

Beischer, N. A., Pepperell, R. J., and Barrie, J. A. (1969). Twin pregnancy and erythroblastosis. *Obstet. Gynecol. 34*:22.

Berkowitz, R. L. (1980). Intrauterine transfusion 1980: An update. *Clin. Perinatol. 7*:285.

Berner, H. W., Seisler, E. P., and Barlow, J. 1972). Fetal cardiac tamponade, a complication of amniocentesis. *Obstet. Gynecol. 40*:599.

Bevis, D. C. A. (1950). Composition of liquor amnii in haemolytic disease of the newborn. *Lancet 2*:443.

Bevis, D. C. A. (1952). The antenatal prediction of haemolytic disease of the newborn. *Lancet 1*:395.

Bevis, D. C. A. (1956). Blood pigments in hemolytic disease of the newborn. *J. Obstet. Gynaecol. Br. Commonw. 63*:68.

Broome, D. L., Wilson, M. G., Weiss, B., and Kellogg, B. (1976). Needle puncture of fetus. A complication of second trimester amniocentesis. *Am. J. Obstet. Gynecol. 126*:247.

Brosens, I. A. (1966). Cytological study of amniotic fluid with Nile blue sulfate staining. *Acta. Cytol. 10*:156.

Bustos, R., Kulovich, M. V., Gluck, L., Gabbe, S. G., Evertson, L., Vargas, C., and Lowenburg, E. (1979). Significance of phosphatidylglycerol in amniotic fluid in complicated pregnancies. *Am. J. Obstet. Gynecol. 133*:899.

Chandra, P., Nitowskyy, H. M., Marion, R., Koenigsberg, M., Taber, E., and Kava, H. W. (1979). Experience with sonography as an adjunct to amniocentesis for prenatal diagnosis of fetal genetic disorders. *Am. J. Obstet. Gynecol. 133*:519.

Copeland, W. Jr., Stempel, L., Lott, J., Copeland, W. Sr., and Zuspan, F. P. (1978) Assessment of a rapid test on amniotic fluid for estimating fetal lung maturity. *Am. J. Obstet. Gynecol. 130*:225.

Cowett, R. M., Hakanson, D. O., Kocon, R. W., and Oh, W. (1976). Untoward neonatal effect of intra-amniotic administration of methylene blue. *Obstet. Gynecol. (Suppl.) 43*:745.

Crandall, B. F., Howard, J., Lebherz, T. B., Rubinstein, L., Sample, W. F., and Sarti, D. (1980). Follow-up of 2000 second trimester amniocentesis. *Obstet. Gynecol. 56*:625.

Cross, H. E., and Maumenee, A. E. (1972). Ocular trauma during amniocentesis. *N. Engl. J. Med. 287*:993.

DiFrancesco, A. (1972). Major intraperitoneal bleeding complicating amniocentesis—Case report. *Aust. N.Z.J. Obstet. Gynaecol. 12*:255.

McBride, J. R., Irwin, J. F., and Wait, R. B. (1975). Major extraperitoneal bleeding complicating amniocentesis—A case report. *Am. J. Obstet. Gynecol. 130*:108.

Doran, T. A., Allen, L. C., Pirani, B. B. K., and Shumak, K. H. (1977). False positive amniotic fluid alpha-fetoprotein levels resulting from contamination with fetal blood: Results of an experiment. *Am. J. Obstet. Gynecol. 127*: 759.

Egley, C. C., Laceration of fetal spleen during midtrimester amniocentesis. *Am. J. Obstet. Gynecol. 116*:582.

Elias, S., Martin, A. O., Patel, V. A., Gerbie, A. and Simpson, J. L. (1979). Analysis for amniotic fluid crystallization in second trimester amniocentesis. *Am. J. Obstet. Gynecol. 133*:401.

Epley, S. L., Hanson, J. W., and Cruikshank, D. P. (1979). Fetal injury with midtrimester diagnostic amniocentesis. *Obstet. Gynecol. 53*:77.

Gluck, L., Julovich, M. V., Borer, R. C., Brenner, P. H., Anderson, G. G., and Spellacy, W. N. (1971). Diagnosis of the respiratory distress syndrome by amniocentesis. *Am. J. Obstet. Gynecol. 109*:440.

Golbus, M. S., Loughman, W. D., Epstein, C. J., Halbasch, G., Stephens, J. D., and Hall, B. D. (1979). Prenatal cytogenetic diagnosis in 3000 amniocenteses. *N. Engl. J. Med. 300*:157.

Gottdiener, J. S., Ellison, R. C., and Lorenzo, R. L. (1975). Arteriovenous fistula after penetration at amniocentesis. *N. Engl. J. Med. 293*:1302.

Harrison, R., Campbell, S., and Craft, I. (1975). Risks of fetomaternal hemorrhage resulting from amniocentesis with and without ultrasound placental localization. *Obstet. Gynecol. 46*:389.

Harvey, D. Parkinson, C. E., and Campbell, S. (1975). Risk of respiratory distress synrome. *Lancet 1*:42.

Hill, L. M., Platt, L. D., and Kellogg, B. (1980). Rh sensitization after genetic amniocentesis. *Obstet. Gynecol. 56*:459.

Hook, E. B. (1981). Rates of chromosome abnormalities at different maternal ages. *Obstet. Gynecol. 58*:282.

Howard, J. A., and Crandell, B. F. (1979). Amniocentesis follow-up: Infant developmental evaluation. *Obstet. Gynecol. 53*:599.

Karp, L. E., and Hayden, P. W. (1977). Fetal puncture during midtrimester amniocentesis. *Obstet. Gynecol. 49*:115.

Karp, L. E., Rothwell, R., Conrad, S. H., Hoehn, H. W., and Hickok, D. E. (1977). Ultrasonic placental localization and bloody taps in midtrimester amniocentesis for prenatal genetic diagnosis. *Obstet. Gynecol. 50*:589.

Kerenyi, T. D., and Chitkara, U. (1981). Selective birth in twin pregnancy with discordancy for Down's syndrome. *N. Engl. J. Med. 304*:1525.

Kerenyi, T. D., and Walker, B. (1977). The preventability of "bloody taps" in second trimester amniocentesis by ultrasound scanning. *Obstet. Gynecol. 50*: 61.

Kirschen, E. J., and Benirsche, K. (1973). Fetal exsanguination after amniocentesis. *Obstet. Gynecol. 42*:615.

Klein, S. A., Young, B. K., Wilson, S. J., and Katz, M. (1981). Continuous fetal monitoring following third trimester amniocentesis. *Obstet. Gynecol. 58*:444.

Kulovich, M. F., Hallman, M. B., and Gluck, L. (1979). The lung profile: I. Normal pregnancy. *Am. J. Obstet. Gynecol. 135*:57.

Kulovich, M. V., and Gluck, L. (1979). The lung profile II. Complicated pregnancy. *Am. J. Obstet. Gynecol. 135*:64.

Leake, R. D., Hobel, C. J., and Lachman, R. S. (1974). Neonatal pneumothorax and subcutaneous emphysema secondary to diagnostic amniocentesis. *Obstet. Gynecol. 43*:884.

Liley, A. W. (1963). Intrauterine transfusion of fetus in hemolytic disease. *Br. Med. J. 2*:1107.

Menees, T. D., Miller, J. D., and Holly, L. E. (1930). Amniography: Preliminary report. *Am. J. Roentgenol. Radium Ther. 24*:363.

Mennuti, M. T., Brummond, W., Crombleholme, W. R., Schwarz, R. H., and Arvan, D. A. (1980). Fetal-maternal bleeding associated with genetic amniocentesis. *Obstet. Gynecol. 55*:48.

Miskin, M., Doran, T. A., Rudd, N., Gardner, H. A., Liedgren, S. and Benzie, R. (1974). Use of ultrasound for placental localization in genetic amniocentesis. *Obstet. Gynecol. 43*:872.

Nadler, H. L. (1976). Prenatal diagnosis of genetic defects. *Adv. Pediatr. 22*:1.

NICHD National Registry for Amniocentesis Study Group (1976). Midtrimester amniocentesis for prenatal diagnosis: Safety and accuracy. *JAMA 236*:1471.

NICHD Consensus Development Conference on Antenatal Diagnosis, Predictors of Fetal Distress (1979). NIH Publication No. 79-1973, pp. III-33.

Pitkin, R. M. (1976). Acute polyhydramnios recurrent in successive pregnancies. *Obstet. Gynecol. 48*:425.

Pitkin, R. M., Zwirek, S. J. (1967). Amniotic fluid creatinine. *Am. J. Obstet. Gynecol. 98*:1135.

Plauche, W. C., Faro, S., and Wycheck, J. (1981). Amniotic fluid optical density: Relationship to L:S ratio, phospholipid content, and desquamation of fetal cells. *Obstet. Gynecol. 58*:309.

Queenan, J. T., and Adams, D. W. (1964). Amniocentesis: A possible immunizing hazard. *Obstet. Gynecol. 24*:530.

Queenan, J. T., and Gadow, E. C. (1970). Polyhydramnios: Chronic versus acute. *Am. J. Obstet. Gynecol. 108*:349.

Report to the Medical Research Council by their working party on amniocentesis (1978). *Br. J. Obstet. Gynaecol. 85* (Suppl. 2).

Rickwood, A. M. K. (1977). A case of ileal atresia and ileocutaneous fistula caused by amniocentesis. *J. Pediatr. 91*:312.

Rhine, S. A. (1976). Prenatal genetic diagnosis and metabolic disorders. *Clin. Obstet. Gynecol. 19*:855.

Sbarra, A. J., Sevaraj, R. J., Cetrulo, C. L., Kennedy, J. L., Herschel, M. J., Knuppel, R., Kappy, K., Mitchell, G. W. Jr., Kelley, E. C. Jr., Paul, B. B., and Louis, F. J. (1978). Positive correlation of optical density at 650 nm with lecithin:splingomyelin ratios in amniotic fluid. *Am. J. Obstet. Gynecol. 130*: 788.

Schatz, F. (1882). Eine besondere Art won ein seihger Polyhydraminie mit anderseitiger Oligohydramnie bei einaguen Zwillingen. *Arch. Gynaekol. 19*: 329.

Schwartz, D. B., Engle, M. J., Brown, D. J., and Farrell, P. M. (1981). The stability of phospholipids in amniotic fluid. *Am. J. Obstet. Gynecol. 141*: 294.

Seller, M. J., Cole, K. J., and Merritt, B. L. (1981). Alphafetoprotein, cholinesterases, and rapidly adhering cells in the prenatal diagnosis of neural tube defects. *Prenatal Diag. 1*:7.

Simpson, J. L. (1979). Antenatal monitoring of genetic disorders. *Clin. Obstet. Gynecol. 6*:259.

Spellacy, W. N., Cruz, A. C., Buki, W. C., and Birk, S. A. (1977). Amniotic fluid L/S ratio in twin gestation. *Obstet. Gynecol. 50*:68.

Steele, M. W., and Breg, W. R., Jr. (1966). Chromosome analysis of human amniotic fluid cells. *Lancet 1*:383.

Strassner, H. T., Golde, S. H., Mosley, G. H., and Platt, L. D. (1980). Effect of blood in amniotic fluid on the detection of phosphatidylgylcerol. *Am. J. Obstet. Gynecol. 138*:697.

Teramo, K., and Sipinen, S. (1978). Spontaneous rupture of fetal membranes after amniocentesis. *Obstet. Gynecol. 52*:272.

Verjaal, M., Leschot, N. J., and Treffers, P. E. (1981). Risk of amniocentesis and laboratory findings in a series of 1500 prenatal diagnoses. *Prenatal Diag. 1*:173.

5
Amniography

PAUL GRECH / Northern General Hospital, Sheffield, England

In certain obstetrical conditions, such as Rh-isoimmunization and hydramnios, all possible information about the fetus and the uterine contents should be gained before heroic procedures are undertaken. Noninvasive techniques should be used whenever possible, but there are few conditions where amniography is the only method available for obtaining conclusive evidence about the fetus in utero. Amniography is the radiological study of the amniotic cavity and its contents after the injection of radiopaque media.

In 1930 Menees et al. injected strontium iodide to localize the placenta. Later other workers used other contrast media but all these substances proved to be too toxic and often led to premature labor. As a result the investigation was more or less abandoned. The introduction of the procedure of intra-uterine transfusion in the management of Rh-isoimmunization and the improvement of the contrast media now available encouraged workers to reassess amniography.

TECHNIQUE

The procedure for performing amniography is essentially the same as for amniocentesis. The placenta is first localized by ultrasonography and amniocentesis is carried out under full aseptic conditions. When enough amniotic fluid is aspirated for analysis, radiopaque substance is injected and, after a suitable interval, an anteroposterior radiograph of the abdomen is taken with the mother supine. Sometimes an oblique view is needed for better visualization of the fetus.

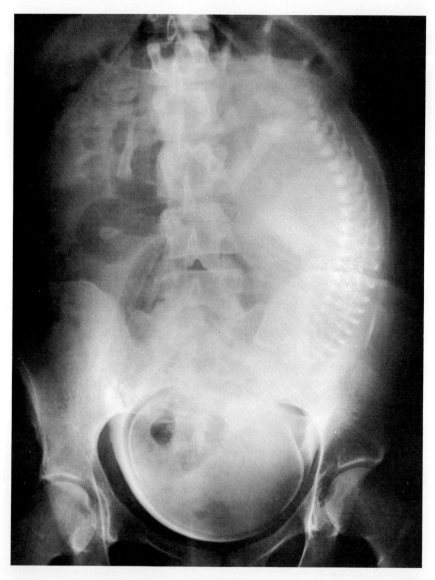

Figure 1. (Legend opposite)

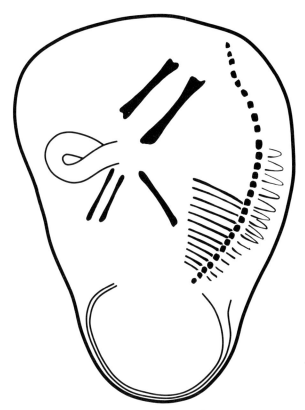

Figure 1. Normal amniogram. Left, an anteroposterior radiograph, and above, an explanatory line drawing showing a normal fetus; a loop of the cord is also visible. Note the normal appearances of the fetal spine and the scalp thickness.

Both water-soluble and fat-soluble media are now being used and it may be worth differentiating between these techniques and comparing the information obtainable using each.

Amniography

This consists of the injection of a water-soluble contrast material such as Hypaque, Renografin, or Conray. We use Conray 280, which is meglumine iothalamate 60% w/v containing 280 mg iodine in combined form per milliliter (May and Baker). Because the contrast is water-soluble it diffuses quickly through the amniotic fluid and renders it radiopaque. The fetus and the uterine contents are demonstrated as negative shadows within the opacified fluid. Figure 1 shows a normal amniogram on a 34-week pregnancy accompanied by line drawing showing the opacified fluid outlining the fetus. The fetal spine is gently flexed and the back and neck show no bumps. The thickness of the scalp on the radiograph measures 2 mm. Even a loop of the umbilical cord is demonstrated. A soft-tissue mass such as a meningocoele which may not produce any bone defects is missed on a plain radiograph but may be revealed by amniography. The detection of fetal malformations by amniography has been reviewed by Queenan and Gadow (1970).

As the fetus swallows the liquor, the radiopaque material shows its gastrointestinal tract and if an intestinal malformation is present, it could be detected. The healthy fetus does not pass meconium in utero; therefore the ingested contrast will remain in the bowel for several weeks; in fact it is still usually present after delivery (Fig. 2).

The amount of water-soluble material used depends on the length of gestation but the general rule is 1 ml/week of gestation. The time of exposure is not critical since opacification of amniotic fluid persists for several hours, but enough time should be allowed for the fetus to ingest the opacified liquor amnii if demonstration of its intestinal tract is required. The opacified fluid can be shown in the fetal gastrointestinal tract within 10-15 min after injection of the contrast medium into the amniotic cavity.

Fetography

This is the delineation of the fetal skin by a fat-soluble contrast medium such as Myodil, which is iophendylate injection containing 30% of organically combined iodine (Glaxo). Erbslöh (1942) published reports of dijoderuca acid isobutylester which has a particular affinity for the vernix caseosa. He was the first to use this technique on living fetuses and proposed the name of fetography. Myodil was first used by Lennon (1967) and remains widely used. The outlining of the soft tissue results as the vernix takes up the liposoluble medium, showing a sharp, shadow as dense as a pencil-line Figure 3 shows a normal fetogram at 36 weeks' gestation when the skin of the whole body is outlined, including the scrotum. The extent of the visualization depends on the presence and extent of the vernix: it first appears about the 32nd week of gestation and at first it is rather patchy. It soon becomes more abundant and between the 36th and 38th week the fetal skin can be completely outlined including the trunk, head, extremities including fingers and toes, and the external genitalia. Vernix starts to decrease after the 38th week and as a result soft-tissue delineation becomes progressively patchy after that.

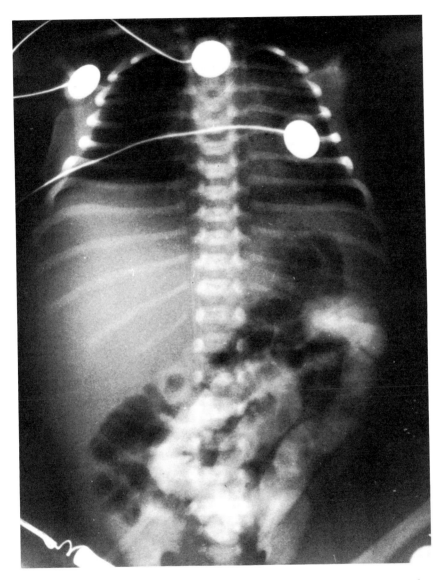

Figure 2. Radiograph of a baby after delivery. An amniogram was carried out 3 weeks earlier to exclude fetal abnormality. A normal fetus was shown. The ingested contrast still opacifies the bowel.

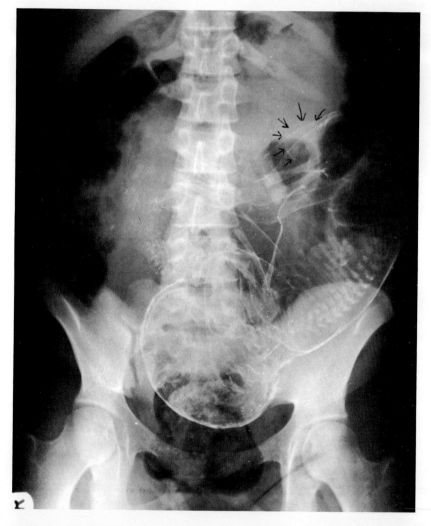

Figure 3. Normal fetogram. The whole fetal skin is well delineated, including the scrotum (arrows).

About 7 ml of iodine-containing substance are injected. Although the vernix starts taking up the contrast soon after the injection, complete visualization is not usually obtained until about 15 hr after the injection, therefore radiography should be deferred until then. The fetus does swallow the fat-soluble contrast but the amount is too little for adequate intestinal opacification.

The relevant details of the techniques are given in Table 1. The variety of information gained is summarized in Table 2; however, the two techniques

Table 1. Comparison of Techniques

	Amniography	Fetography
Contrast medium:	Water-soluble	Liposoluble
Amount:	1 ml/week gestation	7 ml
Action:	Mixes with liquor and renders it opacified	Taken up by the Vernix
Timing for radiography	As required: liquor opacified immediately fetal intestinal tract shown a few hr after injection	About 15 hr after injection

Table 2. Information Obtainable

Sex identification
Uterine outline
Placental localization
Fetal digestive tract
Condition of the fetus
  soft tissue outline
  "vitality test"
Fetal soft-tissue or skeletal abnormaltiies

Table 3. Comparison of the Two Methods

Amniography	Fetography
"Sexing" not too clear	More obvious[a]
Uterine outline clearly shown	Not shown
Placental site identified	Not shown
Fetal digestive tract shown	Less obvious
Condition of the fetus:	
soft-tissue outline shown	More obvious[a]
"vitality test" well-shown	Less obvious
Congenital abnormalities	
soft tissue not too clear	More obvious[a]
skeletal abnormality well-shown	Well-shown
Can be used throughout pregnancy	Used only when vernix is present

[a]Depends on amount of vernix present.

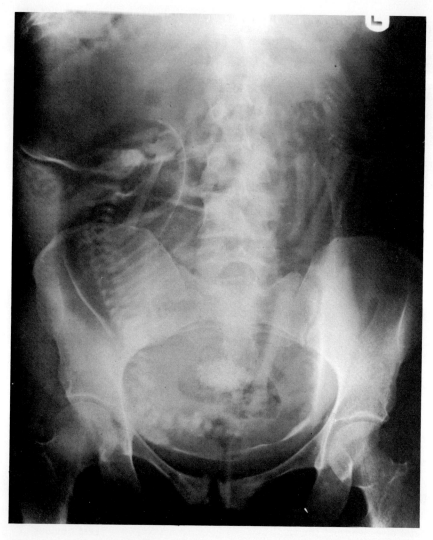

Figure 4. (Legend opposite)

differ considerably. Fetography demonstrates the fetal contour more sharply than amniography; it eliminates the opaqueness of generalized ground-glass appearances given by the opacified amniotic fluid. On the other hand the quantity of contrast injected is much smaller and its affinity for the vernix diminishes fetal ingestion. The radiological findings and the intensity of visualization of the various aspects depend on the method used. These are presented in Table 3. Therefore, in some aspects one technique is superior

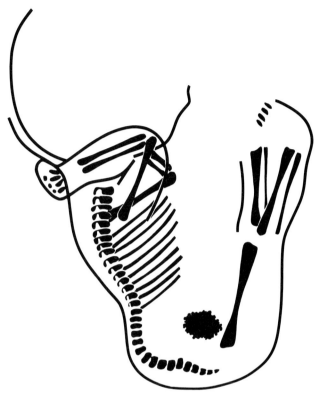

Figure 4. Fetoamniogram (left) with a tracing (above) showing marked fetal abnormalities including hydrocephalus and extensive spina bifida (lumbosacral region). Note that the fetus is alive and the small bowel is opacified by the ingested contrast media.

to the other. The choice of the contrast medium depends on the indication for the procedure or what information is required.

Fetoamniography

To obtain maximum information one can combine both methods; this can be achieved by injecting both fat-soluble and water-soluble media in the same amount as above and then taking one radiograph 12-15 hr after the injection (Fig. 4). Agüero and Zighelboin (1970) first suggested the combined use of fat and water-soluble media; such fetoamniography can give a wide range of information and has proved to be a versatile diagnostic procedure.

INDICATIONS

There are three clear-cut indications for this procedure:

1. In unexplained hydramnios
2. In "high-risk" mothers
3. As a first stage of intrauterine transfusion

Unexplained Hydramnios

The association of hydramnios with congenital malformations is helpful because it alerts the obstetrician to such a possibility. Congenital malformations are usually unsuspected and consequently psychologically traumatic to the parents. They also may lead to difficulty in delivery and possibly to maternal and fetal injuries. Queenan and Gadow (1970) have shown that a third of their patients with unexplained hydramnios had fetuses with congenital abnormality.

Antenatal diagnosis of fetal abnormality starts with ultrasonography and plain radiography; but although these can detect major skeletal abnormality, minor defects are missed. Also sometimes the findings from these preliminary examinations may warrant additional radiological studies using contrast media. Amniography is usually necessary to show soft-tissue malformation or minor spinal abnormalities. Any technique that might help in the detection of such congenital abnormalities prenatally should be encouraged.

"High-Risk" Mothers

Anencephaly and spina bifida cystica are the most common congenital abnormalities of the central nervous system. According to Elwood (1970) and Renwick (1972) the combined incidence in the United Kingdom is about 7:1,000 or 0.7%. The risk of either disorder is increased to 1:20 or 5% in a family with an affected sibling (Carter et al., 1966) and the risk is higher still in a family with two affected siblings. This risk may be as high as 1:10 or greater. Early treatment of correctable malformations is undertaken in several centers and it has been shown that early repair can lead to improved prognosis. Therefore, the advantages of an earliy diagnosis are obvious.

Following the observation by Brock and Sutcliffe (1972) of the connection between raised alpha-fetoprotein (AFP) in the amniotic fluid and fetal neural tube defects, AFP estimations have proved helpful in the prenatal diagnosis of these malformations. These measurements are valuable in the early antenatal diagnosis but after 30 weeks' gestation they may not be distinguishable from normal pregnancies. These measurements can easily be combined with amniography or fetoamniography, especially when the AFP estimation is not so reliable. This can be done at the time of amniocentesis; after the aspiration of the amniotic fluid for the AFP estimation contrast media are injected and followed by radiography. We have done amniography as early as the 15th week of gestation (Fig. 5) but most requests are in more advanced pregnancies.

Amniography, fetography, or fetoamniography gives direct radiographic visualization of the fetal soft tissue. As a result, these techniques are useful in the diagnosis of fetal abnormalities in utero. Obviously, the older the fetus and the larger the lesion, the more obvious the diagnosis. One is particularly interested in detecting spinal abnormalities and some subtle radiological appearances are of significant importance. Special attention should be paid to the alignment of the vertebrae forming a gentle curve; the soft tissue along the back of the normal fetus should show a smooth, unbroken outline and should not reveal any sudden bulge. Fig. 6 shows a soft-tissue "bulge" in the fetal lumbar region which appears as a negative shadow as it displaces the opacified amniotic fluid. This lesion has also "taken up" the fat-soluble contrast showing that there is vernix, indicating that the lesion is covered by skin.

A flat meningocoele may be more difficult to detect than that presenting with a lump. The absence of vernix on the meningocoele or the exposed meninges might cause some difficulty in diagnosis because of the lack of coating of the lesion, but close scrutiny will show certain radiological features which should make one suspicious. Even if the lesion itself is not outlined by the contrast media, the coating of the adjacent fetal skin by the fat-soluble contrast usually gives an indication of such a defect by revealing an oval area of no uptake (Fig. 7); when this is seen in profile the edges of the defect present a V-shaped outline at the upper or lower pole of the lesion (Fig. 8). One should examine closely the vertebrae opposite such a defect for bone abnormality. This is possibly easier to detect in the lateral view but even in the frontal projection there may be evidence of a defect; for example, a sudden increase in the width of a vertebra should raise one's suspicions (Fig. 9).

Finally, amniography might also be needed in a case of binovular twins to assure that amniotic fluid is taken for analytical comparison from both sacs. Figure 10 shows an amniogram carried out on the lower sac showing a normal fetus. The other fetus shows severe skeletal abnormalities including anencephaly. Amniography was performed to ensure that the two specimen of liquor amnii were from both sacs.

First Stage of Intrauterine Transfusion

Before the introduction of Rh-immunoglobulin in the prevention of Rh-hemolytic disease, intrauterine transfusion for affected fetuses was their only chance of survival. With the universal application of passive transfer of anti-D globulin in all Rh-negative gravida at risk and the elimination of incompatible blood transfusion, severe isoimmunization has become a rarity, but the odd case where Rh sensitization has not been prevented or has failed still appears.

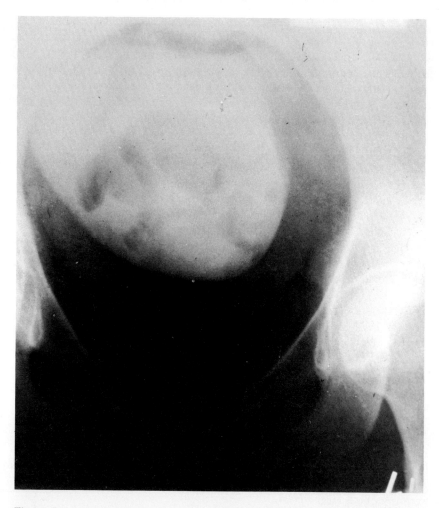

Figure 5. Amniogram of a 15-week pregnancy (above). The fetus can be seen as a negative shadow within the opacified uterus; above right is a line drawing of the amniogram. These show an abnormal flat fetal head suggestive of anencephaly; below right is a clinical photograph of the fetus confirming the diagnosis made by amniography.

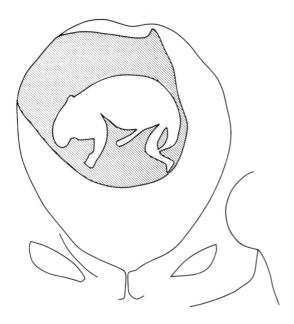

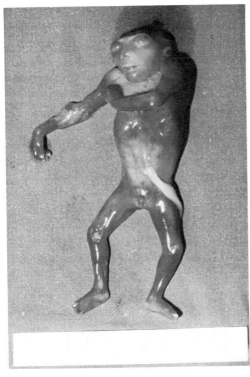

Figure 5. (Continued)

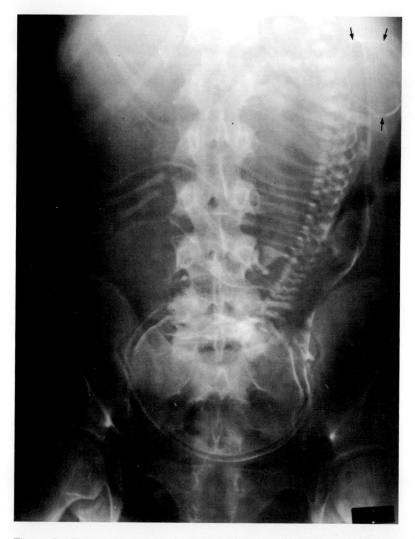

Figure 6. Fetoamniography of a 36-week pregnancy (above) showing a soft-tissue "bulge" in the lumbar region (arrows), as represented in the accompanying line drawing, above right. This is shown as a negative shadow but the skin is well-outlined as it is coated by the fat-soluble contrast medium. The findings were confirmed after delivery (below right).

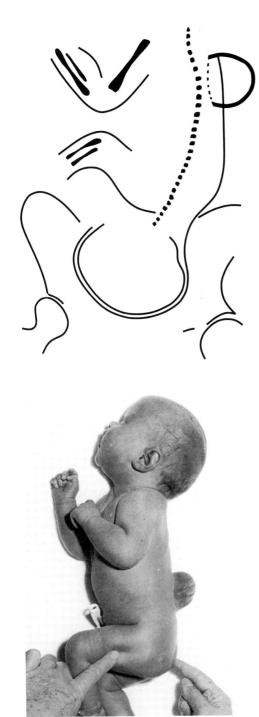

Figure 6. (Continued)

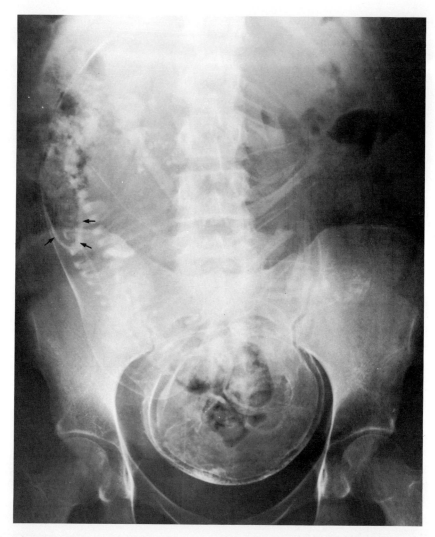

Figure 7. Fetoamniography of a 35-week pregnancy showing a flat meningocoele. The lesion itself is not directly shown since, in the absence of covering skin, no vernix is present. However, the defect is indirectly revealed by the surrounding skin. An oval area of no contrast uptake is demonstrated by the edges of the surrounding skin (arrows) coated by the fat-soluble contrast.

In these cases amniography is used as a first stage in the procedure of intrauterine transfusion to study the state of the fetus and to facilitate the intrauterine process.

To Study the State of the Fetus
From the radiological appearances, one should be able to decide whether it is
salvageable.

Amniography improves our ability to recognize the hydropic fetus. The
fetus seriously affected with hydrops will show Deuel's halo sign, the "Buddha"
sign, and poor vitality.

Deuel's halo sign. Opacification of the amniotic fluid or outlining the fetal
skin surface makes it possible to assess the extent of edema. Deuel's sign is
due to scalp edema which causes an abnormal increase in the width of the gap
between the skull and the scalp skin. In the normal or unaffected fetus this
gap measures not more than 3 mm; if it is more than 3 mm it indicates scalp
edema (Fig. 11).

The "Buddha" sign. The normal fetal attitude shows a gentle flexion; the
hydropic fetus is edematous with loss of such a gentle spinal flexion and the
extent of edema in the rest of the fetus is reflected in its attitude. The
"Buddha" sign includes straightening of the fetal trunk with an enlarged fetal
abdomen and poorly flexed extremities (Fig. 12). Such a presentation would
indicate generalized edema of the fetus.

Vitality test. It has been shown that the normal fetus already swallows by
the age of 15 weeks. The more opacified amniotic fluid the fetus swallows the
more visible its gastrointestinal tract becomes. The opacified amniotic fluid may be
noted in the stomach and small intestine of the fetus within 10 min and the
whole of the intestine is outlined within 15 hr of injection (Fig. 13). Absence
or diminished swallowing is another indication of severe fetal abnormality
and therefore the amount of contrast ingested is a useful gauge for estimating
the fetal "vitality."

To Facilitate the Intrauterine Transfusion Procedure
The opacified fetal intestinal tract provides point of insertion for the
cannula or catheter in the fetal peritoneal cavity through which the intrauterine transfusion is given.

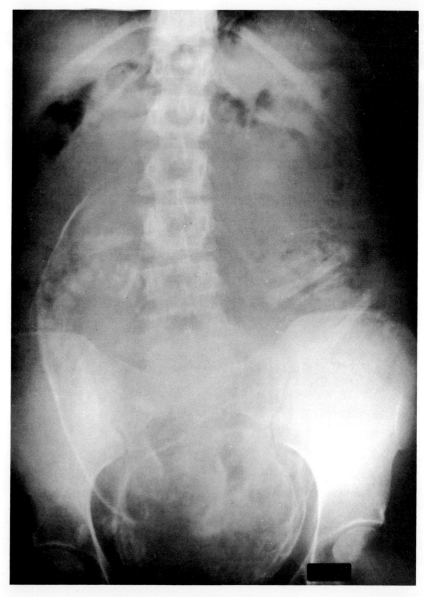

Figure 8. (Legend opposite)

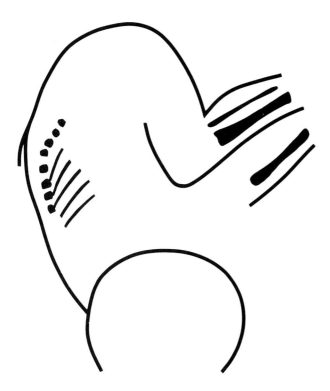

Figure 8. This radiograph (left) accompanied by a line drawing (above) represents a case of flat meningocoele similar to Figure 7. However, the fetus is radiographed in a lateral position and the spinal defect is seen in profile, showing the V-shaped outline in the caudal pole of the lesion, marking the lower edge of the surrounding skin.

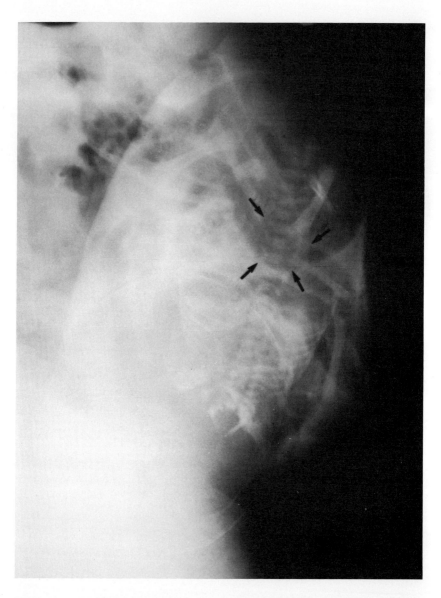

Figure 9. An oblique projection (above) of an amniogram of a 34-week pregnancy where the fetal spine is projected in a frontal position, with a line drawing (above right). The shaded area in the sketch represents the localization of the placenta. The figure along the spine represent the interpedicular distances along the spine as measured in millimeters on the radiograph. Note that there is a sudden increase in width, from 13 to 18 and again back to 14. This raised our suspicion of a spina bifida, although no skin lesion was seen. Clinical photograph of the baby after delivery (below right) shows spina bifida in the lumbar spine.

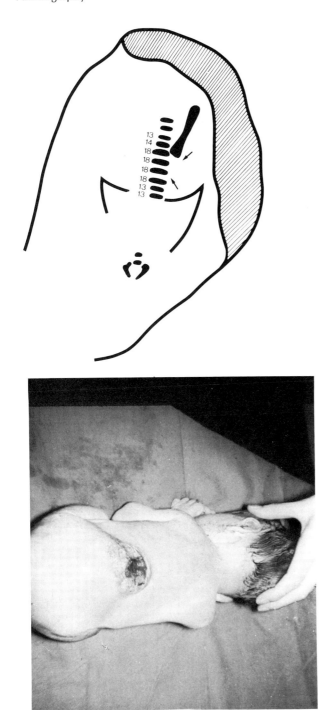

Figure 9. (Continued)

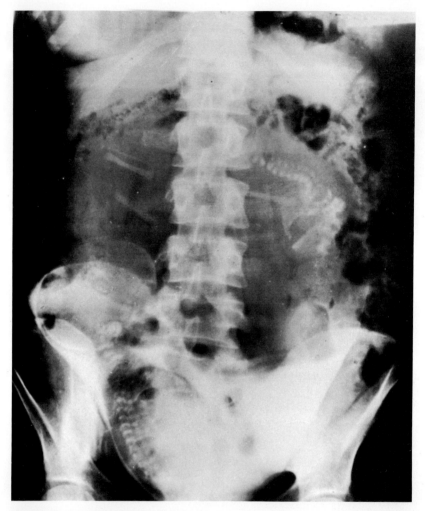

Figure 10. Amniography in a case of twins to ascertain that the amniotic fluid is taken from both sacs for analytical comparison. In this case amniography was carried out on the lower fetus which shows no abnormality; the upper fetus presents extensive skeletal abnormalities. The two samples of amniotic fluid showed markedly differing AFP levels (27 and 81 mg/ml, respectively). On delivery the normal twin weighed 1800 g while the abnormal one, which weighed 700 g, was anencephalic and had an examphalos.

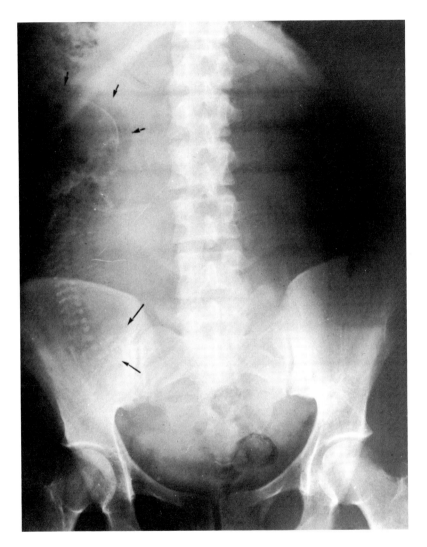

Figure 11. Deuel's halo sign. Amniogram of a 28-week pregnancy in a case of severe Rh-isoimmunization. Hydramnios causes dilution of the contrast. Although the fetus is alive, it shows poor vitality: very little contrast is visible in the bowel (long arrows). The short arrows point to the scalp and there is marked increase in the scalp thickness (11 mm on the radiograph) due to scalp edema. This would indicate that the fetus is severely affected and hydropic.

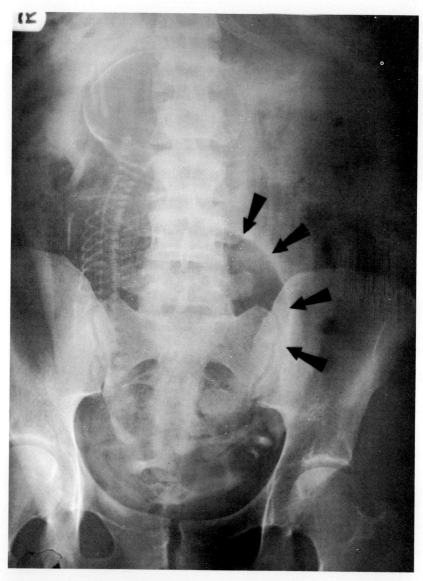

Figure 12. (Legend opposite)

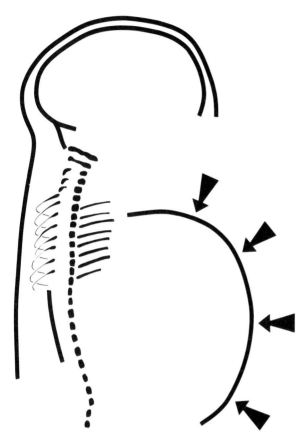

Figure 12. "Buddha" sign. This amniogram (left) was done as a first stage for intrauterine transfusion for Rh-isoimmunization. The fetus is well shown; it is lying in a breech position with a straight spine and presenting an enlarged abdomen (arrows on left and above).

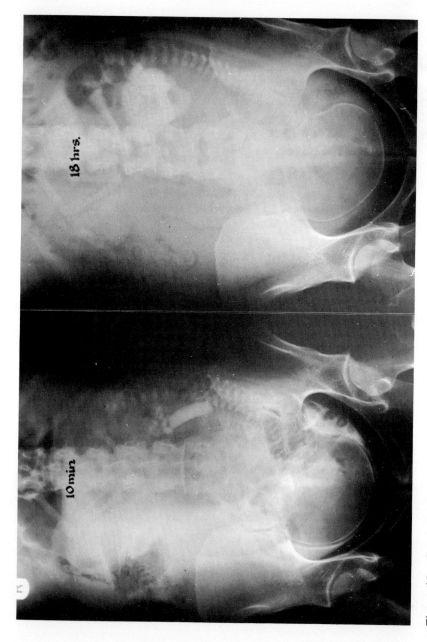

Figure 13. Good "vitality test" on a normal fetus as shown by amniography. The fetal stomach is already opacified 10 min after injection of the contrast. A radiograph taken 18 hr later shows the whole length of the small and large bowel.

PRECAUTIONS TO AVOID COMPLICATIONS

Although several recent reviews (McLain, 1964; Lennon, 1967; Queenan et al., 1968, Spindola-Franco et al., 1969; Grech, 1975) have stressed the relative safety and the low incidence of complications associated with amniography, certain precautions must be taken to minimize potential hazards.

Obviously the greatest hazard is puncturing the placenta. Placental localization must be carried out before amniocentesis; this used to be done by isotope studies but ultrasonography is now widely used.

Secondly, one must ensure that the needle or catheter is properly positioned and that there is a good flow of amniotic fluid. The tip should lie freely in the amniotic sac and there should be unimpeded backflow of liquor amnii on aspiration before the injection of contrast media. Sudden movement of the fetus during the injection or any unexpected increase in resistance to the flow of contrast is an absolute indication to stop the injection and to ascertain that the needle is properly positioned before completing the injection.

The accidental injection of contrast medium in the skin of the fetus may lead to extensive subcutaneous necrosis. Such a potential fetal hazard was highlighted in a report of two cases (Grech and Spitz, 1977) following amniography. This potential hazard was supported by experiments reported by Grainger (1977) from which the following conclusions were drawn:

1. Newborn rabbits are much more sensitive to subcutaneous injection of contrast media than adult rabbits or dogs
2. In newborn rabbits the meglumine ion causes much more subcutaneous necrosis than the sodium ion.

From these conclusions one would deduce that the meglumine cation is much less well tolerated subcutaneously in the newborn or fetus and that perhaps in amniography sodium contrast media are to be preferred to meglumine. However, should the contrast be accidentally injected into the fetal skull or spinal canal, the sodium ion will be less well tolerated than the meglumine (Grech and Bevis, 1969). If the possibility of injection of the contrast medium in the skin of the fetus were eliminated, meglumine is considered to be the safest water-soluble contrast medium. This potential complication of amniography can be prevented by using a teflon cannula instead of a rigid spinal needle to prevent the fetus from stabbing itself on the tip of the needle during a sudden movement.

Apart from this potential hazard, the contrast media used have been found to be free of any toxic effects, either to the mother or fetus.

Finally, one must keep the radiation dose to a safe minimum. The Code of Practice (Department of Health and Social Security, 1972) gives the maximum permissible dose for occupationally exposed persons as not more than 1 rem during that pregnancy after it is diagnosed. This is the only yardstick we have; but oviously if it is permissible for the occupationally exposed mother, it should be acceptable for the rest.

The investigation entails one or two radiographs; it is difficult to compare radiation doses to the fetus since conditions differ from one case to another. This radiation hazard was assessed in 20 cases (Bevis et al., 1972) and it was calculated that the average mother received a skin exposure of 3312 mR during this examination. The average radiation dose to the fetus was estimated at about 200 mrads per exposure. From this study one would conclude that, although the radiation hazard should be considered, it ought not to be over-stated. These limits of radiation should be acceptable if the procedure is indicated because of the information that can be gained and its help in planning management of the case.

REFERENCES

Agüero, O., and Zighelboim, I. (1970). Fetography and molegraphy. *Surg. Gynecol. Obstet. 130*:649-654.

Bevis, D. C. A., Grech, P., and Parsons, R. J. (1972). Radiation hazard in intra-uterine transfusion. *Br. J. Radiol. 45*:193-196.

Brock, D. J. H., and Sutcliffe, R. G. (1972). Alpha-fetoprotein in the ante-natal diagnosis of anencephaly and spina bifida. *Lancet 2*:197-199.

Carter, C. O., Lawrence, K. M., David, P. A. (1966). Genetics of major central nervous system malformations based on South Wales sociogenetic investigation. *Dev. Med. Child Neurol. 9*: [Suppl. 13] , 30-33.

Department of Health and Social Security, (1972). *Code of Practice,* 3rd ed. Her Majesty's Stationery Office, London.

Elwood, J. H. (1970). *Dev. Med. Child Neurol. 12*:582-585.

Erbslöh, J. (1942). Das intrauterine Fetogramm; ein Beitrag zur geburtshilf-licten Rontgendiagnostik. *Roentgenpraxis 14*:28.

Grainger, R. G. (1977). Subcutaneous tolerance of contrast media. *Br. J. Radiol. 50*:447.

Grech, P. (1975). Diagnosis of fetal abnormalities in utero. *Extracts, 3rd European Congress of Radiology.* Churchill Livingstone, Edinburgh, Abstract 257.

Grech, P., and Bevis, D. C. A. (1969). Fetal myelography—An unusual complica-tion in intra-uterine transfusion. *Br. J. Radiol. 42*:389-391.

Grech, P., and Spitz, L. (1977). Fetal complications of amniography. *Br. J. Radiol. 50*:110-112.

Lennon, G. G. (1967). Intrauterine foetal visualization. *J. Obstet. Gynaecol. Br. Commonw. 74*:227.

McLain, C. R., Jr. (1964). Amniography, a versatile diagnostic procedure in obstetrics. *Obstet. Gynecol. 23*:45-50.

Menees, T. O., Miller, J. D., and Holly, L. E. (1930). Amniography. *Am. J. Roentgenol.* *24*:363-366.

Queenan, J. T., and Gadow, E. C. (1970). Amniography for detection of congenital malformations. *Obstet. Gynecol.* *35*:648-657.

Queenan, J. T., Von Gal, H. V., and Kubarych, S. F. (1968). Amniography for clinical evaluation of erythroblastosis fetalis. *Am. J. Obstet. Gynecol.* *102*:264-272.

Renwick, J. H. (1972). Anencephaly and spina bifida are usually preventable by avoidance of a specific but unidentified substance present in certain potato tubers. *Br. J. Prev. Soc. Med.* *26*:67-69.

Spindola-Franco, H., Ceballos-Labat, J., and Cisneros, H. A. (1969). Value of amniography in determining fetal viability. *Acta Radiol.* *8*:17-28.

6

Twin Delivery: Delivery Techniques and Labor Complications

IAN MacGILLIVRAY / University of Aberdeen, Aberdeen, Scotland

There is no doubt that the risks to twins are much greater than to singletons, as shown in the reports on perinatal mortality for twin deliveries compared with singletons (Munnell and Taylor, 1946; Little and Friedman, 1958; MacGillivray and Campbell, 1980). Not only are the death rates increased but so also are the risks of handicap, both physical and mental. Twins are disadvantaged during pregnancy because of complications and also during labor and delivery because of their greater inability to withstand asphyxia and manipulations.

PROGNOSIS FOR TWINS

There are more deaths of second twins than first twins. Most reports consider that the risk is greater to the second twin and a recent report (Sherman and Lowe, 1970), showed that there were 50% more perinatal deaths among second twins than first-borns. There are twice as many deaths due to trauma in firstborn twins compared with singletons and four times as many in second-born twins. Although the stillbirth rate for second twins is much the same as for firstborn, the neonatal mortality rate is twice as high (Little and Friedman, 1958; Sherman and Lowe, 1970). Potter (1963) suggested that the second baby was at greater risk of cerebral anoxia because of the prolonged delivery interval, prolapsed cord, or early separation of the placenta, and the first baby was at greater risk of birth injury because he or she has to dilate the cervix.

129

There may be a competition effect when there are marked weight discrepancies resulting in the death of the smaller child. The second twin is generally smaller than the first and monozygotic twins show a greater discrepancy in birth weight than do dizygotic. The second twin may, however, be at risk because it is larger than the first and this may result in death or be the reason for the trebled incidence of cerebral injury in twins compared with singletons (Dunn, 1965).

DIAGNOSIS

The early diagnosis of twin pregnancies is of great importance not only because of the greater care that has to be taken of the mother but also because it is important to recognize that the physiological changes are more marked than those occurring in the woman with a singleton pregnancy (MacGillivray et al., 1975). Delivery should be planned to take place at a center with full facilities, particularly for neonatal care. The mother should be warned that premature labor may occur and that complications of pregnancy are more common so that she will require more care and attention.

Routine screening tests performed in many centers can alert the obstetrician to the possibility of multiple pregnancy. In many centers a routine ultrasonic scan is performed between 16 and 20 weeks and this, of course, will detect twin pregnancy. Scanning done much earlier in pregnancy will also detect twin pregnancies and it is interesting that there are now several reports of the "disappearing" twin. This occurs when one twin dies and is absorbed. Another routine screening test done at some centers is for neural tube defects, by the estimation of alpha-fetoprotein. When this is raised, twin pregnancy should also be excluded. Routine hormonal assays of, for example, estrogens and placental proteins, will also be likely to give a higher value than for a singleton pregnancy. One of the commonly and easily performed presumptive tests is the assessment of weight gain, which is increased in twin pregnancy compared with singletons. Early diagnosis is also important so that accurate gestation age can be determined ultrasonically and possible postmaturity avoided.

RISKS OF TWIN PREGNANCIES

The risks are increased not only because of the malpositions and malpresentations which can make delivery difficult but also because of the prenatal complications that are liable to occur, such as premature onset of labor, preeclampsia, hydramnios, and poor intrauterine growth of the babies.

Complications of Pregnancy

The method of delivery may be determined to a large extent by the presence of absence of other complications of pregnancy. In particular, these are prepartum hemorrhage, hydramnios, and preeclampsia. Although it is often suggested that the incidence of prepartum hemorrhage is greater in twin pregnancies, no evidence supports this view. Even so, if hemorrhage does occur, and is severe, then the method of delivery will most certainly be by cesarean section.

Hydramnios
This is quite a common feature of multiple pregnancy and is thought to be more common in monozygotic than in dizygotic pregnancies. The hydramnios will predispose to malpositions and malpresentations and prolapse of the cord and will lead to the greater likelihood of interference by cesarean section being necessary.

Preeclampsia
This is well known to be more common in twin pregnancies and this is an important reason for seeing the woman with a twin pregnancy frequently in the latter part of pregnancy. The incidence in an Aberdeen series is shown in Table 1 and it is interesting to note that there is probably no difference in the incidence between monozygotic and dizygotic twinning. The incidence of proteinuric pre-eclampsia is particularly high and, since babies tend to be more poorly grown when proteinuric pre-eclampsia is present, it is not surprising that this makes them more liable to fetal distress in labor. Interference again becomes necessary.

Growth Retardation
Whether this is associated with pre-eclampsia or not can, of course, be difficult to detect and measure in twin pregnancies. Although the combined birth weight of twins is greater than singletons the individual twin is smaller than a singleton at the same gestation. The cause of this poor growth is not known but is probably due to an inadequate uterine blood flow or poor nutrition. There is now some evidence that if one twin dies early in gestation and the pregnancy continues, the other twin will have a low birth weight. More than 50% of deaths in multiple births are accounted for by low birth weight in twins, compared with 10% in singleton pregnancies (Potter, 1963). Expert ultrasonic scanning can be of considerable value in measuring the size of twins and, indeed, in detecting differences in the size of the two babies. Some help may also be obtained by determining the number of placentas present. There is a greater discrepancy in the weights of monozygotic twins and also the risk to the babies is greater than in dizygotic twins. The number of placentas, of course, does not determine the zygosity of the twins, but a single placenta is more likely to indicate a monozygotic twin pregnancy. It has been emphasized, however, that very expert ultrasonic scanning is required to determine the size of the babies; the biparietal diameter will indicate the maturity of the babies but it is not of much help in determining their weight.

Table 1. Incidence of Pre-Eclampsia in 212 Monozygotic and Dizygotic Twin Pregnancies in Aberdeen Primigravidas (%)

	Monozygotic	Dizygotic
Normotensive	44.3	52.1
Late hypertension only	28.6	25.2
Proteinuric pre-eclampsia	27.1	21.1
Total	100% (n=70)	100% (n=142)

This is best done by crown-rump length or cross-sectional scanning of the trunk, but serial biparietal measurements may be halpful. It is not always certain, however, that serial measurements apply to the same baby each time. If the facilities are available it is certainly worthwhile trying to assess the true size of the babies before deciding on the mode of delivery. Ultrasonic scanning is also of value in assessing maturity and in many cases of twin pregnancy there is un-certainty about the length of gestation both because the date of last menstrual period may not be remembered, and because the fundal height does not con-form to the gestational size.

Premature Onset of Labor

This is common in twin pregnancies and, although there are various claims that this can be prevented by rest, beta-sympathomimetic agents, or cervical sutures, there have been no reports of any properly controlled studies of a large series. The amount of physical activity is difficult to assess and the effect of rest is difficult to determine, but complete bed rest is almost certainly unnecessary. On the other hand, increased activity particularly if it is unaccustomed, is best avoided. In any case, most women with twin pregnancies are less inclined to be active in the third trimester. The place of beta-sympathomimetic drugs is still being determined. It has been suggested that cervical sutures in the second and third trimester of twin pregnancies, rather than preventing pre-mature labor, actually do more harm than good (Sinha et al., 1979). If a woman is likely to go into premature labor with a twin pregnancy, she should be in hospital as early as possible so that the delivery can be conducted in a proper manner. Regular examination of the cervix in the last trimester can sometimes be of value in predicting the onset of premature labor.

Relative Risks to First and Second Twins

The size of the two babies is of great importance in determining the date of delivery particularly if it appears that the second baby is smaller than the first. It appears that on balance the prognosis for the second twin is less favorable than for the first. The risks to the two babies are, to some extent, different, for example, the first baby is more likely to be at risk from prolapse of the cord, while the second is more likely to have problems because of mal-presentations. The second baby is also at greater risk because of the likelihood of asphyxia due to malpresentation, from reduced circulation, and som:times placental separation. Ware (1971) found that the Apgar scores in second twins were poor compared with the first twin, particularly when delivered by total breech extraction or version and extraction. The incidence of cerebral injury in twins is three times that in singletons (Dunn, 1965). The risk of cerebral palsy is greater in second twins, especially those delivered by breech. In first-born twins, however, cerebral palsy occurs more often in premature infants presenting by the vertex and the commonest form of palsy is spastic diplegia (Griffiths, 1967). Second-born twins were more often mature and had had ab-normalities of presentations. MacDonald 1962) found that the second twin was more often severely asphyxiated than the first when both babies were delivered by the vertex and in the Aberdeen series of 321 twin babies (MacGillivray and Campbell, 1980), there were twice as many second-born babies with a low Apgar score as first babies. Ware assessed the Apgar scores on the basis of the weight of the babies, but in our Aberdeen series we used gestation length because it is known before the birth of the babies, whereas the weight cannot be known accurately until after birth. The Apgar scores were analyzed for the surviving babies born between 30 and 34 weeks. We believed that after that gestation there was less risk to the babies and if labor started before 30 weeks vaginal delivery would be likely unless circumstances were exceptional. It was found that there were more second twins with a low Apgar score than first twins and that assisted breech delivery resulted in lower Apgar score than in other types of delivery. However, in this series multi-gravid breech deliveries were at greater risk than primigravid, possibly suggest-ing that it is the early gestation as much as the presentation that predisposes to low Apgar scores. In a recent study, Calvert (1980) showed that, on the basis of Apgar scores, delivery by lower-segment cesarean section is more danger-ous when the fetus presents by the breech rather than cephalic even in the best circumstances. He believed that the greater likelihood of a low Apgar score might be due to an inherent abnormality which itself had caused the breech presentation but perhaps was more likely to be due to respiratory efforts before delivery of the head. Calvert stated that a mature, healthy fetus is probably well able to withstand this extra insult, but for a breech-presenting fetus, which becomes distressed during preterm labor, the added hazard might be important. He suggested that if delay in delivery of the fetal head causes the depression, then delivery by classic cesarean section in the case of breech presentation might be preferable where the fetus is already compromised.

ELECTIVE CESAREAN SECTION

Elective cesarean section in twin pregnancy is usually carried out when there are some complications such as pre-eclampsia or hemorrhage. These are, of course, strong indications for cesarean section in many cases irrespective of gestation length. Otherwise, elective cesarean section is reserved for twin pregnancies at or after 38 weeks gestation to avoid possible trauma at delivery if the progress of the pregnancy has been normal up until that time. Although some extremists would suggest that cesarean section should be carried out for the delivery of all twins at this gestation, most would prefer to aim for vaginal delivery unless other circumstances are present. If, for example, the mother is an older primigravida, or has had a previous cesarean section, or if there is a malpresentation, then elective cesarean section might be carried out.

The chances of both babies presenting as cephalic varies between 34.5 and 66.3% (Portes and Granjon, 1946; Guttmacher and Kohl, 1958; Ross and Philpott, 1953) (Table 2) and some obstetricians limit vaginal delivery to cases where both twins are presenting as cephalic. However, others will be quite prepared to deliver at least one of the twins by the breech.

Elective cesarean section at or after 38 weeks when either the first or second twin, or both, is presenting by the breech, is a matter of individual preference for the obstetrician and depends on his or her attitude to delivery of the singleton breech.

There are risks to delivery of twins by cesarean section, particularly of respiratory distress syndrome. Also, the second baby can sometimes suffer

Table 2

	Guttmacher and Kohl (1958)	Portes and Granjon (1946)	Ross and Philpott (1953)	
			Primigravida	Multigravida
Both vertex	46.9	44.3	34.5	37.1
One vertex, one breech	37.0	38.4	30.9	33.1
One breech, one vertex			5.5	12.4
Both breech	8.7	9.9	14.5	7.4
One transverse, one vertex	4.9	5.3		
One transverse, one breech	1.9	1.4		
Both transverse	0.6	0.2		
All cephalic		66.3		
First twin cephalic		74.9		
Second twin cephalic		57.7		
Compound			10.9	4.1
Brow or face transverse lie			3.4	5.7

trauma, especially if it is large and there is a difficult breech extraction through the lower uterine segment incision. There is something to be said for considering the classic or upper segment or the De Lee incision for the delivery of twin breeches. The classic incision is made vertically in the midline through the visceral peritoneum and the upper segment after the dextrorotation of the uterus has been corrected. The De Lee incision is a low longitudinal uterine incision, two-thirds of which is in the lower segment and one-third in the upper uterine segment. The visceral peritoneum is opened transversely and reflected as high up and as low down as possible before making the incision in the uterus. In addition to breech delivery it is also particularly useful in transverse lie. Unfortunately, it is in the primigravida that the strongest case can be made for delivering breeches by cesarean section and it would be undesirable in them to perform a classic or even a De Lee cesarean section. If the pelvis is adequate, the babies are both well-grown, the mother is young, even in primigravidas, and certainly in multigravidas, the author's preference is to aim for vaginal delivery if the baby or babies are presenting by the breech at term.

Brow and face presentations of the first baby will not necessarily be absolute indications for elective cesarean section and some obstetricians may wish to wait and see what progress and conversion occur in labor. Many will, however, prefer in such circumstances to do an elective cesarean section or at most allow only a short trial of labor.

If the first twin is lying transversely or, more particularly, if both are transverse, then delivery should be by elective cesarean section. This should possibly be by the classic or De Lee method if the back of the first baby is presenting. When there is evidence that one or both babies is not fully grown, then, depending on the severity of the growth retardation, cesarean section may be preferred for the delivery. This will obviously apply to pregnancies before 37 weeks as well as after.

The question of elective cesarean sections should then rarely arise except when there are complications such as marked fetal growth retardation of one or both babies, severe pre-eclampsia, or abruption of the placenta. Elective cesarean section for malposition or malpresentation alone should only be considered when the pregnancy has reached 28 weeks at least. Some may prefer to allow the pregnancy to continue beyond 38 weeks before performing elective cesarean section depending on when it is considered that the pregnancy is mature and before postmaturity intervenes.

Postmaturity

This is a subject of considerable controversy and the possible hazards of the pregnancy going past term have not been fully evaluated. If it were possible to detect impending fetal distress from postmaturity by doing such tests as amnioscopy or amniocentesis, cardiotocography or hormone assays, fetal movement counts, or combinations of these, it would be permissible to allow the pregnancy to continue indefinitely. However, since these are difficult enough to do in singleton pregnancies, it becomes obvious that such methods are not applicable in twin pregnancy. Decisions must therefore be made arbitrarily regarding the risks of postmaturity in pregnancy. It is reasonable in the author's opinion to consider that all twins should be delivered by the end of 40 completed weeks. Delivery, of course, will be carried out earlier if there is any growth retardation or other complications.

Interference and delivery will have taken place in the majority of twin pregnancies before term either because of complications arising or because of the onset of spontaneous labor. Elective cesarean section in itself may not be without risk, particularly of respiratory distress syndrome to the babies, as well as to the mother. Therefore, there should be good reason for carrying out an elective section for a twin pregnancy.

CESAREAN SECTION AFTER ONSET OF LABOR

Cesarean section must, of course, be carried out during the course of labor if complications arise, particularly malpresentations. In such cases the labor has often started prematurely and the length of gestation is of great importance in deciding whether to allow it to continue or to do a cesarean section. If the first baby is a transverse lie, cesarean section should be carried out unless the gestation is very short and the twins are considered to be very small. If there is a breech presenting in the first or second twin then, provided there is no obstetric complication, vaginal delivery should be attempted if the pregnancy is of 36 weeks gestation or more. If the pregnancy is less than 30 weeks, it is doubtful if cesarean section should be carried out, no matter what the presentations are, because the baby would be very small and unlikely to survive in any case. Only in units with a highly sophisticated neonatology service would cesarean section be justified in such cases. Between 30 and 34 weeks the risks of vaginal breech delivery, particularly for the second baby, are high and there may be grounds for doing a cesarean section in these cases. There are, however, risks to delivering twins by cesarean section as already referred to by Calvert (1980). This is particularly true of the second breech as this can sometimes be a hazardous breech extraction through a relatively small lower segment incision in cases where the gestation is short.

In the 25 breech deliveries in the Aberdeen series between 30 and 34 weeks of gestation, there were five deaths (20%) and in the remaining 20 there were nine (45%) with an Apgar score between 6 at 1 min and five (25%) below 6 at 5 min. There is not only a risk of perinatal death in breech deliveries, but also of mental handicap among babies born by the breech (Birch et al., 1970). Possibly more might have survived or been in better condition if delivered by cesarean section, particularly by the classic or De Lee method. Evidence of growth retardation, particularly in a second baby, probably strengthens the indication for a cesarean section.

MANAGEMENT OF LABOR

If it has not been possible to prevent or stop premature labor or if labor has started spontaneously after 37 weeks, or, indeed, if labor has been induced, the length of labor in twin pregnancy will be about the same as that in a singleton pregnancy (Bender, 1952; Ross and Phillpott, 1953; Law, 1967). However, unless there is interference in the second stage, labor can be prolonged. Law (1967) suggested that the duration of the second stage should be between 1 and 2 hr.

When the first stage of labor is not progressing quickly enough, oxytocin stimulation is frequently used and is of great value. It is useful to have an oxytocin infusion running before the end of the first stage so that stimulation of the second stage can be achieved readily. Alternatively, an infusion of 5% dextrose can be set up and switched to oxytocin as required in the second stage, particularly after the birth of the first baby.

Anesthesia

It is highly desirable that an anesthetist be available for all twin deliveries, preferably one with particular interest and expertise in obstetric anesthesia. The usual practice now is to give epidural anesthesia. This has several advantages over both pudendal block and general anesthesia. The epidural anesthesia not only gives relief of pain during the first stage of labor but also allows all manipulation required for the delivery of the first and second twins to be carried out, including cesarean section if required. It also ensures that the cervix is fully dilated for the delivery of the first baby; this is particularly important if the first baby is presenting by the breech. The common practice of inducing a pudendal nerve block for the delivery of the first baby, and then the second is in some cases satisfactory, but if a general anesthetic becomes necessary for the delivery of the second, this has to be a hurried and often unsatisfactory and hazardous procedure which is best avoided. Should, however, an epidural anesthetic not be possible, the pudendal block is administered for delivery of the first baby if it is by forceps or assisted breech delivery. The patient should be fully prepared for a general anesthetic in case this is necessary for delivery of the second baby.

Monitoring the Conditions of the Babies

The progress of labor is determined in the usual fashion which nowadays means the use of a partogram. In this way the dilatation of the cervix, the strength of the contractions, and the descent of the presenting part are recorded. Vaginal examination will be performed to determine if there is any pelvic disproportion even if the twins tend to be small. If the facilities are available for cardiotocography, then an electrode is attached to the presenting part of the first baby and the condition of the second baby monitored by an external instrument. If these instruments are not available, the condition of the babies is recorded as accurately as possible by the Pinard stethoscope.

Cardiotocography is well worth attempting although it can be difficult and even, on occasion, misleading as reported by Fehrmann (1980). He described a case in which the electrocardiogram of a live second twin was detected through the scalp electrode attached to a dead first twin. Real-time B scan has been found to be of value in locating the fetal hearts for antepartum monitoring even in a triplet pregnancy (Powell-Phillips et al., 1979) and could be of help in doubtful cases in labor.

DELIVERY OF THE FIRST TWIN

Should fetal distress of either the first or second twin develop during the first stage of labor, a decision will be made about cesarean section depending on various factors, such as degree of dilatation of the cervix and the gestational length. If, however, the condition of the babies is satisfactory and labor progresses well without undue delay, then vaginal delivery can be anticipated.

In most cases a decision will have been made about the type of delivery before the onset of labor, but in some cases an unsuspected malposition or malpresentation of the first twin is found after labor has started. In such cases the delivery is carried out according to the practice usually employed by the obstetrician when dealing with singletons. Generally, when it is a face, brow, or shoulder presentation, delivery will be by cesarean section. Consideration will again have to be given, particularly in the case of a transverse lie, to employing the classic or De Lee incision.

In transverse position of the occiput, the delivery is effected as for a singleton, either by manual rotation and forceps or by Keilland's forceps, according to the obstetrician's usual practice. When labor is allowed to proceed with a breech presentation, the condition of the baby is carefully monitored, preferably with an electrode on the buttock. The delivery may be spontaneous or assisted depending on the progress, but a breech extraction should be avoided. If the breech does not show at the perineum with maternal bearing-down efforts then cesarean section should be performed.

Prolapse of the Cord

This may occur particularly if there is hydramnios. If the cervix is fully dilated, delivery should be effected as quickly as possible. If not, cesarean section is performed.

Obstructed Labor

In a twin pregnancy this is usually due to transverse lie of the first twin and only rarely due to twin-locking. Rupture of the uterus is extremely uncommon in obstructed labor in the primigravid patient and, conversely, fistulas from pressure necrosis are seldom seen in the multigravida. Delay in the rate of cervical dilatation in the primigravida virtually always precedes obstructed labor and is a reliable early warning signal. In the multigravida the obstruction may occur without a preceding change in the normal pattern of cervical dilatation. In those circumstances, the problem is more difficult to detect and is then only recognized by the slow or arrested rate of descent of the presenting part. In the neglected obstructed labor in a primigravida, she will be exhausted, dehydrated, and there may be bowel distention. The liquor will be drained away and the uterus will be molded around the fetus. There may be fetal distress or, in more advanced cases, the fetus or fetuses will be dead. The bladder is often distended and catheterization may be difficult. If there have been prolonged bearing-down efforts the vulva and cervix may be very edematous. In the multigravida the findings are much the same; the lower uterine segment may be tender and a Bandl's ring may be found near the level of the umbilicus. After the rupture of the uterus, there may be little evidence of this because the torn uterine vessels are compressed by the impacted presenting part. On the other hand, there may be more dramatic features, with profound shock. After rupture the contractions are replaced by continuous pain. The abdomen may be grossly distended and the uterus difficult to feel.

This situation is likely to occur where there is poor, or absent, prenatal care, for example, in many parts of Africa. In some of these areas, particularly in Nigeria, the twinning rates are very high, up to 40:1000 births (MacGillivray et al., 1975).

As transport is often difficult in these areas and the women have often been in labor for a prolonged time, they are often in shock on admission to hospital. Active and rapid resuscitation is required before delivery can be undertaken. Since there is often established or potential intrauterine infection an extraperitoneal cesarean section may be indicated. This can be carried out, for example, by the technique described by Crichton (1973) in which the parietal peritoneum is opened transversly. When the visceral peritoneum has been opened and reflected downwards, the upper flap of the visceral peritoneum

is sutured to the upper flap of the parietal peritoneum and the lower flap of
the visceral to the lower flap of the parietal. This renders the lower segment
artificially extraperitoneal. When the lower segment has been closed after
delivery the peritoneum over the uterine wound is left as it is and a drain
placed in the wound.

Destructive Operations

Philpott (1980) recommends these as an alternative to an unnecessary and
hazardous cesarean section. Decapitation is indicated where there is a transverse lie and prolapsed arm. The safest method of performing a decapitation
is to use the Blond-Heidler saw. This is a gigli-type wire saw which is passed
around the fetal neck by attaching a thimble with a ring at one end of the saw.
The ring is attached to a hook at each end of the wire saw and a sawing
motion then severs the head. The trunk of the fetus is then delivered
followed by the decapitated head. If this cannot be done it may be necessary
to use scissors. This must be done extremely carefully and under direct vision
while the prolapsed arm is being brought down as far as possible by an
assistant. The second twin can then be delivered by the breech or by forceps
if it is a cephalic presentation.

A problem sometimes encountered in transverse lie with the membranes
ruptured and the shoulder impacted is that a transverse incision has been made
in the lower segment. In these circumstances, on no account should the arm
be delivered into the wound as subsequent delivery cannot be accomplished by
this manoeuver. Two possible methods of delivery exist, and in deciding which
one to attempt many factors have to be considered. The most important are
the size of the fetus, the presence of a good anesthetist, and an experienced
surgeon. The first method to be tried if the fetus is not very large is to request
the anesthetist to relax the uterus, which is often firmly contracted around
the babies. It may then be possible gently to disimpact the shoulder and push
it upwards until the position of the fetus allows one to grasp a foot and then,
by gentle traction, to complete the delivery. If this proves unsuccessful, the
ends of the transverse incision should be curved upwards to give more access.
The vertical incision, converting the transverse incision into the so-called
T-shaped incision, is best avoided because it causes a weak uterine scar. If
the transverse position with lack of liquor amnii has been recognized in advance,
it is preferable to use either the De Lee or classic incision. The classic cesarean
section is rarely performed today, but it is becoming more common because of
the poorly formed lower uterine segment found when cesarean sections are to
be carried out between 30 and 34 weeks gestation.

DELIVERY OF THE SECOND TWIN

A decision may be m de to do an elective cesarean section if the second twin is presenting by the breech, but this will depend on the preference of the obstetrician, the length of gestation, and other factors. If the second twin is transverse there is usually no problem because it can be turned easily after delivery of the first twin. When the first twin is delivered the lie should be checked and corrected if necessary. This should be done as soon as the first twin is delivered and the fetal heart checked. The membranes should be ruptured within a few minutes of the delivery of the first baby without any undue delay. If the uterus does not start contracting again after a few minutes, an oxytocin drip should be started to stimulate the uterus.

Retention of the second twin for a prolonged time is unlikely to occur, where there is no medical supervision of labor. Adeleye (1972) reviewed 160 case records of retained second twins in Nigeria and found that the perinatal mortality in his hospital delivery group was 23.5%, compared with 50.4% in the emergency admission group. He considered the second twin as being retained when the delivery interval between both twins was 30 min or more. The patients admitted to the hospital from outside however, must have been retained for a much longer period than this, and it is not surprising that the longer the baby is retained the higher the perinatal mortality rate. Malpresentation and uterine inertia were the main causative factors in the retention. Active intervention reduced the length of retention and consequently the perinatal mortality rate.

Spontaneous Delivery

This occurs in many second twin deliveries. In the British Perinatal Mortality Survey (1969) 48.1% of second twins were spontaneous vertex deliveries.

Forceps Delivery

Forceps delivery of the second twin may be necessary if the mother is unable to bear down sufficiently to deliver the baby. This may be either a straight application of the forceps in an occipitoanterior position, or after rotation from a transverse, or alternatively, the application of Keilland's forceps. However, this should only be done when the head is in the pelvis. The application of forceps to a high head above the pelvic rim is dangerous and should not be attempted. Usually, however, when the uterus is made to contract, and possibly with some manual pressure on the head from above, the head will come into the pelvis and forceps can be applied.

Ventouse or Vacuum Extractor

This is preferably used to bring down the head should it remain high, however, rather than apply forceps or do an internal podalic version followed by breech extraction. The ventouse is, however, best avoided in small immature babies. The vacuum cap has to raise a chinon and in the immature baby might cause more tissue damage than is acceptable. The largest cap that will slip through the cervix is held flat against the fetal head as the vacuum is built up. Just enough vacuum is applied ($0.2kg/cm^2$) to hold the cap on the head. It is very important to check around the perimeter to ensure that maternal soft tissues have not been sucked into the rim of the cap. The vacuum should then be increased at one minute intervals to 0.4, 0.6, and then 0.8 kg/cm^2. At each increase of vacuum the operator should again check that no maternal soft tissue is sucked into the rim of the cap. When the maximum vacuum of 0.8 kg/cm^2 has been achieved, the head may be gently pulled at right angles to the line of the pelvis with uterine contractions. The operator can best do this with one hand while pressing the cap onto the head at right angles in the line of traction with the fingers of the other.

Prolapse of the Cord

Prolapsed cord from the second twin is not uncommon but, since the cervix is dilated, there is usually no real problem in delivering the second twin before the prolapsed cord causes asphyxia. If the lie has been corrected to longitudinal before the membranes are ruptured and, therefore, before the cord prolapses, either forceps delivery or breech extraction can be performed quite quickly. However, when the lie is being corrected from transverse occasionally the cord can become tangled around the baby. For example, the cord may be between the baby's legs and around the baby as it is being delivered as a breech. If it seems that there is tension on the cord, it can be clamped and cut before the baby is delivered.

Cesarean Section for the Second Twin

This is seldom required except in neglected cases. The first cesarean section performed in the United States was a self-inflicted operation performed in 1822. The patient was 14 yr of age and illegitimately pregnant with twins. The first twin was born vaginally, and the second was born when she opened her abdomen with a razor. Drs. Bassett and McClellan were called to close the abdominal wound and the patient survived. The fate of the twins, however, is not known (McClellan, 1822). Cesarean section for the second twin is indicated either if the cervix has closed down and there is fetal distress, but delivery cannot be achieved with the ventouse, or in cases of transverse lie where the shoulder has become impacted as described previously for the delivery of the first twin.

Delivery of the Placenta(s)

When there is one placenta, either monochorionic or fused dichorionic, it is delivered after the birth of both babies. This also usually occurs when there are two placentas, but occasionally the first placenta is delivered before the second twin, but without causing any problems. Rarely, there is heavy bleeding in such cases and the second twin must be delivered as expeditiously as possible so that the uterus can then be made to contract and control the bleeding. If oxytocics are given and controlled traction is employed, there is no greater risk of hemorrhage following a twin delivery than a singleton (Wood and Pinkerton, 1966).

FAILURE TO DIAGNOSE TWINS IN LABOR

There is danger to the second twin when there has been failure to diagnose twins in labor, even though an oxytocic has not been given at the delivery of the first. During labor fetal distress in one twin will be likely to go unnoticed and the baby may die in utero or be asphyxiated at birth. There may be undue delay in delivering the second baby after the birth of the first and again asphyxia may occur. As soon as the second twin is diagnosed the fetal heart and the lie should be checked and the membranes ruptured. If an oxytocic has been given with the delivery of the first twin, then there is grave risk to the second twin and considerable urgency in achieving delivery because the placental blood supply will be seriously impeded. The lie is checked and the membranes ruptured, and the babies delivered by forceps or ventouse if the lie is vertex, and by extraction if the breech is presenting.

When the baby is lying transversely and cannot be corrected by external version a general anesthetic will be required to cause relaxation of the uterus and allow either external or internal version followed by a breech extraction. This is usually preferable to performing a cephalic version and forceps or ventous delivery in these circumstances. If sufficient relaxation cannot quickly be achieved, a cesarean section may be performed, but usually by that time the baby will have died and time can be taken to achieve sufficient relaxation for version or a destructive operation. If the cervix has closed down but the baby is still alive, and it is impossible to deliver the baby with the ventouse if it is a vertex presentation, or to do a breech extraction through a partially dilated cervix if the breech is presenting, general anesthesia and cesarean section will be indicated. If the baby has died, time can be taken to allow the cervix to dilate when the effect of the oxytocin has begun to wear off.

LOCKED TWINS

Twin locking or entanglement during labor is extremely rare occurring in perhaps 1:1000 twin deliveries (Nissen, 1958). The m rtality, especially for the
leading twin, is very high due to the complicated manoeuvers required for its
delivery. In Khunda's (1972) series of 74 babies, 21 died at delivery, giving a
fetal mortality of 31%. Twin locking or entanglement causes dystocia when
the delivery of one twin is obstructed by some part or parts of the other twin.
The classic type of twin locking (Fig. 1) is the chin-to-chin locking of two
heads when the first presentation is by the breech and the second by the
vertex. Other types are two heads (Fig. 2) or two breeches trying to enter
the pelvis simultaneously or the after-coming head in a breech being caught
by the trunk of the second twin in a transverse position. Nissen (1958)
described four forms of twin entanglement.

1. Collision: engagement of one twin prevented by the other
2. Impaction: partial engagement of both twins simultaneously
3. Compaction: simultaneous full engagement of the two twins
4. Interlocking: chin-to-chin locking

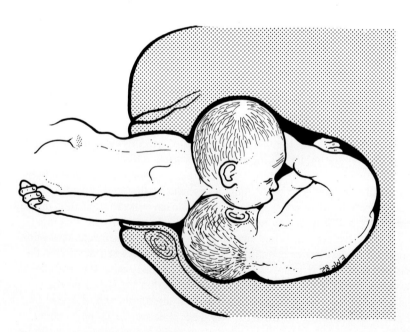

Figure 1. Chin-to-chin locking.

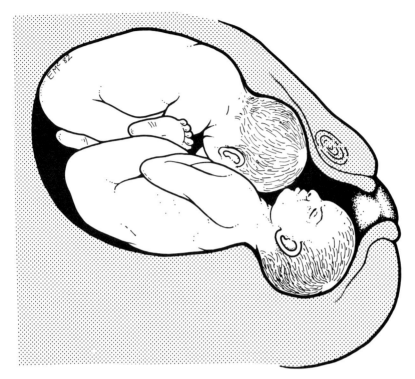

Figure 2. Collision of two heads causing a form of locked twins.

The diagnosis of interlocking cannot be made before labor, but if there is a prolonged labor, or if part of the first baby has been born but delivery cannot be completed, then the condition should be suspected. This would be the case when the first is delivered as breech, but the head cannot be delivered. If two fetal poles are palpable, either partially or fully in the pelvis, the condition can easily be suspected and cesarean section performed. If labor is not progressing satisfactorily and an x-ray is taken it may reveal the condition. In the classic type of locking, however, the diagnosis is not usually made until part of the first baby is born and strenuous efforts have already been made to deliver by traction. General anesthesia is usually required to determine the degree of locking and to decide whether it is possible to disengage the head, but disengagement will be difficult because the liquor will usually have drained away.

In the classic type of chin-to-chin twin locking a technique was described by Kimball and Rand (1950) to effect delivery. Forceps are applied to the head of the second twin and traction and hyperextension are applied to the first twin. The head of the second twin is delivered by flexion. If the first twin is dead then decapitation is carried out and the second twin is born as expeditiously as possible. Cesarean section is unfortunately not of value when there is chin-to-chin interlocking and the first baby is partially born, although it might be possible in some cases to deliver both twins through the classic incision. The Kimball and Rand procedure is dangerous for both the mother and the baby and is only likely to succeed when the babies are small. There is too much risk of damage to the maternal tissue in attempting this manoeuver in normal or large-sized babies. When the babies are small, simultaneous delivery of both twins can be achieved.

CONJOINED TWINS

When obstruction occurs in a twin pregnancy in the presence of active labor, then the possibility of conjoined twins, fetal interlocking, or fetal abnormality must be suspected and, if possible, delivery by cesarean section performed. If

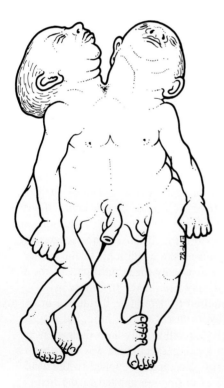

Figure 3. Thoracopagus.

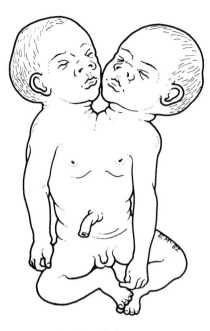

Figure 4. Dicephalus.

this is not done, a difficult destructive operation may be necessary to deliver the twins. This may involve risks to the mother as described in the section on obstructed labor. Conjoined twins occur rarely and were reported only once in 546 twin deliveries by Tan et al. (1971) in their series of seven cases. The imperfect division of the embryo after formation of the two embryonic areas can result in various forms of conjoined twins. These are commonly either joined at the head, craniopagus, or chest thoracopagus, but they may be joined at other parts of the body (Figs. 3-5). The survival of the twins will depend not only on the site and degree of union and sharing of vital organs, but also on the stage at which the diagnosis was made and how delivery was effected. The diagnosis has rarely been made in the past until labor had commenced and was obviously being obstructed. However, with the much greater use of ultrasonic scanning the condition should be suspected more readily because of the position occupied by the twins. Joining of the twins can be suspected if they are facing one another and the fetal heads are at the same plane or if the babies tend to move in unison. Radiological examination can also be helpful. If the diagnosis is made prenatally then the delivery should be by cesarean section. There are now several cases on record of successful surgical separation of conjoined twins, even when the union has been quite extensive.

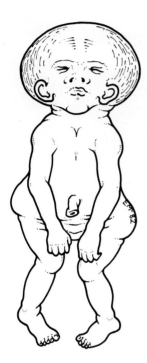

Figure 5. Syncephalus.

DELIVERY OF TRIPLETS AND HIGHER MULTIPLES

Abnormal presentation is very likely to occur in at least one of higher multiples. Intrauterine growth retardation is also more marked the more babies there are. The risks increase to subsequent babies, just as in twin pregnancy the second baby is at greater risk than the first. With triplets, however, provided the presentations are not abnormal, vaginal delivery can be attempted provided also that there are no other contraindications such as length of gestation, obstetric complications, and parity and age of the mother. In quadruplets or more the usual practice nowadays is to deliver by cesarean section unless labor commences at a very early gestation. The delivery of the Dionne quintuplets, who all survived and were delivered spontaneously, was quite remarkable (DaFoe, 1934).

The problem is to know when to perform cesarean section in higher multiple pregnancies because of the likelihood of intrauterine growth retardation. This problem is usually resolved by labor commencing, but the decision has to be made somewhat empirically as it is rarely possible to determine the function of the placenta or placentas in these cases and to assess the condition of the babies. Probably the optimum time would be at 37-38 weeks if the pregnancy progresses as long as this and there are no other complications.

REFERENCES

Adeleye, J. A. (1972). Retained second twin in Ibadan: Its fate and management. *Am. J. Obstet. Gynecol. 114*:204-207.

Bender, S. (1952). Twin pregnancy. A review of 472 cases. *J. Obstet. Gynaecol. Br. Emp. 59*:510-517.

Birch, H., Richardson, S., Baird, D., Horobin, G., and Illsley, R. (1970). *Mental Subnormality in a Community.* Wiliams & Wilkins, Baltimore.

British Perinatal Mortality Survey. (1969). *Perinatal Problems—Second Report of the British Perinatal Mortality Survey.* E. & S. Livingstone Ltd., Edinburgh, London.

Calvert, J. P. (1980). Intrinsic hazard of breech presentation. *Br. Med. J. 281*:1319-1320.

Crichton, D. (1973). A simple technique of extraperitoneal lower segment Caesarean section. *S. Afr. Med. J. 47*:2011-2012.

Da Foe, A. R. (1934). The Dionne quintuplets. *JAMA 103*:673-677.

Dunn, P. M. (1965). Some perinatal observations on twins. *Dev. Med. Child Neurol. 7*:121-134.

Fehrmann, H. (1980). Misdiagnosis of fetal heartrate during a twin labour. *Br. J. Obstet. Gynaecol. 87*1174-1177.

Griffiths, M. (1967). Cerebral palsy in multiple pregnancy. *Dev. Med. Child Neurol. 9*:173.

Guttmacher, A. F., and Kohl, S. G., (1958). The fetus of multiple gestations. *Obstet. Gynecol. 12*:528-541.

Khunda, S. (1972). Locked twins. *Obstet. Gynecol. 39*:453-459.

Kimball, A. P., and Rand, P. R. (1950). A maneuver for the simultaneous delivery of chin-to-chin locked twins. *Am. J. Obstet. Gynecol. 59*:1167.

Law, R. C. (1967). *Standards of Obstetric Care: The Report of the North West Metropolitan Regional Obstetric Survey.* E. & S. Livingstone, Edinburgh.

Little, W. A., and Friedman, E. A. (1958). The twin delivery—factors influencing second twin survival. *Obstet. Gynecol. Surv. 13*:611-623.

MacDonald, R. R., (1962). Management of second twin. *Br. M. J., 1*:518-522.

MacGillivray, I., and Campbell, D. M. (1980). The outcome of twin pregnancies in Aberdeen. *Acta Gemellol.*

MacGillivray, I., Nylander, P. P. S., and Corney, G. (1975). Human Multiple Reproduction. Saunders, London.

McClellan (1822). Quoted by Harley, J. M. G. In *Caesarean Obstetrics,* Vol. 7. MacGillivray, (Ed.). Saunders, London, pp. 529-559.

Munnell, E. W., and Taylor, H. C. (1946). Complications and fetal mortality in 136 cases of multiple pregnancy. *Am. J. Obstet. Gynecol.* *52*:588-597.

Nissen, E. D. (1958). Twins: Collision, impaction, compaction and interlocking. *Obstet. Gynaecol.* *11*:154.

Philpott, R. H. (1980). Obstructed labour. In *Clinics in Obstetrics and Gynaecology.* Vol. 7, *Operative Obstetrics.* I. MacGillivray (Ed.), W. B. Saunders, London, pp. 601-620.

Portes, L., and Granjon, A. (1946). Les présentations au cours des accouchements gemellaires. *Gynecol. Obstet.* *45*:1459.

Potter, E. L. (1963). Twin zygosity and placental form in relation to the outcome of the pregnancy. *Am. J. Obstet. Gynecol.* *42*:870-878.

Powell-Phillips, W. D., Wittmann, and Davison, B. M. (1979). *Br. J. Obstet. Gynaecol.* *86*:666-667.

Ross, R. C., and Philpott, N. W. (1953). Five year survey of multiple pregnancies. *Canad. Med. Assoc. J.* *69*:247-249.

Sherman, G. H., and Lowe, E. W. (1970). Do twins carry a high risk for mother and baby? *JAMA* *62*:217-220.

Sinha, D. P., Nandakumar, V. C., Brough, A. K., and Beebeejaun, M. S. (1979). Relative cervical incompetence in twin pregnancy. *Acta Genet. Med. Gemellol. (Roma)* *28*:327-331.

Tan, K. L., Goon, S. M., Salmon, Y., and Wee, J. H. (1971). Conjoined twins. *Acta Obstet. Gynecol. Scand.* *50*:373-380.

Ware, H. D. (1971). The second twin. *Am. J. Obstet. Gynecol.* *110*:855-873.

Wood, C., and Pinkerton, J. H. M. (1966). Uterine activity following the birth of the first twin. *Aust. N.Z. J. Obstet. Gynaecol.* *6*:95-99.

7
Intrauterine Growth Retardation: Diagnosis and Management

RUDY E. SABBAGHA / Northwestern University Medical School and Northwestern University and Memorial Hospital, Chicago, Illinois

One of the end results of pregnancies complicated by intrauterine growth retardation (IUGR) is the delivery of low-birth-weight (LBW) infants. However, LBW infants may also represent prematurely delivered fetuses whose growth may be appropriate for gestational age. Approximately 40% of all low-birth-weight infants are growth retarded (Bardy, 1970) or small-for-gestational age (SGA) and may be the product of preterm, term, and postterm deliveries. This chapter deals with growth-retarded fetuses, their recognition, medical complications, and obstetric management.

DEFINITION OF IUGR

Some investigators attempt to differentiate fetuses with IUGR from those who are SGA on the basis of causal factors. In this mode of distinction IUGR is thought to result from interference with the nutritional vascular supply to the fetus, and undergrowth in SGA fetuses is attributed to genetic or infectious factors.

It is preferable to define growth retardation according to two parameters that relate to perinatal outcome. The first is a statistical definition including infants whose birth weight is below the 10th percentile for gestational age or 2750 g at 40 weeks' gestation (Brenner et al., 1976). The other is a clinical definition related to fetal malnutrition (FM) which results in a decrease of the subcutaneous tissue and the muscle mass (wasting) of affected neonates

151

(Scott and Usher, 1966). Whereas most of the malnourished neonates are light, (weighing less than the 10th percentile in relation to their maturity), some clearly fall in the normal weight range for gestational age. Nonetheless, regardless of birth weight, FM is associated with an increased incidence of intrauterine fetal death and perinatal asphyxia (Scott and Usher, 1966).

Although these statistical and clinical definitions are very useful for antenatal recognition and monitoring of undergrown fetuses, they are, in fact, simplistic when viewed in relation to:

1. Fetal organ growth at the cellular level
2. Actual versus potential birth weight
3. Actual versus potential cephalic growth

Fetal Growth at the Cellular Level

Investigators (Enesco and Leblong, 1962; Fukuda and Sibatani, 1953; Winick et al., 1967) have shown that fetal organ growth at the cellular level takes place first by cell division or hyperplasia. Subsequently, and in conjunction with hyperplasia, increase in cell size or hypertrophy occurs. Finally, cell division ceases and organ growth continues by cell hypertrophy.

The number of cells constituting any organ is determined by the ratio of the total DNA content to that of the DNA quantity per cell, the latter being constant in diploid cells (Boivin et al., 1948). By contrast, cell size is determined by the ratio between the RNA and DNA content of a particular organ.

A reduction in the total DNA of an organ (i.e., its cell number) implies an arrest in hyperplasia. Because hyperplasia only occurs early in the course of development the diminution in the size of the affected organ can be considered irreversible. By contrast, when an adverse event such as intrauterine malnutrition occurs later in the course of organ development (i.e., during the phase of cell hypertrophy), the insult may be reversible if the nutritional deprivation is corrected.

The biochemical alterations in the DNA and RNA in organs just described, can be applied to human pregnancies. Winnick et al. (1967) have shown that in the human placenta cell division ceases by 34-36 weeks' gestation; after this interval growth occurs only by cell hypertrophy. Thus, examination of the DNA and RNA content of the placenta after birth indicates whether the adverse intrauterine stimulus occurred before or after 34 weeks' gestation. This information is of value in the assessment of the severity and prognosis of IUGR. Naeye (1967) reported a subnormal number of placental cells in infants with both IUGR and chromosomal abnormalities. These data suggest that the condition was related to the inherent genetic composition of the affected neonates and was early in onset and probably irreversible.

Actual Versus Potential Birth Weight

Turner (1971) compared the birth weight of a group of neonates with that of their siblings who were affected by congenital rubella. He showed that 80% of the affected group would be considered growth retarded in comparison with their potential birth weight, exemplified by that of their normal siblings. By contrast, only 46% of the same affected infants fell below the normal birth weight in relation to the population as a whole. Thus, although in a particular neonate birth weight may appear to be normal, the maximum potential of fetal growth may not have been achieved because of varying degrees of IUGR.

Actual Versus Potential Cephalic Fetal Growth

Investigators (Sabbagha et al., 1975; and Sabbagha et al., 1976a) have shown that in at least 90% of normal monkey and human fetuses the biparietal diameter (BPD) measured ultrasonically from midpregancy to term continues to fall· within one of three growth groups: (1) a large fetal bracket with BPDs above the 75th percentile; (2) an average fetal bracket with BPDs ranging between the 25th and 75th percentiles; and (3) a small fetal bracket with BPD less than the 25th percentile. This growth phenomenon is significant because it indicates that fetal cephalic growth can now be assessed in relation to the fetus' own growth potential rather than to a mean value derived from a heterogeneous population of fetuses. For example, a fetus whose BPD falls at the 30th percentile for 36 weeks' gestation is considered normal if its cephalic size was also average in dimension during the second trimester of pregnancy. If, however, the growth potential of the same fetus was expected to be at the 80th percentile rank, its present growth (30th percentile) would be clearly suboptimal.

Table 1. Etiologic Factors in IUGR

Altered growth potential	Maternal factors
Genetic, chromosomal	Heart disease
Antigenic relationship	Chronic hypertension
Congenital anomalies	Pre-eclampsia
Chronic fetal infections (TORCH)	Diabetes mellitus with vascular
Irradiation	complications
Cytotoxic agents	Hyperthyroidism
High altitude	Hemoglobinopathies
Twinning	Cigarette smoking
	Deficient dietary intake

ETIOLOGY OF IUGR

The etiologic factors associated with IUGR are listed in Table 1. Wigglesworth
(1965) and Winick et al. (1967) have shown that interference with the nutritional vascular supply line is more likely to produce asymmetric growth retardation; in these infants fetal organs such as the liver, spleen, and adrenals are
more severely affected than the brain. Clinically, this relative brain sparing
is apt to be associated with third trimester complications such as pregnancy-
induced hypertension.

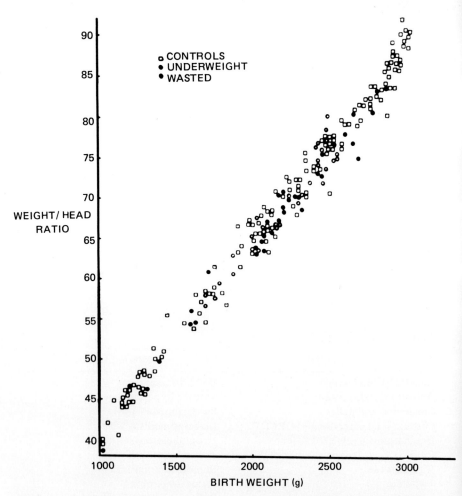

Figure 1. Weight-head ratio of 35 infants with fetal malnutrition who were underweight for gestational age and showed soft tissue wasting, 31 infants who were
underweight but not markedly wasted, and 144 control infants of normal brith
weight for gestational age, plotted against birth weight. (From Usher et al., 1966.)

However, recently Crane and Kopta (1980) challenged these reports by showing that cephalic size was reduced in the majority of SGA fetuses, regardless of the etiology of IUGR.

Sabbagha (1978) showed that in at least 50% of undergrown fetuses, the BPD is small and growth retardation is symmetrical or near symmetrical. Similarly, Usher et al. (1966) have shown that the head and chest circumferences of neonates affected by IUGR are reduced in comparison with those of normal infants of the same gestational age and are similar to those of prematures of the same birth weight (Fig. 1).

OUTCOME OF IUGR

In estimating the relative perinatal risk of all neonates, Yerushalmy (1970) reported an eight-fold increase in perinatal mortality of SGA fetuses. Usher (1970) showed that perinatal mortality is related to the extent to which birth weight is reduced (Table 2). The long-term central nervous system (CNS)

Table 2. Perinatal Mortality in Relation to Severity of Growth Retardation

Underweight for gestational age (%)	Perinatal mortality rate (%)
Less than 15	1.4
20-24	4.3
40 or more	5.4

Table 3. Perinatal and Long-Term Complications Associated with IUGR

Intrauterine fetal death
Asphyxia
Meconium aspiration pneumonitis
Pulmonary hemorrhage
Hypoglycemia
Hypocalcemia
Polycythemia
Hypo- or hypernatremia
Complications of in utero infections
Complications of congenital anomalies
Small stature
Deficient intelligence
Minimal cerebral dysfunction
Speech defects
Learning disabilities

deficits of undergrown infants have been addressed by Fitzharding and Steven (1972b) and are listed in Table 3. The short- and long-term complications associated with SGA infants make it imperative to diagnose the condition in utero.

DIAGNOSIS OF IUGR

With the advent of fetal echography the accuracy of assessment of fetal age, weight, and growth has been enhanced; since all these parameters form the cornerstone of antenatal diagnosis of IUGR, they will be considered separately.

Gestational Age

Gestational age can be estimated ultrasonically in five ways. The first is by measurement of the fetal crown-rump length (CRL) between the 8th and 13th week of pregnancy. Robinson and Fleming (1975) have shown a close correlation between sonar CRL and gestational age. Specifically, they showed that fetal age estimates in the first trimester of pregnancy vary by ±4.7 to ±2 days in 94% of gravidas, depending on whether one or three CRL measurements are obtained respectively. The length of pregnancy in weeks corresponding to mean CRL values is shown in Table 4.

Single sonar BPD measurements between 14 and 26 weeks' gestation may also be used. Campbell (1970) was the first to outline the growth of the fetal sonar biparietal diameter (BPD) relative to weekly intervals of gestation. Subsequently, he showed that 84% of women with uncertain dates, in whom BPD measurements were obtained prior to 30 weeks, delivered within ±9 days of the sonar expected date of delivery (EDD). The results of Campbell's study indicate indirectly that fetal BPD is a reliable predictor of both gestational age and onset of delivery (±9 days). Further, Campbell's observations are consistent with the biologic end-point of pregnancy reported by Yerushalmy (1970) namely: ±2 weeks of the menstrual EDD.

Sabbagha et al. (1976b) showed that the 5th and 95th percentiles of fetal age corresponding to a sonar BPD estimate of 16 weeks' gestation varied by ±7 days; however, in the interval between 17 and 26 weeks' gestation the predictive accuracy of the length of pregnancy by sonar BPD varied by ±11 days (±2SD). This range in fetal age is related to the fact that a single second-trimester BPD measurement groups fetuses into the mean gestational age category regardless of biologic differences in cephalic size. An an illustration (Fig. 2), a fetus with a BPD of 5.0 cm may represent: (1) a 21-week fetus with average cephalic size; (2) a younger fetus (19-3/7 weeks) with a large cephalic size, or (3) an older fetus (22-4/7 weeks) with a small cephalic size. Yet fetal age in all these fetuses is reported as the mean of 21 weeks.

Table 4. Length of Pregnancy and Mean Crown-Rump Length[a]

Menstrual maturity (weeks + days)	Corrected "regressional analysis" (cm) mean values	Menstrual maturity (weeks + days)	Corrected "regressional analysis" (cm) mean values
6 + 2	0.55	10 + 2	3.32
6 + 3	0.61	10 + 3	3.46
6 + 4	0.68	10 + 4	3.60
6 + 5	0.75	10 + 5	3.74
6 + 6	0.81	10 + 6	3.89
7 + 0	0.89	10 + 0	4.04
7 + 1	0.96	11 + 1	4.19
7 + 2	1.04	11 + 2	4.35
7 + 3	1.12	11 + 3	4.51
7 + 4	1.20	11 + 4	4.67
7 + 5	1.29	11 + 5	4.83
7 + 6	1.38	11 + 6	5.00
8 + 0	1.47	12 + 0	5.17
8 + 1	1.57	12 + 1	5.34
8 + 2	1.66	12 + 2	5.52
8 + 3	1.76	12 + 3	5.70
8 + 4	1.87	12 + 4	5.88
8 + 5	1.97	12 + 5	6.06
8 + 6	2.08	12 + 6	6.25
9 + 0	2.19	13 + 0	6.43
9 + 1	2.31	13 + 1	6.63
9 + 2	2.42	13 + 2	6.82
9 + 3	2.54	13 + 3	7.02
9 + 4	2.67	13 + 4	7.22
9 + 5	2.79	13 + 5	7.42
9 + 6	2.92	13 + 6	7.63
10 + 0	3.05	14 + 0	7.83
10 + 1	3.18		

[a] 2 SD limits are ±4.7 days.

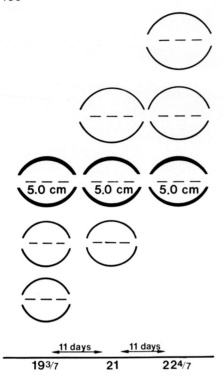

Figure 2. A biologic variation in the length of the BPD is observed at each gestational week. Note: in relation to the mean gestational age, the fetus with the large BPD is less mature and the fetus with the small BPD is more mature. (From Tamura and Sabbagha, 1980.)

By utilizing serial cephalometry, however, the margin of error, (±11 days) can be substantially reduced. This leads to the third method of defining gestational age, the growth adjusted sonar age (GASA).

For this method, two BPD measurements are obtained; the first in the interval of 20-26 weeks of pregnancy and the second between 31 and 33 weeks' gestation. As described in this chapter, Sabbagha et al. (1976b) have shown that 90% of normal fetuses are able to maintain cephalic growth within the confines of a large, average, or small percentile brackets. The majority of the remaining fetuses show a deviation of BPD growth only between two percentile brackets. As a result, if the specific cephalic growth bracket of any fetus is defined, its gestational age can then be adjusted in relation to its BPD growth; thus the term growth adjusted sonographic age (Sabbagha et al., 1977). By using GASA, the variation in assessment of fetal

Table 5. Aphalic Growth Used to Predict Mean Gestational Age

	First sonar[a] (BPD vs fetal age percentile)		Second sonar[b] (BPD percentile range)			
BPD	Range: large fetus vs. small fetus (wk)	Average fetus (age accepted temporarily)	Fetal age (wk)	Average fetus (>25 to <75)	Large fetus (≥75 to 95)	Small fetus (5 to 25)
3.5	± 1	16	29	7.4-7.7	7.8-8.3	6.8-7.3
3.6	± 1.6	16+	29+	7.5-7.8	7.9-8.4	6.9-7.4
3.7	± 1.6	17−	30−	7.6-7.8	7.9-8.5	7.0-7.5
3.8	± 1.6	17	30	7.7-7.9	8.0-8.6	7.1-7.6
3.9	± 1.6	17+	30+	7.8-8.0	8.1-8.7	7.2-7.7
4.0	± 1.6	18−	31−	7.8-8.1	8.2-8.7	7.2-7.7
4.1	± 1.6	18	31	7.9-8.1	8.2-8.8	7.3-7.8
4.2	± 1.6	18+	31+	8.0-8.2	8.3-8.9	7.4-7.9
4.3	± 1.6	19−	32−	8.1-8.2	8.3-8.9	7.4-7.9
4.4	± 1.6	19	32	8.1-8.3	8.4-9.0	7.5-8.0
4.5	± 1.6	19+	32+	8.2-8.4	8.5-9.0	7.6-8.1
4.6	± 1.6	20−	33−	8.3-8.4	8.5-9.1	7.6-8.2
4.7	± 1.6	20	33	8.4-8.5	8.6-9.1	7.6-8.3
4.8	± 1.6	20+	33+	8.5-8.6	8.7-9.2	7.8-8.4
4.9	± 1.6	21−	34−	8.5-8.7	8.8-9.2	7.8-8.4
5.0	± 1.6	21	34	8.6-8.8	8.9-9.3	7.9-8.5
5.1	± 1.6	21+	34+	8.7-8.9	9.0-9.4	8.0-8.6
5.2	± 1.6	22−	35−	8.7-8.9	9.0-9.5	8.1-8.6
5.3	± 1.6	22−	35	8.8-9.0	9.1-9.6	8.2-8.7
5.4	± 1.6	22	35+	8.9-9.0	9.2-9.6	8.2-8.8
5.5	± 1.6	22+	36−	8.9-9.1	9.3-9.6	8.2-8.8
5.6	± 1.6	23−	36	9.0-9.2	9.3-9.7	8.2-8.8
5.7	± 1.6	23	37	9.1-9.3	9.4-9.8	8.4-8.9
5.8	± 1.6	23+	38	9.2-9.4	9.5-9.9	8.5-9.1
5.9	± 1.6	24−	39	9.3-9.5	9.6-10.0	8.7-9.2
6.0	± 1.6	24	40	9.5-9.6	9.7-10.1	8.9-9.4
6.1	± 1.6	24+				
6.2	± 1.6	25−				
6.3	± 1.6	25				
6.4	± 1.6	25+				
6.5	± 1.6	26−				
6.6	± 2	26				
7.5	± 3	29−				
8.5	± 3	33				
9.5	± 3	37+				

BPD = biparietal diameter, measured from outer to inner aspects of fetal head; + = + 1-3 days; − = 1-3 days.

[a]First sonar is done prior to 26 weeks because of small variation in fetal age of ±11 days.

[b]Second sonar must be done between 30 and 33 weeks because of maximal variation in fetal BPD size in this interval and prior to onset of IUGR in most cases; must be done at least 6 weeks after first BPD.

Table 6. Method of Assigning Growth Adjusted Sonar Age (GASA) to Fetuses

First sonar 18-26 weeks[a]			Second sonar 30-33 weeks[b]						
Date[c]	BPD (cm)	Average fetal age accepted temporarily (Table 5)[d] (wk)	Date[c]	Interval between scans (wk)	Age of average fetus (wk)	BPD expected for fetus of average size (Table 5)	BPD obtained	GASA	BPD percentile for GASA
8-12	4.2	18+	11-11	13	31+	8.0-8.2	8.2 (Same as expected)	31+ no change	25th-75th
1-10	5.8	23+	3-10	9−	32−	8.1-8.2	8.5 (Larger than expected)	31− 1 week younger	75th-95th
2-15	5.1	21+	5-10	12	33+	8.5-8.6	9.1 (Much larger than expected)	32 approximately 10 days younger	>95th
1-10	6.0	24	5-30	7+	31+	8.0-8.2	7.5 (Much smaller than expected)	33 fetus is very small	<5th

BPD = biparietal diameter. + = 1-3 days. − = 1-3 days.

[a]First sonar is done prior to 26 weeks because of small variation in fetal age of ±11 days.

[b]Second sonar must be done between 30 and 33 weeks because of maximal variation in fetal BPD size in this interval and prior to onset IUGR in most cases and must be done at least 6 weeks after first BPD.

[c]Gestation disc calculator is first rotated to show the date in relation to the 50th percentile fetal age accepted temporarily. If this fetal age is qualified by a plus or minus sign, the disc is rotated an average of 2 days to the left or right, respectively. The calculator will then show the date on which fetal age is approximately 30-33 weeks.

[d]In comparison to fetuses with average BPDs those with larger BPDs are 1 week younger while those with smaller BPDs are 1 week older. If the BPD is very large or very small, the fetus is up to 11 days younger or older than an average fetus.

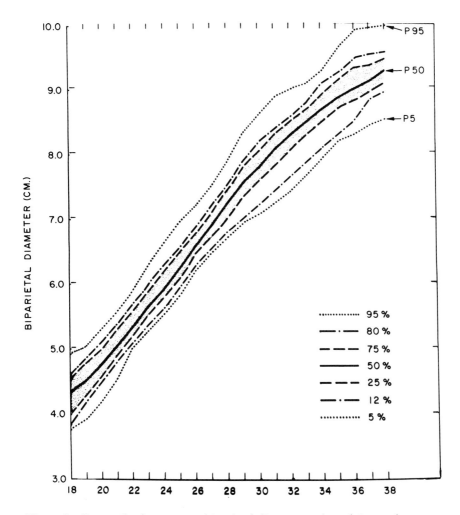

Figure 3. Percentile chart: sonar biparietal diameter at 1-week intervals.

age is reduced from ±11 days to: (1) ±3 days in fetuses (90%) who maintain their cephalic growth; and (2) ±5 days in fetuses (10%) who show a deviation in the BPD from one bracket to the next.

The precise cephalic growth bracket of any fetus is determined by two BPD measurements. The first is used to predict the mean gestational age (Table 5). The second BPD is obtained by approximately 31 weeks' gestation because of the maximal spread of large versus small BPDs observed during this interval (Fig. 3) and prior to any change in BPD size secondary to IUGR occurring in the third trimester of pregnancy. The specific fetal growth bracket (large, average or, small) is then determined by the second BPD measurement (Table 5). The actual procedure of assigning fetuses GASA is presented in Table 6.

The fourth method of defining dates is by measuring the femur length of the fetus from 14 to 23 weeks' gestation; the accuracy of this method is similar to that of the BPD.

If the estimate of fetal age based on a sonar CRL measurement or an early BPD or femur length falls within 1 week of menstrual dates, then the latter dates can be considered reliable. In this way the ultrasonic exam is used to confirm menstrual dates and is the fifth method of detemrining gestational age.

Composite BPD Chart

A variety of different charts relate BPD to gestational age. Sonographers must select a reliable BPD chart for the estim tion of the length of pregnancy.

Sabbagha and Hughey (1978) examined the variation in the mean BPD values at each week of gestation reported by four major studies and these were not statistically significant. Additionally Sabbagha et al. (1976b) showed that BPD growth in a large number of black and Caucasian pregnant women of similar socioeconomic status was markedly similar. Because of these observations a composite mean BPD chart (Table 7) was constructed. This has universal applicability and leads to overall uniformity and reliability in the definition of gestational age.

Fetal Weight

Campbell and Wilkin (1975) have shown that fetal weight predictions can be derived from the measurement of the fetal abdominal circumference (AC) at the level of the liver using the umbilical vein or the ductus venosus as an ultrasonic marker (Table 8). This is understandable since the AC includes the liver and the subcutaneous tissue layer in that area, both of which are sensitive indices of normal or altered fetal growth. In the presence of IUGR, the liver is small (Gruenwald, 1964) and the layer of subcutaneous tissue is thin (Scott and Usher, 1966). Similarly in the presence of macrosomia, the fetal AC falls in an upper percentile bracket, reflecting the large size of the liver and an increase in the width of the subcutaneous tissue (Ogata et al., 1980). According to Campbell and Wilkin (1975) the accuracy of fetal weight prediction by the AC is related to the actual size of the fetus (Table 9). Other investigators (Warsof et al., 1977) reported a wider variation in the estimate of fetal weight using both fetal BPD and AC: ±212 g/1000 g, or ±636 g in a 3000 g infant. From these studies it is apparent that the smaller the fetus the closer is the prediction of birth weight from the AC or from the BPD and the AC.

Estimates of fetal weight are particularly useful in pregnant women at high risk for delivery of LBW infants (in the weight range of 750 g to 1000 g) because such data enable the obstetrician to use sound clinical management

Table 7. Composite Mean of 7059 Fetal Sonographic Biparietal Diameters (BPD) from 14 to 40 Weeks' Gestation at Different Assumed Speeds of Sound in Tissue

Weeks	Speed of sound (m/sec)		
	1540[a]	1529[b]	1600[c]
14	2.8	2.8	2.9
15	3.2	3.2	3.3
16	3.6	3.6	3.7
17	3.9	3.9	4.1
18	4.2	4.2	4.4
19	4.5	4.5	4.7
20	4.8	4.8	5.0
21	5.1	5.1	5.3
22	5.4	5.4	5.6
23	5.8	5.8	6.0
24	6.1	6.1	6.3
25	6.4	6.4	6.6
26	6.7	6.7	7.0
27	7.0	6.9	7.3
28	7.2	7.1	7.5
29	7.5	7.4	7.8
30	7.8	7.7	8.1
31	8.0	7.9	8.3
32	8.2	8.1	8.5
33	8.5	8.4	8.8
34	8.7	8.6	9.0
35	8.8	8.7	9.1
36	9.0	8.9	9.4
37	9.2	9.1	9.6
38	9.3	9.2	9.7
39	9.4	9.3	9.8
40	9.5	9.4	9.9

[a]BPD given in centimeters from leading edge of the near-skull table to the leading edge of the far-skull table, i.e., from outer to inner aspects of fetal head (0-1 BPD).
[b]BPDs given in centimeters from outer to outer aspects of fetal head (0-0 BPD).

to prevent asphyxia. This is the first step in preparing for effective intensive neonatal care.

However, using the BPD and AC or the AC alone to predict a mean birth weight of, for example, 3000 g carries some hazards because the variation of the estimate is approximately 500 g and the fetus in question may be growth retarded, weighing only 2500 g. Because, in such pregnancies, the possibility of missing IUGR is real, it is far preferable to use the BPD, AC, and other

Table 8.   Relationship between Fetal Abdominal Circumference Measurements from 21 to 40 cm and Birth Weight Centiles

Abdominal circumference (cm)	Estimated birth weight centiles (g)		
	5	50	95
21	780	900	1040
22	900	1030	1190
23	1030	1180	1360
24	1170	1340	1540
25	1320	1510	1730
26	1470	1690	1940
27	1640	1880	2150
28	1810	2090	2380
29	1990	2280	2610
30	2170	2490	2850
31	2350	2690	3080
32	2530	2900	3320
33	2710	3100	3550
34	2880	3290	3760
35	3030	3470	3970
36	3180	3640	4160
37	3310	3790	4330
38	3420	3920	4490
39	3510	4020	4610
40	3570	4190	4720

Source: Campbell and Wilkin (1975).

Table 9.   Variation in Weight Predicted by Abdominal Circumference (AC) Measurements

Variation (g)	[a]Weight (g)
160	1000
290	2000
450	3000
590	4000

[a]Weight predicted by AC.
Source: Campbell and Wilkin (1975)

ultrasonic methods to delineate fetuses whose growth is altered and who are, thus, at high risk for IUGR.

Fetal Growth

Once gestational age is established, fetal growth can be assessed by ultrasonic evaluation of the head-to-abdomen (H/A) ratio, total intrauterine volume (TIUV), fetal cephalic size using the BPD, and fetal growth pattern using both BPD and AC.

H/A Ratio
The fetal head circumference can be measured from the same echogram displaying the plane from which the BPD is obtained. Similarly, the abdominal circumference can be measured from echograms obtained perpendicular to the longitudinal fetal lie in the area of the fetal liver where a small segment of the umbilical vein is apparent. These measurements are obtained by a variety of methods including:

1. An electronic caliper which can be displayed on the face of the cathode ray tube or television monitor and manually controlled. The oscillations of such calipers, however, may be too wide and lead to incorrectly large measurements.
2. A mapwalker carefully rolled along the outer margin of the echogram showing the plane of the cephalic or the abdominal circumference.
3. A digitizer arm moved along the outer perimeter of the head or abdominal circumference. Tamura and Sabbagha (1980) showed that the accuracy of this method is <2% of the AC measurements. They used the digitizer to construct the sonar AC percentile ranks from 18 to 41 weeks' gestation (Table 10).

Campbell and Thoms (1977) showed that a comparison of the circumferences of the fetal head and body or the H/A ratio should normally fall below unity in the latter part of pregnancy (Table 10). The same investigators subsequently showed that approximately 70% of asymetrically growth-retarded fetuses have a H/A ratio > 2SD above the mean (Table 11).

The H/A ratio may be of particular value in the recognition of asymmetrical IUGR in those women who develop complications in the third trimester of pregnancy and in whom dates and fetal size have not been established by an ultrasound examination in midpregnancy.

TIUV
Gohari et al. (1977) compared the pregnant uterus to an ellipse and measured the total intrauterine volume (TIUV) at different weeks of gestation.

Table 10. Head-Abdomen (H-A) Circumference Ratio
Versus Gestational Age (GA)

GA (weeks)	Mean H-A ratio	+ SD
28	1.13	1.21
32	1.075	1.17
34	1.04	1.13
36	1.02	1.12
38	0.99	1.06
40	0.97	1.05

Source: Campbell and Thoms (1977).

Table 11. Fetal Abdominal Circumference Measurements (cm)[a]

Weeks of gestation	Percentile								
	2.5	5	10	25	50	75	80	95	97.5
18	9.8	10.3	10.9	11.9	13.1	14.2	14.5	15.9	16.4
19	11.1	11.6	12.3	13.3	14.4	15.6	15.9	17.2	17.8
20	12.1	12.6	13.3	14.3	15.4	16.6	16.9	18.2	18.8
21	13.7	14.2	14.8	15.9	17.0	18.1	18.4	19.8	20.3
22	14.7	15.2	15.8	16.9	18.0	19.1	19.4	20.8	21.3
23	16.0	16.5	17.1	18.2	19.3	20.4	20.7	22.1	22.6
24	17.2	17.7	18.3	19.4	20.5	21.6	21.9	23.3	23.8
25	18.0	18.5	19.1	20.2	21.3	22.4	22.7	24.1	24.6
26	18.8	19.3	19.9	21.0	22.1	23.2	23.5	24.9	25.4
27	20.4	20.9	21.5	22.6	23.7	24.8	25.1	26.5	27.0
28	22.0	22.5	23.1	24.2	25.3	26.4	26.7	28.1	28.6
29	23.6	24.1	24.7	25.8	26.9	28.0	28.3	29.7	30.2
30	24.1	24.6	25.2	26.3	27.4	28.5	28.8	30.2	30.7
31	24.7	25.2	25.8	26.9	28.0	29.1	29.4	30.8	31.3
32	25.4	25.9	26.5	27.6	28.7	29.8	30.1	31.5	32.0
33	25.7	26.2	26.8	27.9	29.0	30.1	30.4	31.8	32.3
34	26.8	27.3	27.9	29.0	30.1	31.2	31.5	32.9	33.4
35	28.9	29.4	30.0	31.1	32.2	33.3	33.6	35.0	35.5
36	30.0	30.5	31.1	32.2	33.3	34.4	34.7	36.1	36.6
37	31.1	31.6	32.2	33.3	34.4	35.5	35.8	37.2	37.7
38	32.4	32.9	33.5	34.6	35.7	36.8	37.1	38.5	39.0
39	32.6	33.1	33.7	34.8	35.9	37.0	37.3	38.7	39.2
40	32.8	33.3	33.9	35.0	36.1	37.2	37.5	38.9	39.4
41	33.8	34.3	34.9	36.0	37.1	38.2	38.5	39.9	40.4

[a]Circumference measurements are obtained from the outer aspect of the fetal abdomen at the area of the liver that shows the ductus venosus or umbilical vein.

Source: Tamura and Sabbagha (1980).

Table 12. Total Intrauterine Volume (TIUV) at 1.5 SD[a] below
Mean in Relation to Gestational Age

Weeks' gestation	TIUV, 1.5 SD below mean
16	450
18	600
20	750
22	900
24	1100
26	1250
28	1500
30	1750
32	2000
34	2350
36	2550
38	2850
40	3000

[a]Figures rounded to approximate numbers. TIUV in 75% of growth-re-
tarted fetuses falls below 1.5 SD of mean value in relation to a specific
week of gestation.

Source: Gohari et al. (1977).

Specifically, TIUV was calculated by multiplying 0.5233 by the maximum
dimensions of the uterine length, width, and height obtained from appropriately taken echograms.

Low TIUVs are used to predict IUGR because, in a large proportion of pregnancies associated with undergrown fetuses, oligohydramnios is also present.
Estimates of TIUV, however, are indirect indices of fetal size and weight,
because the fetus is not examined directly. In fact, Warsof et al. (1977)
showed that determination of fetal weight by BPD and AC was not improved
by using TIUV. Nonetheless, if TIUV is < 1SD of the mean for gestation,
the chance of the fetus being growth retarded is about 50% (Hobbins, 1980)
(Table 12).

BPD
Sabbagha (1978) defined the specificity and sensitivity of cephalometry in
the detection of IUGR. He showed that when the fetal BPD in the third
trimester of pregnancy is normal (i.e., consistently falling in an upper or
average percentile bracket) the proportion of normal neonates (weight
>10th percentile) is quite high; 96.5 and 90%, respectively (Fig. 4). In
other words, fetal BPD is a highly specific test ruling out IUGR in the
majority of such fetuses. The small percentage of growth-retarded fetuses

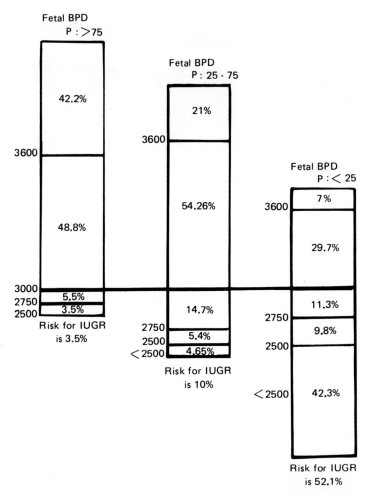

Figure 4. Percentage distribution of neonatal weights (g) according to fetal BPD growth patterns.

in whom the BPD is normal (Fig. 4) are characterized by being asymmetrically growth retarded with relative sparing of brain growth.

By contrast, when third-trimester BPDs are abnormal (i.e., <25th percentile), the proportion of growth-retarded fetuses (weight < 10th percentile) is approximately 50% (Fig. 4). Thus, the sensitivity of the fetal BPD, in the diagnosis of IUGR is 50%. Fetuses with a small BPD in whom birth weight is also < 10th percentile are characterized by being symmetrically or near symmetrically small. Finally, when the BPD drops from a particular percentile bracket to a

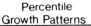

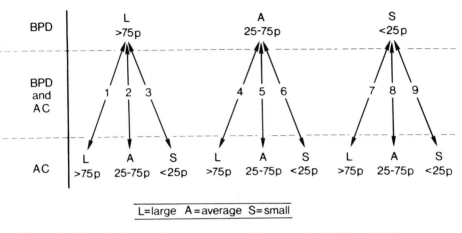

Figure 5. Nine fetal growth patterns noted by using both BPD and AC percentiles (p).

lower one, the incidence of IUGR is 20%. The specificity and sensitivity of cephalometry is improved by measurement of the fetal AC.

AC
By obtaining one or two fetal ACs during the latter part of the third trimester of pregnancy and interpreting the result in concert with the BPD, it is possible to place fetuses in one of nine growth patterns (Fig. 5). Growth patterns 3 and 6 characterize the fetus at high risk for asymmetrical IUGR. Growth pattern 9 characterizes the fetus at high risk for symmetrical or near symmetrical IUGR.

   Preliminary data indicate that with this approach, all IUGR fetuses will fall into one of these three growth patterns: 3, 6, or 9. However, in each category there will be some false positives, the frequency of which remains to be defined. Nonetheless, since the incidence of IUGR in high-risk pregnancies is small, it is cost-effective to monitor further fetuses in growth patterns 3, 6, and 9 by other methods as discussed below.

MANAGEMENT OF IUGR

Obstetricians who recognize that they are dealing with a fetus at high risk for IUGR are able to direct attention towards preventing prenatal death, intrapartum asphyxia, and possibly future CNS deficits. The plan of management should include:

1. Evaluation of the need for hospitalization, particularly in the presence of maternal medical complications
2. Examination of the feasibility of bed rest at home
3. A review of the nutritional status of the mother
4. Careful monitoring of fetal well-being based on the following parameters:
   a. Weekly or biweekly nonstress tests (NSTs)
   b. Contraction stress test (CST) if the NST is nonreactive
   c. Biochemical determination of maternal estriol values in selected cases
   d. Consultation iwth a high-risk obstetrical and neonatal center regarding perinatal management, including assessment of pulmonary maturity (Gluck, 1976)

The optimal time delivery of the growth-retarded fetus has not been scientifically determined. Tejani et al. (1976) and others believe that there is no need to delay delivery appreciably beyond 36 weeks' gestation, particularly if pulmonary maturity is attained. By contrast, Cetrulo and Freeman (1977) and others believe that delivery should not be effected unless there is evidence of abnormal bioelectric and biochemical tests. It appears that the management of each of these fetuses should be individualized depending on the duration of growth retardation, severity of maternal medical complications, cervical dilation and effacement, and the results of the battery of biophysical and biochemical tests.

REFERENCES

Bard, H. (1970). Intrauterine growth retardation. *Clin. Obstet. Gynecol. 13*:3, 511.

Boivin, A., Vendrely, R., and Vendrely, C. (1948). L'acide desoxyribo-nucleique du noyau cellulaire, depositaire des caractères hereditaires; arguments d'ordre analytique. *C. R. Acad. Sci. (Paris) 226*:1061.

Brenner, W., Edelman, D., and Hendricks, C. (1976). A standard of fetal growth for the United States of America. *Am. J. Obstet. Gynecol. 126*:555.

Campbell, S. (1970). Ultrasonic fetal cephalometry during the second trimester of pregnancy. *J. Obstet. Gynaecol. Br. Commonw. 17*:12.

Campbell, S. (1974). The assessment of fetal development by diagnostic ultrasound. *Clin. Perinatol. 1*:507.

Campbell, S., and Thoms, A. (1977). Ultrasound measurement of fetal head to abdomen ratio in the assessment of growth retardation. *Br. J. Obstet. Gynaecol. 84*:165.

Campbell, S., and Wilkin, D. (1975). Ultrasonic measurement of fetal abdomen circumference in the estimation of fetal weight. *Br. J. Obstet. Gynaecol. 82*:689.

Cetrulo, C., and Freeman, R. (1977). Bioelectric evaluation in intrauterine growth retardation. *Clin. Obstet. Gynecol.* 20:4, 979.

Crane, J. P., and Kopta, M. (1980). Comparative newborn anthropometric data in symmetric versus asymmetric intrauterine growth retardation. *Am. J. Obstet. Gynecol. 138*:518.

Enesco, M., and Leblong, C. P. (1962). Increase in cell number as a factor in the growth of the organs of the young male rat. *J. Embryol. Exp. Morpho. 10*:530.

Fitzhardinge, P. M., and Steven, E. M. (1972a). The small-for-date infant: I. Later growth patterns. *Pediatrics 49*:671.

Fitzhardinge, P. M., and Steven, E. M. (1972b). The small-for-date infant: II. Neurological and intellectual sequelae. *Pediatrics 50*:50.

Fukuda, M., and Sibatani, A. (1953). Biochemical studies on number and composition of liver cells in postnatal growth of the rat. *J. Biochem. (Tokyo) 40*:95.

Gluck, L. (1976). Fetal maturity and amniotic fluid surfactant determinations. In *Management of the High-Risk Pregnancy*. W. N. Spellacy (Ed.), University Park Press, Baltimore, 1976.

Gohari, P., Berkowitz, R. L., and Hobbins, J. C. (1977). Prediction of intrauterine growth retardation by determination of total intrauterine volume. *Am. J. Obstet. Gynecol. 127*:255.

Gruenwald, P. (1964). Infants of low birth weight among 5,000 deliveries. *Pediatrics 34*:157.

Hobbins, J. C. (1980). Use of ultrasound in complicated pregnancies. *Clin. Perinatol. 7*:2, 397-411.

Naeye, R. L. (1967). Prenatal organ and cellular growth with various chromosomal disorders. *Biol. Neonate 11*:248.

Ogata, E. S., Sabbagha, R. E., Metzger, B. D., Phelps, R. L., Depp, O. R., and Freinkel, N. (1980). Ultrasonography to assess evolving macrosomia in pregnant diabetics. *JAMA 243*:2405.

Robinson, H. P., and Fleming, J. E. E. (1975). A critical evaluation of sonar crown-rump length measurements. *Br. J. Obstet. Gynaecol. 82*:702.

Sabbagha, R. E. (1978). Intrauterine growth retardation: Antenatal diagnosis by ultrasound. *Obstet. Gynecol. 52*:252.

Sabbagha, R. E., Barton, F. B., and Barton, B. A. (1976a). Sonar BPD I: Analysis of percentile growth differences in two normal populations using same methodology. *Am. J. Obstet. Gynecol. 126*:479-484.

Sabbagha, R. E., Barton, B. A., Barton, F. B., Kingas, E., Orgill, J., and Turner, J. H. (1976b). Sonar biparietal diameter II. Predictive of three fetal growth patterns leading to a closer assessment of gestational age and neonatal weight. *Am. J. Obstet. Gynecol. 126*:485.

Sabbagha, R. E., Hughey, M., and Depp, R. (1977). Growth adjusted sonographic age: A simplified method. *Obstet. Gynecol. 51*:3, 386.

Sabbagha, R. E., Turner, J. H., and Chez, R. A. (1975). Sonar biparietal
diameter standards in the rhesus monkey. *Am. J. Obstet. Gynecol. 121*:371.

Scott, K. E., and Usher, R. H. (1966). Fetal malnutrition: Its incidence, causes
and effects. *Am. J. Obstet. Gynecol. 94*:951.

Tamura, R. K., and Sabbagha, R. E. (1980). Percentile ranks of sonar fetal
abdominal circumference measurements. *Am. J. Obstet. Gynecol. 138*:5,
475-479.

Tejani, N., Mann, L. I., and Weiss, R. R. (1976). Antenatal diagnosis and management of the small-for-gestational-age fetus. *Obstet. Gynecol. 47*:31.

Turner, G. (1971). Recognition of intrauterine growth retardation by considering comparative birth weights. *Lancet 2*:1123.

Usher, R. H., McClean, F., and Scott, K. E. (1966). Judgement of fetal age.
II. Clinical significance of gestational age and an objective method for its
assessment. *Pediatr. Clin. North Am.*

Usher, R. H. (1970). Clinical and therapeutic aspect of fetal malnutrition.
Pediatr. Clin. North Am. 17:169.

Warsof, S., Gohari, P., Berkowits, R., and Hobbins, J. (1977). The estimation
of fetal weight by computer-assisted analysis. *Am. J. Obstet. Gynecol.
128*:881.

Wigglesworth, J. S. (1964). Experimental growth retardation in the foetal rat.
J. Pathol. Bacteriol. 88:1.

Winick, M., Coscia, A., and Noble, A. (1967). Cellular growth in human
placenta. I. Normal placental growth. *Pediatrics 39*:248.

Yerushalmy, J. (1970). Relation of birth weight, gestational age, and the rate
of intrauterine growth to perinatal mortality. *Clin. Obstet. Gynecol. 13*:
307.

8
Nonstress Testing

MAURICE L. DRUZIN / New York Hospital-Cornell Medical Center, New York, New York

RICHARD H. PAUL / Los Angeles County/University of Southern California School of Medicine, Los Angeles, California

HISTORICAL PERSPECTIVE

The 1970s will be remembered as the period in which a conscious assessment of fetal well-being within the concept of the high-risk pregnancy became a new challenging part of the practice of obstetrics.

The term "high-risk pregnancy" had previously applied to maternal conditions known to be associated with an increased incidence of perinatal complications. Today, the term applies equally to pregnancy in which the fetus may exhibit compromise in the absence of maternal complications. The integration of the recognition of both maternal and fetal factors has given rise to the subspeciality referred to as "perinatology" or maternal-fetal medicine.

The acknowledgement of the fetus as a complex, dynamic, independent, and yet dependent entity has been made possible by technological advances making it practical to examine fetal condition without imposing unacceptable maternal or fetal risks.

Electronic monitoring of the fetal heart rate (FHR) is one of the most (if not the most) widely used methods of assessing fetal condition in Europe and the United States, as well as in other parts of the world.

Intrapartum monitoring of the fetus may be accomplished by noninvasive external methods of determining FHR and uterine activity. In labor, invasive methods, requiring amniotomy and insertion of devices measuring FHR and intrauterine pressure, are often necessary to obtain optimal recordings for interpretation.

In the antepartum period, use of electronic heart rate monitoring is restricted to the noninvasive methods.

Hon and Wohlgemuth (1961) proposed the concept of fetal "stress testing" when he evaluated the effects of maternal exercise on fetal heart rate. It was thought that maternal exercise might alter uterine blood flow, decrease fetal oxygenation, and possibly be reflected by changes in the fetal heart rate. The use of maternal hypoxemia as a fetal stress was described by Copher and Hurber (1967) and in 1969, Pose and colleagues described the use of oxytocin-induced uterine contractions as a stress that might identify the fetus with poor oxygen reserve. The use of contraction stress tests (CST) or oxytocin challenge tests (OCT) was introduced in the early 1970s throughout the United States and South America (Freeman, 1974, Freeman and James, 1977). These tests, attempting to mimic labor, were based on the observation of late decelerations of the FHR as indicative of uteroplacental insufficiency provoked by the stress of uterine activity. Thus, the fetus which, before labor, could not tolerate uterine contractions would be judged to be compromised in utero.

The concept of nonstress testing (NST) was proposed by Hammacher and Kubli in Europe (Hammacher, 1969; Kubli et al., 1969). This approach utilized characteristics of the FHR in response to fetal movements. The presence of fetal movements as a sign of fetal well-being has been utilized for many years. Maternal perception of decreased fetal movement has been thought indicative of probable fetal compromise. This has been extensively studied by Sadowsky et al. (1974) in Israel and in the United Kingdom. Sadowsky proposed the concept of a "fetal alarm signal" when the total number of fetal movements is less than 10 in a 24-hr hperiod. Although subjective evaluation of movement by the mother may be subject to error, this approach has proved to be a useful screening procedure. When combining the subjective assessment of FM with the objective evaluation of the FHR in response to FM, a picture of fetal condition emerges which reflects many complex and interrelated physiological mechanisms. Lack of accelerations of the heart rate associated with movements seemed to identify a high-risk group of fetuses. The use of this approach was combined with the use of the stress test following observations by numerous investigators of the higher incidence of abnormal stress tests when accelerations were absent (Lee et al., 1976, Sadowsky et al., 1974; Trierweiler et al., 1976).

This information has lead to the present approach of use of the NST as the primary test with the CST used only in the face of an abnormal NST (Evertson et al., 1979; Keegan and Paul, 1980; Schifrin et al., 1979).

PHYSIOLOGICAL BASIS OF ANTEPARTUM FETAL HEART RATE TESTING (AFHRT)

Fetal metabolism depends on the transport of oxygen and other substance across the placenta. The main source of fuel for fetal metabolism is glucose. The mechanism of transport of glucose is facilitated diffusion. Alterations in maternal glucose blood levels are rapidly reflected in the fetus. Profound alterations in maternal levels, such as in diabetes mellitus, may have adverse effects on the fetus as evidenced by the occurrence of fetal death following hyperglycemic-ketoacidotic episodes. However, the fetus would appear to receive adequate amounts of substrate in the form of glucose or use other energy sources irrespective of hypoglycemic maternal levels. Thus, the rate-limiting factor in terms of fetal aerobic metabolism is oxygen. Impairment of oxygen transport leads to anaerobic metabolism which can result in fetal compromise and, ultimately, fetal death.

Intervillous-space blood flow can be reduced during uterine contractions. This is usually tolerated by the healthy fetus. However, in the fetus with inadequate placental reserve, the stress evoked by uterine contractions leading to a reduction in blood flow may be manifested clinically in the form of late decelerations of the fetal heart rate (Caldeyro-Barcia, 1966; Myers et al., 1973). Late decelerations (LD) are a result of transient fetal hypoxemia. It has been suggested that LD develop when the fetal oxygen levels are reduced below critical levels of oxygen tension. It has not been conclusively determined whether this FHR response is a reflection of central or peripheral effects. In the initial stages, late deceleration is apparently mostly a reflex-mediated response whereas in later evolution with fetal deterioration a direct depressant effect on the myocardium emerges. Late deceleration appears to be an early indicator of fetal compromise and in the early reflex stage it can be seen in both abnormal and normal fetuses. These decelerations are a reflection of the mechanism of physiological insult, that is, impaired uterine blood flow.

The fetal reserve or tolerance to stress would appear to be reflected in the variability of the FHR which presumably is mediated by the autonomic nervous system. When present, it is thought to indicate intact CNS function. Variability is the term used to describe the beat-to-beat variation of the FHR. Normally each successive interval between clinical heart beats or on the electrocardiagram (ECG) is different in terms of duration from both the preceding and the subsequent intervals. By measuring the R-R interval of each successive fetal EKG, the duration of that cardiac cycle can be precisely calculated. This interval, expressed in milliseconds, can be mathematically converted to a rate in terms of beats per minute

(BPM). When displayed on a moving strip chart, the difference in rate between each beat will be seen as a jagged line. The visual impression of these variations or "jiggle" is referred to as "variability." Beat-to-beat variability is mediated by the counterbalancing actions of the parasympathetic) and sympathetic nervous system. Activation of the vagus (parasympathetic) slows the fetal heart rate (increases the R-R interval) while activation of the sympathetic branch causes the FHR to increase (decreases the R-R interval). The constant interaction of these two components of the autonomic nervous system leads to the appearance of FHR beat-to-beat variability. The function of the autonomic nervous system is ultimately dependent on the level of oxygenation. Initially, hypoxemia will provoke increased variability of the FHR and apparently reflects a "normal" response to the stimuli or stress. Finally, the loss of variability may denote a reduction of oxygen content below the critical level at which presumed cellular dysfunction within the CNS has occurred. Presence of FHR variability is the most important clinical sign of the ability of a given fetus to withstand repeated stress. Late decelerations with normal variability denote a fetus able to withstand repeated stresses (impaired uteroplacental blood flow) whereas absent variability reflects a fetus more likely to be compromised (Schifrin, 1977). The external methods of measuring FHR used in AFHRT preclude accurate measurement of variability because of artifacts introduced by instrumentation logic or averaging techniques, and thus a valuable commentary of fetal condition is unavailable. Accurate measurement of the low voltage fetal ECG by external methods has been difficult because of interference by the relatively higher voltage maternal ECG and concurrence of maternal and fetal ECG. If these problems were solved, much valuable information concerning variability would become available and allow the clinician to interpret fetal condition more accurately.

The function of AFHRT should be to identify those fetuses at risk for intrauterine death so that intervention can be undertaken before irreversible fetal compromise occurs. The rationale for the use of the NST as an effective method of prepartum assessment of fetal well-being is based on the relationship between the presence of FHR accelerations and fetal movements. The mechanisms involved in these FHR responses require the integrated neurological function of peripheral receptors, spinal cord, brain, sympathetic and parasympathetic systems as well as a responsive myocardium (Timor-Tritsch et al., 1978).

Normal physiologic variations in heart rate and the frequency and character of fetal movements may be influenced by an intrinsic rest/activity state of the fetus, gestational age, hypoxia, acidosis, congenital anomalies, and certain medications. Fetal "rest states" are characterized by a decrease in the number of fetal movements, decreased FHR variability, and minimal accelerations. The average length of the rest/activity cycles is 40-60 min but the rest state can be prolonged and the frequency and amplitude of the accelerations can be diminished with the use of certain narcotics or sedatives (Keegan et al., 1979; Manning et al., 1980; Timor-Tritsch et al., 1980).

INDICATIONS FOR AFHRT

These include: diabetes mellitus, postterm pregnancy, hypertensive disorders of pregnancy, intrauterine growth retardation, history of previous stillbirth, anemia, hemaglobinopathies, decreased fetal movement, cyanotic heart disease, and other disorders associated with increased perinatal loss.

Most of the reported experience with the CST has been based on evaluations starting at 34 weeks gestation (Freeman, 1974; Freeman and James, 1977). However, the reliability of the CST before 33 weeks has been shown in one study (Gabbe, 1978). In general, the decision on when to start AFHRT should be based on the risk of intrauterine death and at a point in gestation where therapy or intervention by delivery give the infant a reasonable chance of survival. The latter will depend on available neonatal facilities.

Current clinical experience with the NST has been primarily based on evaluations starting at 34 weeks of gestation and later. Meager experience before 34 weeks would seem to indicate that a nonreactive test is more frequent in earlier gestation.

CONTRAINDICATIONS FOR AFHRT

There are no contraindications to the use of the NST. The CST is contraindicated in those patients considered at risk for uterine rupture or premature labor. These include patients who have experienced previous classic cesarean section, incompetent cervix, history of premature labor, placenta previa, multiple gestation, and premature rupture of the membranes.

It has been suggested that all pregnant women undergo AFHRT at least once in late pregnancy. The cost-effectiveness of this approach has yet to be conclusively proved in the low-risk gravida but this may be a more specific method of risk assessment than those currently used which are merely based on statistical methods.

PERFORMANCE OF AFHRT

Antepartum fetal heart rate testing is performed using an external system to monitor fetal movement, uterine contractions, and fetal heart rate (FHR). Uterine activity and fetal movements are obtained with a tocodynamometer strapped to the abdomen in conjunction with manual

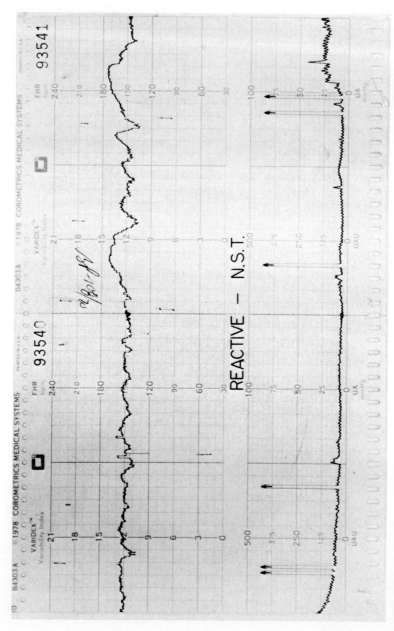

Figure 1. A reactive pattern in a nonstress test, showing fetal heart rate accelerations of at least 15 beats/min.

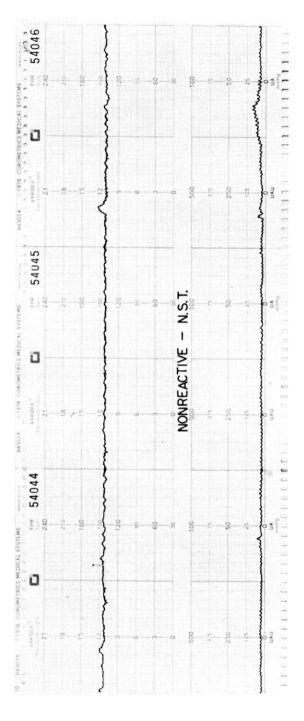

Figure 2. A nonreactive pattern in a nonstress test.

palpation of the uterus by the examiner. This method will register the frequency and duration, but not the actual strength, of contractions. The patient is given an "event marker" with which she can register perceived fetal movements on the strip chart. Thus the patient and the examiner may both record fetal movements.

The FHR can be derived from ultrasonic, phonocardiogram, or abdominal wall electrocardiogram signals. Ultrasound will provide an adequate FHR tracing in up to 95% of the cases, while the success rate of the other two methods has been reported in 40-60% of cases (Martin and Schifrin, 1977).

In an attempt to reduce the high incidence of nonreactive NST, various methods of stimulation have been employed to alter fetal rest/activity states in utero. Miller et al. (1979) studied the effect of maternal blood glucose levels on fetal activity. They observed a significant increase in fetal activity following maternal ingestion of glucose. Since the NST associates FHR response and fetal movements, the increase in fetal activity induced by glucose ingestion may enhance the chances of observing FHR accelerations. Read et al. (1977) evaluated FHR accelerations in response to acoustic stimulation as a measure of fetal well-being. They concluded that, since the presence of acceleration of the FHR in response to an auditory stimulus has a high correlation with a negative OCT, this response should obviate the need for an OCT.

At our institution, abdominal-wall manipulation has been employed as a method of fetal stimulation, but its absolute quantitative effectiveness has not been demonstrated.

INTERPRETATION OF THE NST

At Los Angeles County/University of Southern California Medical Center, Women's Hospital, a reactive pattern is defined as the presence of two accelerations equal to or greater than 15 beats/min, lasting 15 sec, associated with fetal movements in a 10-min interval (Fig. 1). A nonreactive pattern is one showing either one or no FHR accelerations, or accelerations of less than 15 beats/min lasting less than 15 sec (Evertson et al., 1979) (Fig. 2).

PERFORMANCE OF THE CST

The CST is performed while the patient is in the semi-Fowler's position to avoid the supine-hypotensive syndrome. A baseline period of 10-15 min is used to assess fetal heart rate (FHR) characteristics and the possibility of periodic changes. Blood pressure should be monitored every 10 min to identify supine hypotension that might provoke an abnormal CST. Uterine activity is evaluated for spontaneous contractions. If recurrent late decelerations occur with spontaneous contractions, the test is interpreted as positive irrespective of the frequency of the uterine contractions. In patients having less than three spontaneous contractions in 10 min in which no decelerations are noted, an oxytocin infusion is begun at a rate of 0.5 mll/min. This rate of infusion is doubled every 15 min until three contractions of moderate intensity, lasting 40-60 sec are achieved within 10 min. Uterine activity with these characteristics is believed to be similar to that expected in labor and thus an adequate stress. Once adequate stress test criteria are achieved the oxytocin infusion is stopped and the patient should be monitored until uterine activity diminishes to pretest levels.

INTERPRETATION OF THE CST

There are two schemes of interpretation of the CST as described by Freeman and Schifrin. The scheme proposed by Freeman can be described as follows (Garite and Freeman, 1979).

1. *Negative*

   A test is interpreted as negative if no late decelerations appear any time in the test period including the observation period and the period after the completion of the test. There must be a minimum of three contractions lasting longer than 40 sec in a 10-min period to qualify as an OCT (Fig. 3).

2. *Positive*

   A test is interpreted as positive when it demonstrates persistent or consistent late decelerations associated with more than half of the uterine contractions, provided there is no evidence of uterine hyperstimulation. A test may also be interpreted as positive if repetitive late decelerations occur with less uterine activity than required in the definition of the negative CST (Fig. 4). Thus, a test result showing repetitive late decelerations with uterine activity, either spontaneous or oxytocin-induced, of less than three contractions in 10 min may be interpreted as positive, and further uterine stimulation should not be undertaken.

3. *Suspicious*

   This test result demonstrated late decelerations that do not persist throughout the tracing. It is considered inconclusive.

4. *Hyperstimulation*

   This defines FHR decelerations occurring with excessive uteirne activity as defined by contractions lasting more than 90 sec or occurring more frequently than every 2 min. When FHR decelerations are present, the test is considered inconclusive. In the absence of periodic changes of the FHR, in spite of uterine hyperstimulation, the test is interpreted as negative.

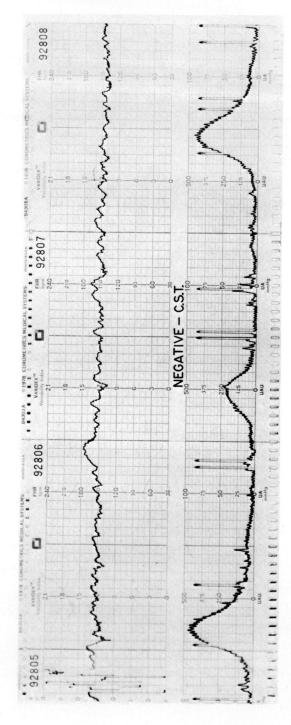

Figure 3. Negative results in a contraction stress test; there are no late decelerations of the fetal heart rate.

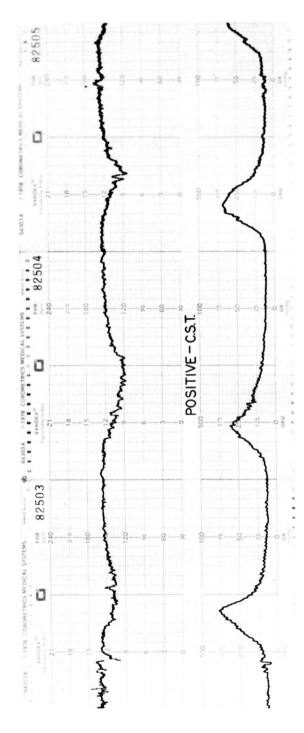

Figure 4. Positive results in a contraction stress test; there are repetitive late decelerations.

183

5. *Unsatisfactory*

In certain instances adequate duration and/or frequency of the uterine contractions is not achieved, or the FHR tracing is not of a quality to be adequately interpreted.

An alternative interpretation of the CST, based on the concept of the "10-min" window, has been proposed by Schifrin (Schifrin, 1977; Schifrin et al., 1975). When interpreting the test, an attempt is made to identify a 10-min segment of the tracing that satisfies the criteria for a positive or a negative test, which requires three uterine contractions in the 10-min segment. Using this scheme he describes the following:

1. *Negative.* A negative test shows a stable FHR without evidence of periodic heart rate decelerations.
2. *Positive.* This test shows repeated late decelerations. In cases showing both a positive and a negative window, the test is considered positive. Using this scheme, positive tests may be found in 3-10% of the cases.
3. *Equivocal.* In this test neither a positive nor a negative window can be identified. This is considered inconclusive.
4. *Unsatisfactory.* Those tests in which either the FHR cannot be monitored satisfactory or adequate uterine activity cannot be elicited within 2 hr of beginning the test.

According to this scheme of interpretation, occasional decelerations are disregarded in the presence of a negative window.

CLINICAL APPLICATION

Nonstress Test

A reactive test is obtained in approximately 90% of the cases and is a reliable indicator of fetal well-being. The false negative rate of the NST, defined as fetal death within a week of a reactive NST, is less than 1%. Suspected causes of false negative tests include: umbilical cord accidents, abruptio placenta, and sudden changes in metabolic status of the mother.

The nonreactive test lacks specificity. Its false abnormal rate has been reported as high as 60-80% (Schifrin et al., 1979). This can be significantly reduced with repeat testing; 75% of the initial nonreactive tests will then become reactive. The possible reasons for these "false" nonreactive results are: fetal rest and activity cycles (Sterman and Hoppenbrouwers), maternal drug ingestion, and maternal hypoglycemia.

Contraction Stress Test

A negative test result is obtained in 85-90% of the cases and is a reliable indication of fetal well-being. The false negative rate of the CST, defined as
fetal death within a week of a negative CST, is less than 1% (Caldeyro-Barcia
et al. 1966). Suspected causes of false negative tests are the same as listed
above.

A positive CST identifies a group of patients with an increased rate of
perinatal mortality and morbidity. The incidence of false positive results,
defined as patients with positive CSTs with no evidence of fetal distress in
labor, has been reported as 25-50% (Gauthier et al., 1979). Known causes of
false positive tests include undiagnosed supine hypotension and excessive
uterine activity. Maternal postural changes may reduce uterine blood flow
without the clinical manifestation of the supine hypotensive-syndrome, but
still constitute a possible cause for a false positive CST.

MANAGEMENT OF AFHRT

Reactive tests are repeated at weekly intervals. Persistent nonreactive tests
are followed by a CST. If the CST is negative, the test is considered inconclusive and is repeated in 24 hr (Druzin et al., 1980). If the CST is
positive, one should consider delivery in the presence of a mature fetus.
In the case of prematurity it would seem wise to consider other methods
of antenatal assessment, such as estriols, before a decision to deliver is
made.

Currently, the following working scheme (Fig. 5) is being employed at
Los Angeles County/University of Southern California Medical Center, Women's
Hospital. A combined NST-CST approach is followed. The CST is performed
only in the hospital setting whereas the NST can be accomplished in the outpatient facilities. Testing is performed by specifically trained nurses using
the NST as the primary approach. A reactive pattern, as previously defined,
is retested on a weekly basis or more often if there are marked changes in
the clinical situation of the mother. When a nonreactive pattern is observed
for 40 min the patient is scheduled for a repeat NST during the same day.
If, on repeat testing, a persistent nonreactive pattern is seen, a CST is performed. If two accelerations in any 10-min period during the CST are noted,
the pattern is considered reactive and the CST is terminated. If no accelerations are noted, the CST is continued until three contractions in 10 min are
noted. Patients with negative, suspicious, or equivocal CSTs are retested
within 24 hr beginning with the NST. Positive CSTs are evaluated for
delivery particularly when the fetus is mature.

Garite and Freeman have proposed the use of a lecithin-sphingomyelin ratio
determination in patients with a positive CST. If the ratio is equal to or greater

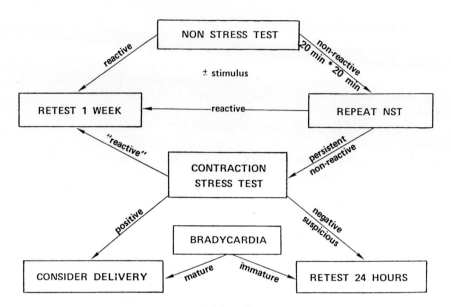

Figure 5. Working scheme for testing antepartum fetal heart rate used at Los Angeles County/University of Southern California Medical Center, Women's Hospital.

than 2, delivery is recommended (Garite and Freeman, 1979). Because of the test's high false positive rate, premature delivery may not be indicated on the basis of a positive CST alone. In such cases the addition of other forms of antenatal fetal surveillance such as estriol determinations may prevent unnecessary premature intervention.

The route of delivery following a positive CST has been controversial. Farahani et al. (1976) recommended cesarean delivery on the assumption that a fetus showing evidence of distress during the CST will probably not tolerate labor. On the other hand, in a recent report from our institution, Gauthier described that 75% of the fetuses with a positive CST, showed no evidence of intrapartum fetal distress during labor. Vaginal delivery was achieved in 55% of the patients who had a positive CST (Gauthier et al., 1979). Based on this data, he recommended that a trial of labor should be attempted in the face of a positive CST whenever obstetrical factors are favorable and careful intrapartum monitoring could be performed.

A problem that may be encountered, particularly in the postterm pregnancy, is the occurrence of fetal bradycardia. Recent data from our institution

(Druzin et al., 1981) have shown that bradycardia during AFHRT denotes a fetus at high risk of developing fetal distress in labor. Consideration should be given to possible intervention when the fetus is mature, irrespective of whether the NST is reactive or nonreactive.

ADVANTAGES AND DISADVANTAGES OF NST AND CST

Both CSTs and NSTs have been reliable in the prevention of antenatal death and the prediction of perinatal morbidity and mortality (Evertson et al., 1979; Freeman, 1974; Freeman and James, 1977; Keegan and Paul, 1980).

The false negative rate for the prevention of antenatal deaths, a major goal of AFHRT, is less than 1% using either method (Evertson et al., 1978).

Prepartum fetal death is the definitive endpoint against which these methods might be judged. However, fetal distress in labor and neonatal outcome are also used in assessing the reliability of the various approaches. The endpoints are subject to factors not within the predictive capability of AFHRT.

The disadvantages of the CST are: (1) the need for a hospital setting to conduct the test; (2) the need for an intravenous infusion for the administration of oxytocin; (3) the presence of some relative contraindications which preclude its use in some high risk pregnancies; (4) its time-consuming nature (mean time 90-120 min) makes it impractical as a routine screening test, and; (5) advanced stages of fetal compromise may not show evidence of late decelerations.

The advantages of the NST include: (1) applicability in an outpatient setting; (2) less complex and thus more rapid (mean 12 min); and (3) the absence of contraindications.

The disadvantage of the NST is its high false positive rate (nonreactive), reported to be 60-80%. However, this can be significantly reduced with repeat testing on the same day. After repeated observation of a persistent nonreactive pattern, a CST is performed. In our experience this reduces the need for the CST to less than 3%. The reactive test appears to be the most reliable and practical evaluator of fetal well-being.

CONCLUSIONS

1. Both NST and CST have played an important role in the prenatal surveillance of high-risk pregnancies.
2. Consistency in performance and interpretation of the tests by experienced personnel is of the utmost importance.
3. Normal AFHRT (reactive NST) is a reliable predictor of fetal well-being. The false negative rate for the preventing of antenatal death is less than 1%.

4. Abnormal AFHRT (nonreactive NST or positive CST) is inconclusive. It identifies a patient population at higher risk. However, the high false positive rate reduces specificity.
5. The controversy over which testing method detects compromise earlier remains unresolved.
6. Because the NST can be more simply applied to a larger patient population, the overall impact in minimizing fetal losses would appear greater than that of the CST.

FUTURE DEVELOPMENTS

Using biophysical methods of fetal assessment such as real-time ultrasonography, it has been shown that AFHRT is only one aspect of judging fetal condition in utero. Observation of other parameters such as fetal breathing, fetal tone, amniotic-fluid volume, and bladder function may be equally reliable predictors of the fetus' status at any time. Currently, investigations are underway to determine the optimal means of detecting the fetus at risk.

Manning and associates (1980) have reported on the assessment of multiple biophysical variables to determine fetal condition with greater accuracy. Fetal breathing movements can be seen on real-time ultrasound scanning as episodic movements of the fetal chest wall. Using real time ultrasonography, they demonstrated that the false positive rates for both the NST and CST were significantly reduced when "fetal breathing movements" (FBM) were demonstrated. The presence of FBM is considered a sign of fetal well being.

The investigators have shown that using five biophysical variables, the NST, FBM, fetal movement, fetal tone and amniotic fluid volume, a greater accuracy of prediction of outcome is possible than using one variable alone. Studies in progress will demonstrate the practicality and clinical usefulness of this approach.

REFERENCES

Caldeyro-Barcia, Mendez-Bauer, C., Poseior, J. J., Escarcena, L. A., Pose, S. V., Arnt, I. C., Gulin, L., Althabe, O., and Bierniarz, J. (1966). Control of human fetal heart rate during labor. In *The Heart and Circulation in the Newborn and Infant*. E. E. Cassels (Ed.), Grune & Stratton, New York, pp. 7-36.
Copher, D. E., and Hurber, C. P. (1967). Heart rate response of the human fetus to induces maternal hypoxia. *Am. J. Obstet. Gynecol. 98*:320.
Druzin, M. L., Gratacos, J., and Paul, R. H. (1980). Antepartum fetal heart rate testing: VI. The predictive reliability of "normal" tests in the prevention of antepartum death. *Am. J. Obstet. Gynecol. 137*:746.

Druzin, M. L., Gratacos, J., and Keegan, K. A. (1981). Antepartum fetal heart rate testing: VII. The significance of fetal bradycardia. *Am. J. Obstet. Gynecol. 139*:2.

Evertson, L. R., Gauthier, R. J., Schifrin, B. S., and Paul, R. H. (1979). Antepartum fetal heart rate testing. I. Evolution of the nonstress test. *Am. J. Obstet. Gynecol. 133*:29.

Evertson, L. R., Gauthier, R. J., and Collea, J. V. (1978). Fetal demise following negative contraction stress tests. *Obstet. Gynecol. 51*:671.

Farahani, G., Vasudeva, K., Petrie, R. H., and Fenton, A. (1976). Oxytocin challenge test in high-risk pregnancy. *Obstet. Gynecol. 47*:159.

Freeman, R. K. (1974). Clinical value of antepartum fetal heart rate monitoring. In *Modern Perinatal Medicine*. L. Gluck (Ed.), Year Book Med. Pub. Inc., Chicago, p. 163.

Freeman, R. K., and James, J. (1977). Clinical experience with the oxytocin challenge test. II. An aminous atypical pattern. *Obstet. Gynecol. 46*:255.

Gabbe, S. G. (1978). Application of scientific rationale in the management of the pregnant diabetic patient. *Semin. Perinatol. 2*:361.

Garite, T. J., and Freeman, R. K. (1979). Antepartum stress test monitoring. In *Clinics in Obstetrics and Gynecology*. E. J. Quilligan (Ed.), Saunders, p. 295.

Gauthier, R. J., Evertson, L. R., and Paul, R. H. (1979). Antepartum fetal heart rate testing. II. Intrapartum fetal heart rate observation and newborn outcome following a positive contraction stress test. *Am. J. Obstet. Gynecol. 133*:34.

Hammacher, K. (1969). The clinical significance of cardiotocography. In *Perinatal Medicine*. P. M. Huntington, K. A. Huter, and E. Saline (Eds.), George Shieme Verlag, K. G. Stuttgart, pp. 80-93.

Hon, E. H., and Wohlgemuth, R. (1961). The electronic evaluation of fetal heart rate IV. The effect of maternal exercise. *Am. J. Obstet. Gynecol. 81*: 361.

Keegan, K. A., Paul, R. H. (1980). Antepartum fetal heart rate testing. IV. The nonstress test as a primary approach. *Am. J. Obstet. Gynecol. 136*: 75-80.

Keegan, K. A., Paul, R. H., Broussard, P. M., McCart, D., and Smith, M. A. (1979). Antepartum fetal heart rate testing. III. The effect of pheonobarbital on the nonstress test. *Am. J. Obstet. Gynecol. 133*:579-580.

Kubli, F. W., Kaeser, O., and Kinselman, M. (1969). Diagnostic management of chronic placental insufficiency. In *The Foeto-Placental Unit*. A. Pecile and C. Finzi (Eds.), Excerpta Medica Foundation, Amsterdam, pp. 323-339.

Lee, C. Y., DiLoreto, P. C., and Logrand, B. (1976). Fetal activity acceleration determination for the evaluation of fetal reserve. *Obstet. Gynecol. 48*: 19.

Linzey, E. M., and Freeman, R. K. (1978). Fetal monitoring. In Antepartum
Fetal Monitoring. *Yearbook of Obstetrics and Gynecology.*

Manning, F. A., Platt, L. D., and Sipos, L. (1980). Antepartum fetal evaluation development of a fetal biophysical profile. *Am. J. Obstet. Gynecol.*
136:787.

Martin, C. B., and Schifrin, B. S. (1977). Prenatal fetal monitoring, perinatal
intensive care. S. Aladjem and A. K. Brown (Eds.), C. V. Mosby, St. Louis,
pp. 155-173.

Miller, F. C., Skiba, H., and Klapholz, H. (1979). The effect of maternal
blood sugar levels on fetal activity. *Obstet. Gynecol. 52*:662.

Myers, R. E., Mueller-Heubach, E., and Adamsons, K. (1973). Predictability
of the state of fetal oxygenation from a quantitative analysis of the
components of late deceleration. *Am. J. Obstet. Gynecol. 115*:1083.

Pose, S. V., Castillo, J. B., Mora-Rojas, E. O. et al. (1969). Test of fetal tolerance to induced uterine contractions for the diagnosis of chronic distress.
In *Perinatal Factors Affecting Human Development.* Pan Am Health Organ-
ization Scientific Publication No. 185.

Read, J. A., and Miller, F. C. (1977). Fetal heart rate acceleration in response
to acoustic stimulation as a measure of fetal well-being. *Am. J. Obstet.*
Gynecol. 129:513.

Sadowsky, E., Yaffe, H., and Polishuk, W. Z. (1974). Fetal movement monitoring in normal and pathologic pregnancy. *Int. J. Gynaecol. Obstet. 12*:75.

Schifrin, B. S. (1977). Antepartum fetal heart rate monitoring. In *Intrauterine
Asphyxia and the Developing Fetal Brain.* L. Gluck (Ed.), Year Book
Med. Pub. Inc., Chicago, pp. 205-224.

Schifrin, B. S., Lapidus, M., and Doctor, G. (1975). Contraction stress test
for antepartum fetal evaluation. *Obstet. Gynecol. 45*:433.

Schifrin, B. S., Foye, G., Amato, J., Kates, R., and McKenna, J. (1979).
Routine fetal heart rate monitoring in the antepartum period. *Obstet.*
Gynecol. 54:21.

Sterman, M. B., and Hoppenbrouwers, T. (1971). The development of sleep-
walking and rest activity patterns from fetus to adult in man. In *Brain
Development and Behavior.* M. B. Sterman, D. J. McGinty, and A. M.
Adinolfi (Eds.), Academic Press, New York, pp. 203-227.

Timor-Tritsch, I. E., Dieker, L. J., Hertz, R. H., et al. (1978). Studies of
antepartum behavioral state in the human fetus at term. *Am. J. Obstet.*
Gynecol. 132:524.

Trierweiler, M. W., Freeman, R. K., and James, J. (1976). Baseline fetal heart
rate characteristics as an indicator of fetal status during the antepartum
period. *Am. J. Obstet. Gynecol. 125*:618.

9

Is Pelvimetry Worthwhile?

RICHARD L. BERKOWITZ* / Yale University School of Medicine and
Yale-New Haven Medical Center, New Haven, Connecticut

EMILY A. FINE / Yale-New Haven Hospital, New Haven, Connecticut

A safe vaginal delivery depends in part on a maternal pelvis that is large enough
to permit a fetus to pass through it atraumatically. Pelvimetry has been used
for more than 40 yr to provide objective measurements of the pelvis when
fetomaternal disporoportion was suspected. It has been used to make management decisions in cephalic presentations with floating heads before labor or
failure to progress during the active phase of labor, and in breech presentations
where vaginal delivery is being considered.

Numerous techniques for taking and interpreting pelvimetry films have been
developed. This has created a rich, albeit confusing, literature with many reported series that cannot easily be compared. Some authors believe that
pelvimetry should continue to play an important role in the management of
difficult labors (Friedman, 1976). Others claim that more accurate information
can be obtained by well-directed trials of labor (Barton and Garbaciak, 1979;
Schifrin, 1974). Controversy also exists over the long-term effects of exposure
to x-radiation in utero, with some authorities citing significantly increased
risks of leukemia and other malignancies in childhood following even low
levels of radiation (Stewart, 1958).

Since x-ray pelvimetry may not be innocuous, and its efficacy in making
sound decisions has been questioned, it seems worthwhile to review the risks
and benefits of this modality in modern obstetrical management. A comprehensive review of the voluminous literature on this subject is not possible here.

*Present affiliation: Mt. Sinai School of Medicine, New York, New York.

An attempt will be made, however, to sample a variety of studies and then to present a viewpoint reflecting the accumulated experience from many centers, as well as the authors' work in this field.

PELVIC ANATOMY AND MORPHOLOGY

The pelvis encloses a complex three-dimensional space which has been described as a slightly tapering cylinder with an obliquely cut top. It has traditionally been divided into three planes. The inlet is bounded anteriorly by the upper inner posterior margin of the superior rami of the pubic bones, laterally by the iliopectineal lines, and posteriorly by the posterior extensions of these lines and the anterior surface of the sacral promontory at the level where the iliopectineal lines converge. The dimensions of obstetrical importance in this plane include the anteroposterior (AP), the widest transverse, and the posterior sagittal (PS), which is the portion of the AP diameter lying posterior to its intersection with the transverse diameter (Figures 1a,b).

The midplane is referred to as "the plane of least dimensions" (Pritchard and MacDonald, 1976). It is bounded interiorly by the inner lower border of the symphysis pubis, laterally by the ischial spines, and posteriorly by the lower third of the sacrum (usually the junction of S4 and S5). The dimensions of obstetrical importance in this plane include the bispinous, AP, and PS (Fig. 1a,b).

The outlet is composed of two triangular planes which share a common base: the bituberal diameter. The anterior triangle is bounded by the descending rami of the pubis and its size is determined by the subpubic angle. The configuration of the posterior triangle is a function of the size and shape of the sacrosciatic notch and the inclination of the sacrum. Despite earlier controversy, the current consensus of opinion seems to be that dystocia from pelvic outlet contraction is very rare and, if present, is invariably associated with disproportion in one or both of the other planes.

Numerous descriptions of pelvic morphologic variations have been published but the most widely accepted is that of Caldwell and Moloy (1933). They defined four pure types of pelvis (gynecoid, android, anthropoid, and platypelloid) and described a system for classifying mixtures of these basic types (Fig. 2). Their descriptive scheme is taught to most obstetricians in training who are advised to utilize it when making manual pelvic assessments as well as in their interpretation of pelvimetry films. Delivery outcome is reportedly related to morphology as follows.

In the pure android pelvis, if engagement occurs in a transverse position, the anteriorly inclined sacrum and narrow posterior pelvis force the fetal head into the equally narrow anterior segment. The fetus then adopts an occipito-posterior position which permits the smaller frontal diameter to use

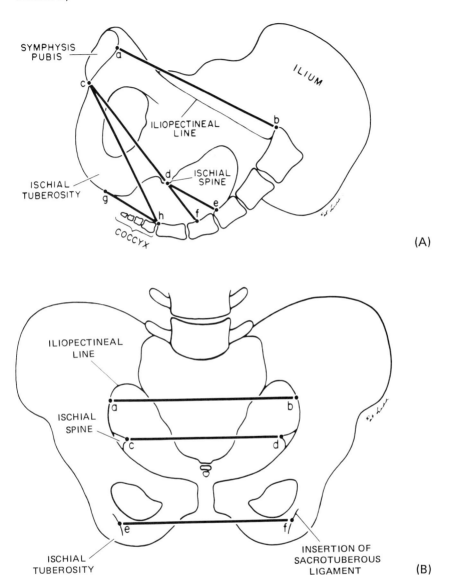

Figure 1. (A) Anteroposterior view of pelvic dimensions (above): ab, obstetric conjugate; cf, anteroposterior diameter of the midplane; df, posterior sagittal of the midplane (Caldwell and Moloy); df, posterior sagittal of the midplane (Thoms); ch, anteroposterior diameter of the outlet; and gh, posterior sagittal of the outlet. (B) Lateral view of pelvis dimensions (below); ab, inlet transverse; cd, interspinous; ef, intertuberous. (From Aiman, J. (1976). X-ray pelvimetry of the pregnant adolescent: Pelvic size and frequency of contraction, *Obstet. Gynecol. 48*:282.

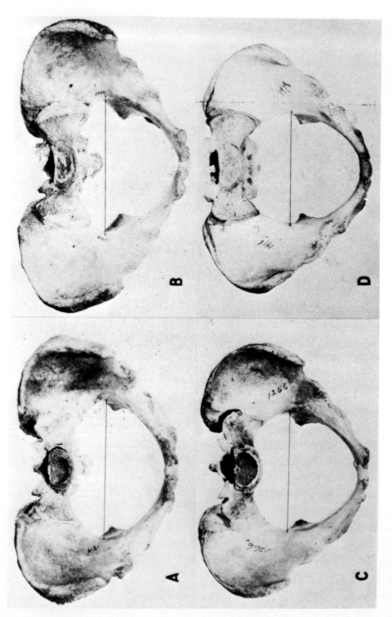

Figure 2.   Pelvic classifications with respect to the inlet: (A) Platypelloid; (B) android; (C) gynecoid; (D) anthropoid. (From Caldwell, W. D., and Moloy, H. C. (1933). Anatomical variations in the female pelvis and their effect in labor with a suggested classification. *Am. J. Obstet. Gynecol. 26*:488.

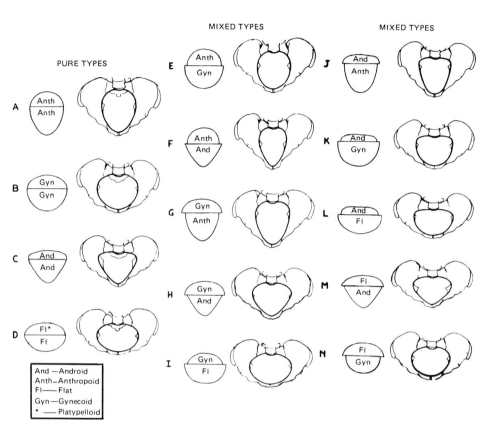

Figure 3. Pelvic inlet classifications of mixed types. (From Thoms, H. (1940). Roentgen pelvimetry as a routine prenatal procedure. *Am. J. Obstet. Gynecol. 40*:900.

the available space in the anterior segment. The head meets increasing resistance as it descends due to progressive convergence of the side walls, and pelvic arrest may occur. A wide subpubic arch may improve the prognosis, since it can partially overcome the effects of a narrow sacrosciatic notch and forward sacrum.

Problems with anthropoid pelves are related to the degree of transverse diameter contraction. The fetal head may be unable to engage and be found floating at term. If, however, the baby is small enough, engagement can occur in the AP diameter. Persistent occiput posterior positions may result, in which case mechanical rotation is contraindicated.

The platypelloid pelvis is usually only associated with difficult deliveries
when the subpubic angle is narrow, which causes the ischial spines to be
relatively prominent. The fetal head often engages easily and descends in
the transverse position to the pelvic floor. Rotation to the occiput anterior
position should obviously not be attempted.

The gynecoid pelvis has the optimal shape for easy passage of the fetus.
In this case problems only arise in the symmetrically contracted pelves of
small women. These women, however, often have constitutionally small
babies which can successfully negotiate the compromised birth canal. Even
when the ischial spines are relatively prominent or the subpubic angle is
narrow, the posterior segment is frequently large enough to provide an
adequate compensatory space.

Various combinations of these four basic shapes cause their own unique
problems (Fig. 3). It should be pointed out, however, that pelvic architecture is only one variable in the complex phenomenon of fetal passage through
the maternal pelvis. Other factors which may affect outcome include fetal
size, cranial position and attitude, cranial molding potential, fetomaternal
soft-tissue relationships, and adequacy of uterine contractile forces. The
various techniques designed to evaluate pelvic morphology give minimal insight into many of these latter variables. The information they provide is,
therefore, necessarily limited in its scope.

MANUAL ASSESSMENT

Manual assessment has long been considered a useful way to estimate pelvic
size and shape. The diagonal conjugate is the distance from the lower margin
of the symphysis pubis to the sacral promontory. By subtracting 1.5-2.0 cm
from this measurement, an approximation of the AP of the inlet is obtained.
Thoms (1938) has noted, however, that the height and width of the pubic
bone is variable, as is the position of the sacral promontory in relation to the
true inlet. Further limitations of this determination are that minimal values
are dependent on the length of the clinician's fingers and to some extent on
patient compliance. The inclination of the sacrum can be determined by
manual assessment, but the transverse diameter of the inlet can only be
measured by x-ray pelvimetry.

Prominent ischial spines and convergent side walls on vaginal examination
suggest midpelvic contracture (Pritchard and MacDonald, 1976). The
presence of thick pubic rami and tubercles, in association with a straight
anteriorly inclined sacrum, suggests android tendencies (Caldwell and Moloy,
1933). The posterior portion of the midpelvis can be evaluated by examining
the relationship between the sacrosciatic notch (SSN) and the sacrum. A
short SSN or anteriorly inclined sacrum suggests an android midpelvis, while
a broad SSN is more consistent with anthropoid morphology.

The outlet is best evaluated manually by measuring the bituberous diameter and the subpubic angle.

X-RAY PELVIMETRY TECHNIQUES

Because x-rays are dispersed from a point source, the image on the film of the object being studied is necessarily distorted. The degree of distortion is a function of the object's distance from both the x-ray source and the film and, therefore, differs significantly for various landmarks within a three-dimensional space such as the maternal pelvis. Numerous x-ray pelvimetry techniques have been described since the pioneer work done by Thoms, and by Caldwell and Moloy during the 1930s. Each approach has attempted to provide a technically feasible and easily reproducible solution to the problem of image distortion. The large number of methods reported reflects the ingenuity of the investigators as well as the difficulty of the problem.

Thoms (1929) devised the "frame" or "position" approach to x-ray pelvimetry. In this method, the patient is placed in a semirecumbent position with her pelvic inlet parallel to the x-ray plate. After taking an AP x-ray the film is re-exposed with a lead grid of centimeter markings placed at the precise level of the patient's pelvic inlet (Fig. 4). Since the centimeter markings on the grid are distorted in exactly the same fashion as the points at the level of the inlet, direct measurements in the plane of the inlet can be made from the film by using the superimposed markings on the grid. A correction table for measurements at the level of the midpelvis was developed, which was based on the distance below the inlet at which this plane occurred. This depth is determined from the lateral film (Thoms, 1940). The problem of distortion on the lateral film was eliminated by placing a lead centimeter marker between the patient's buttocks (Fig. 5). The notches on this ruler are subjected to the same distortions as the midline AP diameters and can be used for direct measurements of these dimensions.

Thoms (1941) subsequently modified his grid so that the interspinous and outlet dimensions can be measured directly off the AP film without resorting to correction tables. The top row of perforations, still 1 cm apart, continue to represent the level of the inlet. The five rows of marks below this level, however, are spaced at progressively smaller distances and correspond to the 5-, 6-, 7-, 8-, and 9-cm levels below the inlet. To measure diameters in planes below the inlet, the depth of that level is determined from the lateral film, and the appropriate row of markers on the AP film are then used for making direct measurements.

The original Thoms method required placing the patient in a semirecumbent position so that the inlet is as parallel to the x-ray plate as possible. This, however, results in passing x-rays through the long axis of the fetal body.

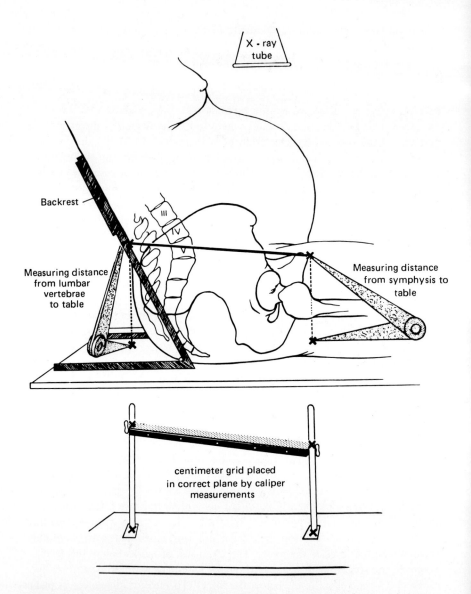

Figure 4. Positioning of patient and markers for the Thoms' anteroposterior pelvic x-rays. (From Eastman, N. J., and Hellman, L. M. (1966). The normal pelvis. In *Williams Obstetrics,* 13th ed., Appleton-Century-Crofts, New York, p. 298).

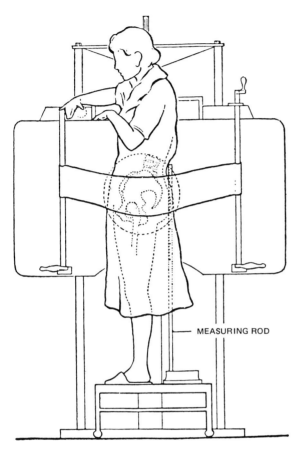

MEASURING ROD

Figure 5. Positioning of the patient, standing, for lateral x-ray of pelvis to obtain anteroposterior diameters by Thoms' technique. (From Eastman, N. J., and Hellman, L. M. (1966). The normal pelvis. In *Williams Obstetrics,* 13th ed. Appleton-Century-Crofts, New York, p. 296).

Inlet measurements obtained with the patient lying on her back have been shown to be comparable to those taken in the position originally recommended. (Colcher and Sussman, 1944). The Thoms' technique has, therefore, been modified at many institutions, including our own, by AP films being taken with the patient placed in a near-prone position (75° from the upright) before superimposing the distorted centimeter grid. This greatly reduces fetal radiation exposure without significantly compromising the accuracy of the method.

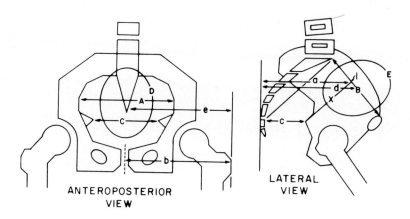

ANTEROPOSTERIOR
VIEW

LATERAL
VIEW

Designation	Dimension	View*
A	Widest transverse inlet diameter	AP
B	Anteroposterior diameter of inlet	LAT
C	Interspinious diameter	AP
D	Head circumference	AP
E	Head circumference	LAT
a	Object-film distance for widest transverse inlet diameter	LAT
b	Object-film distance for AP inlet diameter	AP
c	Object-film distance for interspinous diameter	LAT
d	Object-film distance for AP head circumference	LAT
e	Object-film distance for LAT head circumference	AP

*AP, anteroposterior; LAT, lateral

Figure 6. Schematic representation of a fetal head in a maternal pelvis with required dimensions for the Ball technique. (From Klapholz, H. (1975). A computerized aid to Ball pelvimetry. *Am. J. Obstet. Gynecol. 121*:1067.

Unlike the "frame" approach, the stereoscopic or "parallax" type of pelvimetry introduced by Caldwell et al. (1939) emphasized the importance of the type and amount of space available in the pelvis. Four views of the pelvis were taken and a special precision stereoscope was necessary to interpret the films. The shortcomings of this approach include its complexity, the subjectivity involved in the readings, and the excessive irradiation required.

Ball and Marchbanks (1933) introduced a method which permits comparison of fetal head size with that of the various pelvic planes. Only two films taken from perpendicular views are necessary to obtain all pelvic and fetal measurements (Ball, 1936). Fetal head volume is calculated from head circumferences measured in both AP and lateral films. This value is then compared with the areas of the inlet and midpelvis, which are calculated from formulas utilizing AP and transverse diameters of these planes. Ball's method utilizes a simple principle of physics to handle the problem of distortion. Given that linear magnification of an object as projected on a film will vary with the tube-film distance, the degree of magnification can be calculated when that distance is known by using the geometric axiom that parallel sides of similar triangles are proportional to each other. As long as the x-ray tube-to-film distance, the object-to-film distance, and the image size of an object are known, the true object size can be calculated. With the Ball technique, image size is read directly off one film and its object-to-film distance is measured from the x-ray taken at right angles to it (Fig. 6). The true object size can then be calculated, or read off a nomogram (Friedman and Taylor, 1969) or computer program printout (Klapholz, 1975). This clever method only involves two x-rays, can be interpreted without complex hardware, and, most importantly, considers fetal head size as a variable in determining the presence of disproportion.

PROGNOSTIC USEFULNESS OF X-RAY PELVIMETRY

Cephalic Presentations

The literature is replete with studies describing the relationship between x-ray pelvimetry results and obstetric outcome. A number of difficulties arise when trying to interpret this data. Virtually none of these series presents a uniform approach to the management of patients in labor or objective criteria for performing cesarean sections. In most cases, the women studied were considered to be at risk for cephalopelvic disproportion (CPD) because of the clinical impression of a compromised pelvis on manual assessment, a floating head at term, or failure to progress in labor. The bias of the referring obstetrician was, therefore, likely to be in favor of finding a compromised fetopelvic relationship. Without a predetermined protocol for the management of labor, it is possible that x-ray pelvimetry can be used to "confirm" a subjective clinical bias of disproportion and result in the performance of cesarean sections which might not have occurred had proper trials of labor been permitted. A series in which disproportion by x-ray correlates well with delivery by cesarean section, therefore, may be the result of self-fulfilling prophesies. On the other hand, the demonstration of the lack of disproportion by x-ray might lead to a trial of labor in a situation where clinically this would be pointless. The question raised in reviewing these series is whether x-ray pelvimetry alters obstetrical management by providing information that could not be accurately obtained with less invasive methods.

Schwarz et al. (1956) using the Ball method, reported that the cesarean section rate in their series was 1% when "no disproportion" was found, 33% where "borderline disproportion" was present, and 80% when "absolute disproportion" was detected. They noted a better correlation between inlet disproportion and route of delivery than between midpelvic disproportion and outcome.

In 1958 Steer published a review of the experience at Columbia University with 1,636 cases of pelvimetry, utilizing a variety of techniques. A review of the material at his institution did not reveal a "single best technique." He concluded that pelvimetry could provide a statistical statement of the probability of serious arrest in an individual case and that this could be used as one factor in determining the optimal method of delivery. If, however, a "yes or no" prognosis was desired, x-ray studies were of no value. Steer recommends that elective cesarean section should only be considered for that small group of women in whom the diameter of a circle that fits the inlet is 1 cm or less greater than the fetal head circumference. Even among these women, 24% delivered vaginally, but with a perinatal mortality of 23%.

Russell and Richards (1971) compared obstetrical outcome in 833 patients who underwent pelvimetry for suspected CPD with that of 110 controls who were referred for radiological assessment of maturity. Their findings illustrate how the selection process may affect outcome. No significant differences were noted in fetal size, pelvic measurements, and contracted pelvic planes between the two groups. Despite these similarities the patients selected for pelvimetry because of suspected disproportion had a cesarean section rate of 29%, more than three times the hospital control rate. In addition, the forceps delivery rate in the suspected CPD group was four times that of the controls. Interestingly, the mean birth weight of infants born to the women with suspected disproportion was actually lower than that for the controls.

Joyce and colleagues (1975) reviewed the experience at their institution over a 4-year period using a single erect lateral view to measure the obstetrical conjugate and sacral angle. Their conclusion was that for cephalic presentations pelvimetry was rarely helpful and that a trial of labor was almost always warranted in women who had not undergone previous cesarean sections. They stated that pelvimetry might influence management in a subsequent pregnancy in patients with a poor obstetric history or previous cesarean section. In those cases, however, they recommended that it be performed in the puerperium to avoid irradiating the fetus.

Kelly et al. (1975) analyzed clinical data from 16 hospitals for 67,078 deliveries of singletons weighing 1000 g or more. Pelvimetry was performed on 6.9% of these patients. The authors found that indications for performing this procedure varied from one institution to another and also from doctor to doctor within a given institution. They found no consistent relationship between pelvimetry and cesarean section rates at the hospitals in the study. Of those patients undergoing abdominal delivery, 41% had received pelvimetry. The incidence of cesarean sections was 27% in women whose pelvimetry was interpreted as normal. The authors point out that in this latter group the decision regarding route of delivery was the same, on clinical grounds, as would have been made if pelvimetry had never been used.

Kelly and colleagues also compared two groups of primiparas delivering infants weighing more than 2500 g by cesarean section for CPD. One group had undergone pelvimetry, while the other had not. Essentially no difference was found in the duration of labor experienced by each group. In other words, the use of pelvimetry did not significantly shorten labor in women with CPD when compared with the use of clinical judgment alone. When the duration of labor before cesarean section was examined in those patients having unsuccessful elective oxytocin stimulation, again no significant difference could be demonstrated between those who had pelvimetry and those who did not.

Hannah (1965) retrospectively studied 300 patients who underwent x-ray pelvimetry using a single erect lateral film. He found that a decision to permit or prohibit a trial of labor was based on x-ray assessment of the pelvic architecture in only 5% of cases. In the remaining 95% sufficient clinical information was available at the time the film was taken to allow a precise and sensible plan of management without the necessity of taking an x-ray.

A problem addressed by Kriewall and McPherson (1980) at the University of Michigan was that of individual interpretation of a set of pelvimetry films. When 15 pelvimetry studies were retrospectively examined by a "mixed" group who did not know the pregnancy outcomes, the route of delivery (vaginal versus cesarean section) was correctly predicted in 49% of cases by the clinical faculty, 44% by the house officers, 51% by the medical students, and 53% by the nonclinical personnel. Since it was recognized that delivery by cesarean section may not be due to proven CPD, the analysis was repeated for a group of patients who all had delivered vaginally. In that situation the correct prediction for route of delivery was made in 58% of cases by the faculty, 53% of cases by both the house officers and medical students, and 63% of cases by the nonclinical personnel. Kriewall states that "statistically the results from viewing x-rays alone were no different than if the group had all flipped coins with each patient and made a determination according to the coin flip." He further adds that no consistency of response was found when each subgroup was analyzed separately.

In a study at Yale-New Haven Hospital 100 pelvimetry studies of cephalic presentations were retrospectively analyzed (Fine et al., 1980). The Thoms method of interpretation was compared with the modified Ball technique and both were then contrasted with manual assessment of the pelvis as prognostic indicators for safe vaginal delivery. Uneventful, nonsurgical deliveries occurred in 28.6% of patients with either inlet or midpelvic disproportion by the Thoms method and 22.5% of women with absolute disproportion in either plane by the modified Ball method. Furthermore, neither of these two pelvimetry techniques was significantly more accurate than manual assessment of the pelvis in predicting obstetrical outcome. The authors of this study note that since there was no consistent protocol for the management of labor or operative intervention, conclusions cannot be drawn from the group of patients who underwent cesarean section. Some abdominal deliveries may have been performed for reasons unrelated to proven CPD in patients who would have had an uneventful vaginal delivery if given an adequate trial of labor. On the other hand, the existence of a group of infants who were delivered spontaneously with good Apgar scores despite x-ray evidence of frank disproportion indicates that pelvimetry results may certainly be falsely positive.

As mentioned earlier, all of these studies have serious design flaws. The existing data, however, strongly suggest that x-ray pelvimetry, as utilized clinically, has not been proven to be of significant prognostic usefulness in patients with cephalic presentations.

Breech Presentations

Bony dystocia may be a major cause of fetal morbidity and mortality in term breech presentations. After delivery of the body, an unmolded, aftercoming head must rapidly traverse the birth canal. The types of adjustment made by a fetus in vertex presentation to overcome borderline cephalopelvic disproportion often cannot be made by a breech of comparable size. Precise knowledge of the size of the bony pelvis would, therefore, seem to be a variable of great importance when a patient with a term-sized breech is to be delivered vaginally. For this reason, x-ray pelvimetry has been recommended for any woman with a breech at term who is not going to have an elective cesarean section.

No prospective studies examining pregnancy outcome as a function of pelvimetry results obtained before breech delivery are available. Interestingly, in a large retrospective study of term breech deliveries, Rovinsky et al. (1973) found that the incidence of traumatic excess perinatal mortality was "very significantly higher" among patients who had x-ray pelvimetry as compared with those who did not. They reported this to be more true for multiparas than primiparas. When the cases of traumatic mortality in patients who had received pelvimetry were reviewed, however, all of the fetal deaths were found to have been avoidable. The authors attributed these unhappy outcomes to three errors in clinical judgment: applicability of concepts of adequate pelvic capacity derived from vaginal delivery of vertex presentations; underestimation of fetal weight; and reliance on clinical evidence of pelvic capacity, such as birth weight of largest infant delivered vaginally, albeit as a vertex. The author's conclusions, therefore, were the opposite of initial impressions derived from their data. They believed that x-ray pelvimetry should be performed before the onset of labor in every patient with a breech presentation at term regardless of maternal parity, size of infants previously delivered vaginally, or present estim: ted fetal weight. They emphasized that for vaginal delivery to be feasible without undue trauma to mother or infant, all pelvic measurements must be at least mean normal values. Since most textbooks define borderline pelvic capacity, these authors presented data from the older literature which listed mean *normal* pelvic dimensions (Table 1). Given measurements larger than average, they believed that pelvic configuration was of secondary relevance. The inlet dimensions were found to be of paramount importance. No case of significant midpelvic or outlet contraction was encountered when measurements of the inlet were adequate.

While Rovinsky et al. did not recommend that specific pelvic measurements be utilized as lower limits of acceptability, other authors have. Andros has advocated the use of pelvimetry in all cases of term breech deliveries and has recommended the demonstration of a very large pelvis as a prerequisite for safe vaginal delivery (Chez, 1977) (Table 2). He has stated in several articles (Zatuchini and Andros, 1965; 1967) that pelvic diameters adequate for a cephalic presentation may be inadequate for the same fetus in breech presentation. This is true not only because the aftercoming head has no opportunity to mold, but also because the fetocervical extension and rotation inherent in every vaginal breech delivery may introduce cranial dimensions larger than the biparietal diameter for descent through the pelvis.

Collea and colleagues (1978) have reported a randomized prospective study of vaginal versus cesarean delivery of term frank breeches. In all cases, the fetus was a singleton at 36 weeks gestation or older and had an estimated weight of 2500-3500 g. In the group selected for vaginal deivery, x-ray pelvimetry was obtained and 35 of 70 patients were found to have one or more measurements which were inadequate according to a predetermined set of minimal requirements (Table 2). These 35 patients were delivered by elective cesarean section. Of the remaining 35 patients, 30 delivered vaginally. All of these neonates survived; however, two sustained brachial plexus injuries. The authors concluded that there is a role for vaginal delivery in carefully selected cases of term frank breech presentations.

In his series of term frank breech deliveries, O'Leary (1979) required normal gynecoid morphology on pelvimetry and utilized minimal inlet measurements slightly larger than those used by Collea et al. (1978) (Table 2). He also

Table 1. Mean Normal Dimensions of the Adult Female Pelvis (cm)

Pelvic Dimension	Berman (1956)	Thoms and Greulich (1940)	Young and Ince (1940)
Anteroposterior diameter of inlet (obstetric true conjugate)	12.0	11.9	11.8
Transverse diameter of inlet	13.5	12.8	13.1
Interspinous diameter	10.5	10.4	9.9
Intertuberous diameter	10.5	–	10.1
Subpubic angle (degrees)	85.0	–	93.5

Source: Rovinsky, J. J., Miller, J. A., and Solomon, K. (1973). Management of breech presentation at term. *Am. J. Obstet. Gynecol. 115:*497.

Table 2. Minimal Acceptable Pelvimetry Data for Vaginal Delivery of a Term-Sized Breech (cm)

	Chez (1977)	Collea et al. (1978)	O'Leary (1979)
Inlet			
AP	11.0	10.5	11.0
Trans	13.0	11.5	12.0
Midpelvis			
AP	13.0	11.5	–
Bispinous	11.0	10.0	10.0
Other			
	–	–	Sacrum: hollow Subpubic arch: normal

insisted on the presence of a hollow sacrum and a normal subpubic arch. Using these pelvimetry criteria, as well as a number of other objective determinants, he found that vaginal delivery can be safe for breech infants at term.

In an earlier study, Todd and Steer (1963) using the same inlet criteria adopted by O'Leary, found that vaginal delivery was possible in 85% of patients with a radiologically adequate pelvis. The perinatal mortality in this group was 0.5%. When, however, the inlet had an AP diameter of less than 11 cm, and/or a transverse diameter of less than 12 cm, vaginal delivery was accomplished in only 40% of cases with an accompanying perinatal mortality of 5%.

Joyce et al. (1975), using a single standing lateral film, measured the "obstetric conjugate" from the inner edge of the pubic symphysis to the sacral promontory. They found that this measurement should be at least 11.4 cm for a fetus at 38 weeks, and 11.7 cm for a fetus at term to pass through safely as a breech. A graph in their paper, however, shows three failed vaginal deliveries for obstetric conjugates of 12.5-13.3 cm for fetuses weighing 3500 g or less.

Kauppila (1975) has reported that, in a series of full-term breech infants delivered vaginally, when the radiographically determined "conjugata vera" (CV) was 11.5 cm or greater, 15.4% of cases had difficult partial breech extractions. When the CV was less than 11.5 cm this incidence rose to 25.5%, but the difference was not statistically significant. He also found that, in a group of 205 patients with conjugate veras of 12 cm or greater, regular gynecoid inlets, and normal outlets, 17% experienced difficulties in partial extraction, while 19.4% of controls who had not had pelvimetry had similar difficulties. The author concluded that even a roentgenologically normal pelvis does not guarantee an easy vaginal delivery.

Beischer (1966) presented a series in which 65 patients with term breech fetuses were demonstrated to have some degree of pelvic contracture on pelvimetry. Fifty-one of these women were given a trial of labor and 36 delivered vaginally. The perinatal mortality rate was 11% in those delivered vaginally and an additional 14% had difficult deliveries of the aftercoming head. The criteria of critical pelvic contraction in this series was found to be 10 cm for the "true conjugate," 12 cm for the transverse of the inlet, 20 cm for the interspinous plus available AP diameters of the outlet, and 9.5 cm for the available AP of the outlet. Beischer concluded that a trial labor is contraindicated in breech presentation when significant pelvic contraction exists, even though the fetus is considered to be of below-average weight.

IS PELVIMETRY WORTHWHILE?

Controversy continues to exist about the value of pelvimetry, but more and more reports have concluded that it is no longer needed for the management of dysfunctional labor in a patient with a vertex presentation. The issue of x-ray hazard has not been addressed in this discussion, but there is evidence that any radiation of the fetus may have serious long-term effects (Stewart, 1958; Rugh, 1958; MacMahon, 1962; Natarajan and Bross, 1973; Gauldin, 1974). As Schifrin (1974) has stated, despite continuing dispute, there is no evidence to suggest that x-ray is not without at least a potential risk.

When a patient with a vertex presentation has failed to make progress in labor, the question posed by the clinician who orders pelvimetry is "Will this baby fit through this pelvis?" Many of the reports cited in this chapter suggest that an x-ray study simply cannot answer that question with enough accuracy to base a rational management decision on the information provided. When disproportion is so severe that vaginal delivery is clearly impossible, as in cases of rickets, traumatic pelvic deformities, dwarfism, etc., the evidence will be obvious on clinical examination. When this is not the case, most authors today believe that a well-controlled trial of labor is indicated. Schifrin has stated that increases in fetal morbidity and mortality associated with various patterns of dysfunctional labor essentially disappear if midforceps deliveries are abandoned and all deliveries are either spontaneous vaginal or cesarean (Schifin, 1974). This statement is based on the observation that it is the technique of delivery and not, within limits, the labor pattern itself that so drastically alters perinatal outcome.

Friedman (1976), on the other hand, advocates the use of Ball pelvimetry for patients with vertex presentations who develop secondary arrests of dilatation, arrests of descent, or prolonged deceleration phases. If disproportion is demonstrated by this technique, he advocates immediate cesarean section to prevent the morbidity associated with further labor. In the study by Fine et al. (1980), however, it has been demonstrated that absolute disproportion by the Ball method may be associated with an uneventful vaginal delivery in more than 20% of cases. Furthermore, in that series, the Ball method was not found to be any more accurate in predicting obstetrical outcome than the Thoms method or manual assessment of the pelvis. We, therefore, agree with Schifrin and others who advocate a trial of labor in women with vertex presentations who develop dysfunctional patterns during the active phase of labor. This, of course, must be accompanied by objective monitoring of continued fetal well-being, as well as evidence of effective uterine contractions.

At Yale-New Haven Hospital a trial of labor is conducted with an intrauterine catheter in place to measure directly the pressure generated by contractions. Intravenous pitocin is administered by infusion pump, at increasing doses, until 50 mmHg contractions occurring every 2-3 min are obtained. The fetal heart rate is continuously monitored with an EKG electrode attached to the fetal scalp. If, after 2-3 hr of this type of stimulation, no progress has been made, a cesarean section is performed. Midforceps deliveries are assiduously avoided in this group of patients, and failure to bring the head down to the perineum is further indication for abdominal delivery. By utilizing this approach, and steadfastly avoiding difficult vaginal deliveries, we have been impressed with the lack of associated fetal morbidity. Furthermore, each woman is given an optimal opportunity to deliver vaginally, while fetal exposure to x-radiation is entirely eliminated. In our opinion, advocates of x-ray pelvimetry are obligated to show, in a properly constructed randomized prospective study, that the use of that potentially dangerous modality offers clear-cut advantages over our approach.

The usefulness of pelvimetry in patients with breech presentations is different. Schifrin (1974) has argued that it has no place in the management of patients with breech delivery because it cannot predict difficulties which will occur at the time of delivery. Commenting on the results of the study by Rovinsky et al. (1973), he points out that when disproportion was demonstrated in that series, elective cesarean section was performed. When the pelvic measurements were considered adequate, however, vaginal delivery was undertaken and this group of infants suffered excessive traumatic morbidity. Kauppila (1975) has also noted, in his large series, that women with pelves demonstrated to be normal by x-ray may have difficulty at the time of delivery. These observations, however, are oversimplifications of the data. More than pelvimetry measurements must be considered before deciding whether a patient should deliver a term breech vaginally. The estimated fetal weight, type of breech presentation, progress in labor, and attitude of the fetal head must be considered, in addition to other variables. Collea et al. (1978) and O'Leary (1979) have demonstrated that carefully selected breeches can be delivered safely at term if attention is paid to appropriate screening procedures. In both series, evaluation prior to delivery included an objective assessment of the pelvic bony architecture. Beischer (1966), and Todd and Steer (1963) have all shown that when pelvimetry measurements are suboptimal, an increased risk of perinatal morbidity and mortality exists. If an obstetrician decides that the risk associated with the vaginal delivery of *any* breech at term is unacceptable, the argument becomes academic. If, however, selection criteria are used to screen a population of candidates for vaginal delivery, we believe that the objective demonstration of a roomy gynecoid pelvis should be part of that evaluation.

REFERENCES

Ball, R. P. (1936). Roentgen pelvimetry and fetal cephalometry. *Surg. Gynecol. Obstet. 62*:798.

Ball, R. P., and Marchbanks, S. S. (1933). Roentgen pelvimetry cephalometry: A new technique. *Radiology 24*:77.

Barton, J. J., and Garbaciak, J. A. (1979). Is x-ray pelvimetry necessary? *Contemp. Ob./Gyn. 13*:27.

Beischer, N. A. (1966). Pelvic contraction in breech presentation. *J. Obstet. Gynaecol. Br. Commonw. 73*:421.

Caldwell, M. E., and Moloy, H. C. (1933). Anatomical variations in the female pelves and their effect in labor with a suggested classification. *Am. J. Obstet. Gynecol. 26*:479.

Caldwell, M. E., Moloy, H. C., and Swenson, P. C. (1939). The use of the roentgen rays in obstetrics. I. Roentgen pelvimetry and cephalometry: technique of pelvioroentgenography. *Am. J. Roentgenol. 41*:305.

Chez, R. A. (1977). Management of breech presentation. Symposium. *Contemp. Ob./Gyn. 10*:118.

Colcher, A. E., and Sussman, W. (1944). A practical technique for roentgen pelvimetry with a new positioning. *Am. J. Roentgenol. 5*:207.

Collea, J. V., Rabin, S. C., Weghorts, G. R., and Quilligan, E. J. (1978). The randomized management of term frank breech presentation: Vaginal delivery versus cesarean section. *Am. J. Obstet. Gynecol. 131*:186.

Fine, E. A., Bracken, M., and Berkowitz, R. L. (1980). An evaluation of the usefulness of x-ray pelvimetry: Comparison of the Thoms and modified Ball methods with manual pelvimetry. *Am. J. Obstet. Gynecol. 137*:15.

Friedman, E. A. (1976). Evaluation and management of pelvic dystocia. *Contemp. Ob./Gyn. 7*:155.

Friedman, E. A., and Taylor, M. B. (1969). A modified nomographic aid for x-ray cephalopelvimetry. *Am. J. Obstet. Gynecol. 105*:1110.

Gauldin, M. E. (1974). Possible effects of diagnostic x-ray on human embryo and fetus. *J. Ark. Med. Soc. 70*:424.

Hannah, W. J. (1965). X-ray pelvimetry—a critical appraisal. *Am. J. Obstet. Gynecol. 91*:333.

Joyce, D. N., Giwa-Osagie, F., and Stevenson, G. W. (1975). Role of pelvimetry in active management of labour. *Br. Med. J. 4*:505.

Kauppila, O. (1975). The perinatal mortality in breech deliveries and observations on affecting factors. *Acta Obstet. Gynecol. Scand. [Suppl.] 39.*

Kelly, K. M., Madden, D. A., Arcarese, J. S., Barnett, M., and Brown, R. F. (1975). The utilization and efficacy of pelvimetry. *Am. J. Roentgenol. Radium Ther. Nucl. Med. 125*:66.

Klapholz, H. (1975). A computerized aid to Ball pelvimetry. *Am. J. Obstet. Gynecol. 121*:1067.

Kriewall, T. J., and McPherson, G. K. (1980). Effects of uterine contractility on the fetal cranium: Perspectives from the past, present and future. In *Advances in Perinatal Medicine.* S. Milunsky, E. A. Friedman and L. Gluck (Eds.), Plenum Press, New York.

MacMahon, B. (1962). Prenatal x-ray exposure and childhood cancer. *J. Natl. Cancer Inst. 28*:1173.

Natarajan, N., and Bross, I. D. J. (1973). Preconception radiation and leukemia. *J. Med. 4*:276.

O'Leary, J. A. (1979). Vaginal delivery of the term breech. *Obstet. Gynecol. 53*:341.

Pritchard, J. and MacDonald, P. (1976). *Williams Obstetrics,* 15th ed. Appleton-Centruy-Crofts, New York.

Rovinsky, J. J., Miller, J. A., and Kaplan, S. (1973). Management of breech presentation at term. *Am. J. Obstet. Gynecol. 115*:497.

Rugh, R. (1958). X-radiation effects on the human fetus. *J. Pediatr. 52*:531.

Russell, J. G. B., and Richards, B. (1971). A review of pelvimetry data. *Br. J. Radiol. 44*:780.

Schifrin, B. S. (1974). The case against pelvimetry. *Contemp. Ob./Gyn.* *4*:77.

Schwarz, G. S., Kirkpatrick, R. H., and Tovell, H. M. M. (1956). Correlation of cephalopelvimetry to obstetrical outcome with special reference to radiologic disproportion. *Radiology* *67*:854.

Steer, C. M. (1958). X-ray pelvimetry and the outcome of labor. *Am. J. Obstet. Gynecol.* *76*:118.

Stewart, A. M. (1958). Survey of childhood malignancies. *Br. Med. J.* *2*: 1495.

Thoms, H. (1929). A new method of roentgen pelvimetry. *JAMA* *92*:1515.

Thoms, H. (1940). Roentgen pelvimetry as a routine prenatal procedure. *Am. J. Obstet. Gynecol.* *40*:891.

Thoms, H. (1941). The clinical application of roentgen pelvimetry and a study of the results in 1,100 white women. *Am. J. Obstet. Gynecol.* *42*:957.

Todd, W. D., and Steer, C. M. (1963). Term breech: Review of 1006 term breech deliveries. *Obstet. Gynecol.* *22*:583.

Zatuchni, G. I., and Andros, G. J. (1965). Prognostic index for vaginal delivery in breech presentation at term. *Am. J. Obstet. Gynecol.* *93*:237.

Zatuchni, G. I., and Andros, G. J. (1967). Prognostic index for vaginal delivery in breech presentation at term—Prospective study. *Am. J. Obstet. Gynecol.* *98*:854.

10
Methods of Induction of Labor

IAN RICHARD JOHNSON / University Hospital, Queen's Medical Centre, Nottingham, England

METHODS OF INDUCTION OF LABOR

Induction of labor is a procedure that has been used for hundreds of years for various indications. Many techniques have been employed and in recent years, as these techniques have become safer, induction has been used more widely than ever. The basic requirements of any induction technique are that it should be:

1. Safe for the mother
2. Safe for the fetus
3. Acceptable to the patient
4. Easy for the doctor to perform
5. Lead to a short induction-delivery interval

Ideally the method should, in physiological terms, closely mimic the onset of natural labor, or quickly put the patient in the same position as if she had entered labor naturally.

The history of the methods used for induction of labor has been reviewed by Nixon and Smyth (1959). These methods can be divided into six major groups:

1. Drugs such as castor oil or quinine
2. 'Physiological' drugs such as oxytocin and prostaglandins

213

3. "Physiological" physical methods such as breast massage
4. Dilatation of the cervix, instrumentally or with osmotic dilators
5. Artificial rupture of the membranes
6. Local irritation of the uterus or its contents, through injection of irritant solutions into the amniotic sac or extraamniotic space.

The more extreme methods have been abandoned because they were either unsafe or ineffective. Methods used in the last decade include:

Mechanical:
    Laminaria tents
    Enema
    Rupture of the membranes
    Membrane sweep

Pharmacological:
    Castor oil
    Oxytocin: buccal
                  intravenous
    Prostaglandins: oral
                  intramuscular
                  intravenous
                  extra-amniotic
                  vaginal
                  intracervical

Although all of these methods are still in use, either singly, or in combination, the most commonly employed technique is that of artificial rupture of the membranes.

ARTIFICIAL RUPTURE OF THE MEMBRANES

Artificial rupture of the membranes (amniotomy or ARM) is one of the oldest methods of induction of labor. It has remained popular because of its relative efficiency and safety when used with proper care.

Because an indication to induce labor automatically places the patient in an "at risk" group, the possibility of operative intervention after ARM is increased and it is prudent to restrict the ingestion of food and drink immediately before ARM. The patient may be starved overnight and induced early in the morning, or, alternatively, be given a light breakfast at least 2 hr before the procedure. To facilitate descent of the presenting part and to reduce the risk of fecal contamination during labor, the patient is given an enema before ARM.

Amniotomy should only be performed for induction of labor in well-equipped obstetric units, prepared to proceed to cesarean section immediately if required. The procedure is usually performed in the delivery suite. It involves the introduction of surgical instruments into the uterine cavity, together with the removal of an important barrier to fetal infection. Consequently, care must be taken to avoid the introduction of infection into the uterus and the operator should observe normal aseptic precautions, "scrubbing-up," draping the patient, and using sterile instruments. The procedure is often uncomfortable for the patient and may be painful. It is usually performed in the lithotomy position and this may increase the patient's embarrassment, discomfort, and anxiety. It is important, therefore, that a full explanation be given to the patient before the procedure begins as to why it is being performed and exactly what will be done. In the majority of cases an experienced obstetrician will be able to perform the amniotomy without the patient requiring any sedation. A midwife or nurse reassuring anxious patients is a great help, but occasionally some form of analgesia is required. Inhalation agents such as nitrous oxide and oxygen mixtures are the safest and easiest drugs to use. Parenteral or oral sedatives can be used, but their effects will last long past the time of ARM; because of their long half-life and their effects on the newborn, benzodiazepines are best avoided. General anesthesia has been employed in the past, but the risks of a general anesthetic in pregnancy are such that this is only rarely justified for amniotomy (Brant, 1970).

It is almost invariably possible to perform an ARM in late pregnancy by passing a sharp instrument through the cervical os. The procedure is only performed safely, however, when a finger can be pushed through the cervical os sufficiently far to feel the presenting part. The finger is used to sweep around the lower segment of the uterus, separating the membranes and forming a discreet bag of amniotic fluid, the forewaters (Fig. 1). These are then broken by any of a large variety of instruments, some specially designed for the purpose. Commonly used instruments are the amniotomy hook and Gelder forewater amniotomy forceps, but probably the most straightforward are Kocher's forceps (Fig. 2). Puncture of the membranes with any of these instruments leads to drainage of the forewaters.

The alternative to straightforward rupture of the forewaters is to use a Drew-Smythe catheter to break the hindwaters. This instrument (Fig. 3) is passed through the cervical canal and around the fetal head in the extra-amniotic space. Once the catheter is in position, a trocar is used to puncture the membranes behind the head. The trocar is withdrawn and liquor drained from the main body of the amniotic cavity (Fig. 4).

It has been claimed (Drew-Smythe, 1931) that use of the Drew-Smythe catheter to drain the hindwaters has distinct advantages over forewater rupture.

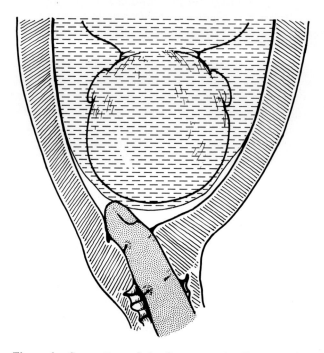

Figure 1. Separation of the forewaters by "sweeping" the membranes.

Because the hole in the sac is further from the vagina there may be less risk of infection spreading to the amniotic fluid. The release of the hindwaters avoids allowing a sudden gush of fluid to prolapse the umbilical cord, and, when the fetal head is high, less disturbance may be caused by hindwater rupture than forewater, with consequently less likelihood of the head floating away and an abnormal presentation developing. A cleaner sample of amniotic fluid may be obtained, not contaminated with vaginal debris or blood, which may be of use in the estimation of surfactant levels. Liquor obtained from the hindwaters will always be stained with meconium if any has been passed by the fetus, whereas the forewaters, being isolated by an engaged fetal head, may be clear.

Despite these postulated advantages, hindwater rupture is not commonly performed. Passage of the Drew-Smythe catheter around the fetal head is not always easy, and forewater rupture often results. Hindwater rupture is less successful than forewater in inducing labor, possibly because the amnion and chorion override each other and effectively seal off the opening. There is a risk of pushing the catheter into the edge of the placenta and causing bleeding, or even of rupturing the uterus. The Drew-Smythe catheter may be used

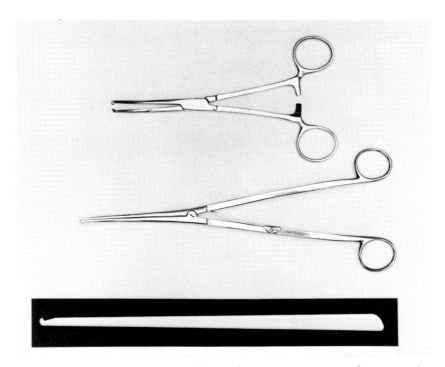

Figure 2. The amniotomy hook, Gelder forewater amniotomy forceps, and Kocher's forceps.

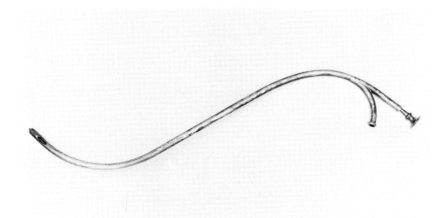

Figure 3. The Drew-Smythe catheter.

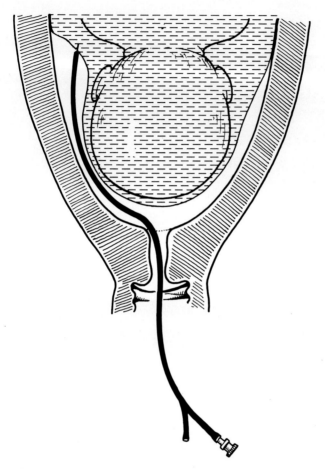

Figure 4. Rupture of the hindwaters with a Drew-Smythe catheter.

for obtaining a clear specimen of liquor from the forewaters for culture or surfactant estimation. Use of the catheter to rupture the membranes through a cervix that will not allow passage of a finger or larger instrument is to be avoided, unless the operator is absolutely certain of the attitude of the presenting part. The dangers of such a blind procedure to a face or brow presentation are obvious.

Forewater rupture is the usual procedure. The presenting part should ideally be engaged, although, if the cervix is safely applied to the presenting part, the station is not necessarily important. The floating, mobile presenting part, above the brim of the pelvis, is dangerous and more likely to become unstable or to lead to a prolapsed cord after amniotomy. If care is taken to avoid these cases it is probable that the incidence of prolapsed cord is greater in cases of spontaneous rupture of the membranes than at amniotomy. It is certainly safer to have the cord prolapse into the vagina when the operator's hand is also there, rather than when the patient is in the community or prenatal ward. The fetal presenting part can be prevented from pushing on the cord, cesarean section can be performed immediately, and the fetus should not be put in any danger. The risks of infection after forewater rupture are minimized by attention to aseptic techniques, a short induction-delivery interval, and the use of prophylactic antibiotics in those few cases in which the membranes have been ruptured for longer than 24 hr.

The advantages of forewater rupture as a method of induction are several. The color of the draining liquor can be inspected for the presence of meconium, a sign of fetal distress and an indication to take a fetal blood sample, itself only possible because of the ARM exposing the presenting part. The volume of liquor draining can also be estimated. Scanty loss indicates potential fetal problems as it may be associated with growth retardation or postmaturity. In some cases no liquor is found and a hair plucked from the fetal scalp is the only evidence of successful amniotomy. The exposure of the fetal presenting part allows an electrode to be attached to the fetus, to monitor accurately the fetal heart rate throughout labor. An intrauterine catheter connected to a pressure transducer may also be put in position to monitor uterine contractions. Drainage of the forewaters allows descent of the fetal head onto the cervix and increases the efficiency of labor.

The major disadvantage of ARM is the possibility of infection. Spread of bacteria from the vagina and ectocervix to the amniotic cavity is largely prevented by intact membranes. Once broken, the membranes cease to be an effective barrier and the spread of infection is further enhanced by introduction of surgical instruments through the cervix at ARM and the fingers at vaginal examination. The longer the induction-delivery interval, the longer the organisms have to spread through the cervix and, generally, the more vaginal examinations are performed to assess progress, adding to the risks. Consequently, the performance of an ARM automatically puts a deadline on delivery. The length of time allowed for delivery to take place after ARM varies from center to center, but if labor continues to progress, as measured by cervical dilatation and descent of the presenting part, the patient may be allowed to continue in labor for up to 24 hr.

It is not clear why amniotomy is ever effective in inducing the onset of labor. Reducing the volume held in the uterus may be important. If this were so the procedure would not be effective in cases of oligohydramnios, which it is, and would be even more effective when large quantities of fluid are drained at hindwater rupture, which it is not. Ocytocin release from the posterior pituitary is promoted by stimulation of the cervix and vagina, such as occurs at vaginal examination. Since the half-life of oxytocin in the circulation is very short it is unlikely that the release of this hormone during examination plays a substantial role in the onset of labor. The concentrations of prostaglandin $F_{2\alpha}$ and 13,14 dehydro-15-keto prostaglandin F, a prostaglandin metabolite, are both increased after amniotomy (Mitchell et al., 1976), an increase that, in humans, is not dependent upon transient release of oxytocin (Sellers et al., 1980). Fetal membranes contain enzymes capable of prostaglandin synthesis (Kierse and Turnbull, 1976) and disruption of the membranes at amniotomy may cause a release of prostaglandins locally in the uterus, leading to the onset of labor.

Whatever the physiological basis, ARM has been shown to be a safe and easily performed procedure. Its efficiency in inducing labor in late pregnancy, however, is not acceptable. Turnbull and Anderson (1967) showed that only 75% of a mixed group of primigravidas and multigravidas were in labor 24 hr after ARM. Factors of importance in determining the patients' response to ARM included the favorability of the cervix, parity, and gestational age. The greater the favorability of the cervix, the nearer the patient to term, and the less the number of previous pregnancies, the faster the onset of labor. Of these factors, ripeness of the cervix appeared to be the most important (Turnbull and Anderson, 1967).

Amniotomy, therefore, carries advantages in terms of accessibility of the fetus and liquor, but is not, of itself, efficient enough in causing the onset of labor, particularly when the cervix is unripe. It follows that some other agent or agents must be used to improve the efficiency of induction of labor. This agent could be employed in one of three ways:

As a preliminary to amniotomy (a ripening agent)
Instead of amniotomy
In conjunction with amniotomy

Some drugs have been used in all three ways.

CERVICAL RIPENING

Cocks (1955) discussed the significance of the initial condition of the cervix to the subsequent course of labor and classified degrees of ripeness of the cervix. He showed that an unripe cervix at the onset of induction led to a long induction-delivery interval. In a similar study, Friedman (1962) stated that if the cervix was unripe at the time of induction there was an increase in both the number of forceps deliveries and cesarean sections.

When faced with an unfavorable cervix, the obstetrician should reconsider the need to induce labor, particularly if postmaturity is one of the indications for induction. While it is quite possible for a patient to be postmature with an unripe cervix it is more likely that an error has been made in the calculation of her expected date of delivery. If delivery is really necessary, the combination of the indication for delivery and the prospect of a long induction-delivery interval may warrant elective cesarean section. When these points have been considered, those patients still requiring induction of labor are given a ripening agent as a preliminary to normal induction. The attempt to ripen the cervix has the advantage that it does not necessarily commit the patient to delivery within a certain set period. Because the procedure may stress the fetus it should still be treated as seriously as formal induction. Consequently the indication for ripening and induction should be sufficiently important to warrant operative delivery should that become necessary.

The agents that have been used for cervical ripening fall into two groups:

Osmotic dilators, such as laminaria tents
Pharmacological agents, oxytoxics such as oxytocin and the prostaglandins, and estrogens

Laminaria Tents

Laminaria tents are made of the dried stems of a seaweed. When immersed in water they swell considerably and if placed, in their dry state, in the cervix, absorb water, swell, and cause cervical dilatation. Their use originally led to problems with intrauterine infection because of the difficulty of sterilizing them. Now that they are sterilized by radiation they have once again become popular. By ripening the cervix prior to induction of labor they have been shown (Tohan et al., 1979) to shorten the induction-delivery interval and reduce the operative delivery rate. They may work by slowly swelling and stretching the cervix, making it dilate. Consideration must be given, however, to the high concentrations of arachidonic acid, a precursor of prostaglandins E_2 and $F_{2\alpha}$, in the seaweed. Arachidonic acid stimulates collagen breakdown in the cervix (Ellwood et al., 1980) and consequently laminaria may soften the cervix by changing the nature of its ground substance. Some patients given laminaria to ripen the cervix will go into labor spontaneously (Tohan et al., 1979) and it has been suggested (Agress and Benedetti, 1981) that synthesis of prostaglandins from the arachidonic acid in the laminaria leads to an increase in uterine activity. Alternatively, stretching of the cervix may itself increase the release of both prostaglandins and oxytocin. Because uterine activity may be increased the fetus is put under stress. An intrauterine fetal death has been reported (Agress and Benedetti, 1981) associated with the use of laminaria for cervical ripening. Consequently, the fetal heart rate should be monitored throughout the ripening process, to prevent intrapartum asphyxia.

Oxytocin

Oxytocin, or its synthetic form syntocinon, has been used for many years in attempts to ripen the cervix or to induce labor. Embrey (1962) found that the range of individual response to intravenous oxytocin was very variable and depended to a large extent on the state of the cervix. If the cervix was unfavorable the response to oxytocin was poor; hardly a recommendation for the use of the drug as a ripening agent. Buccal oxytocin can be used, but the rate of absorption is unpredictable and there is a risk of uterine hypertonicity. Once again, oxytocin by this route is not effective when the cervix is unripe (Dillon et al., 1960). Oxytocin is inactivated in the gut and therefore cannot be given orally; intramuscular oxytocin has been abandoned because of the dangers of overstimulation of the uterus. Although intravenous syntocinon has been used before amniotomy in attempts to ripen the cervix (Anderson, 1965; Beazley and Gillespie, 1971) the results have, in general, been poor. Ripening does not take place and the patient is inconvenienced with an infusion. Because of the danger of uterine activity occurring and leading to fetal asphyxia, the fetal heart rate must be continuously monitored. There is a small risk of amniotic fluid embolism. Because of these problems oxytocin should be, and largely has been, abandoned as a ripening agent.

Prostaglandins

Cervical ripening has been produced successfully using prostaglandins E_2 and $F_{2\alpha}$ by a variety of routes. Comparison of intravenous oxytocin and oral prostaglandin E_2 (Valentine, 1977) showed that the prostaglandin improved the favorability of the cervix and shortened the subsequent induction-delivery interval. Prostaglandins have also been given intramuscularly and intravenously (Karim et al., 1968), but the half-lives of these substances are such that the dose required to achieve a significant local concentration in the uterus is high enough to cause unwanted effects such as vomiting and diarrhea, limiting the acceptability of the technique to the patient.

Local application of prostaglandins to the uterus has allowed a higher concentration to be achieved without unacceptable side effects. In a trial of prostaglandin E_2 in viscous gel applied in the extra-amniotic intrauterine space (Calder et al., 1977) there was a 25% reduction in the length of induced labor. A simpler technique, application of 5 mg of prostaglandin E_2 in a 4% viscous cellulose gel into the upper vagina (Mackenzie and Embrey, 1977) caused nearly 50% of the patients to go into spontaneous labor. Comparison of the methods of ripening in a small series (Wilson, 1978) showed that extra-amniotic prostaglandin E$_2$ gel was the most efficient ripening agent and led to a shorter induction-delivery interval and a lower cesarean section rate than the others. Intravaginal prostaglandin E$_2$ gel was nearly as effective and was slightly more acceptable to the patient. Oral prostaglandins and intravenous syntocinon were much less effective.

The mode of action of the prostaglandins is uncertain. It has been assumed that the prostaglandins cause uterine contractions to increase in intensity and frequency, consequently ripening the cervix. Recent investigations (Ekman et al., 1980) have shown that changes occur in the ground substance of the cervix, including a 30% increase in the mucopolysaccharide concentration. It is possible that these agents work by two methods: increasing uterine activity and directly softening the cervix.

Because uterine activity is increased during ripening by prostaglandins, the fetus is put under stress. Consequently, the fetal heart rate must be monitored continuously. Fetal intrapartum deaths have been reported when this has not been done (Quinn et al., 1981). This seriously limits the usefulness of prostaglandins, since the patient, after a relatively noninvasive procedure such as having vaginal gel inserted, has to be immobilized by an external fetal heart recorder. Clearly an agent that caused cervical ripening by a direct effect upon the cervix without any increase in uterine activity would be of great benefit. The patient would be much more comfortable and could walk around without being attached to machinery. The search for such an agent has recently concentrated upon the estrogens.

Estrogen Gels

Estrogens increase the excitability of the uterine muscle and cause an increase in myometrial activity throughout pregnancy. Direct application of estradiol in gel to the cervix, however, ripens the cervix, but causes only a slight increase in uterine activity (Gordon and Calder, 1977). In a comparison of estriol and prostaglandin F$_{2\alpha}$ gels (Quinn et al., 1981), the ripening effect of both gels was similar when they were given into the extra-amniotic space, but the estriol caused significantly less uterine activity than prostaglandin F$_{2\alpha}$. Comparison of estradiol and prostaglandin E$_2$ gels showed similar results (Stewart et al., 1981). The prostaglandin E$_2$ was slightly more effective in ripening the cervix, but estradiol caused only minimal uterine activity.

Unfortunately, although estrogen gels cause cervical ripening with less uterine activity than prostaglandins, some activity and potential stress to the fetus seems inevitable. Consequently, patients receiving these forms of treatment still require continuous fetal heart rate monitoring. A clear advantage of estrogens over prostaglandins remains to be demonstrated.

INDUCTION OF LABOR WITHOUT AMNIOTOMY

Although one occasionally hears of the combination of castor oil, an enema, and a bath used in an attempt to induce labor, this technique has largely fallen into disuse because it is unpleasant for the patient and ineffective. In recent years induction of labor without amniotomy has depended upon oxytocic drugs, oxytocin, and prostaglandins.

Oxytocin

Oxytocin used alone is effective in inducing labor in a few patients near term. The response of the uterus is estrogen-dependent and increases with advancing gestational age as the number of oxytocin receptors in the uterus increases (Soloff, 1975). Although several different routes of administration have been used, (sublingual, intramuscular, intranasal, and intravenous), all have been abandoned except for the last because of unreliable absorption and the dangers of hyperstimulation.

Intravenous oxytocin is administered to the patient in gradually increasing doses until efficient contractions are established. A typical regime would begin at 1 mU/min and be increased logarithmically, doubling the dose every 15 min until the patient begins contracting adequately, perhaps three contractions every 10 min. This type of regime is best managed with an infusion pump such as the Ivac (see Fig. 5) which delivers a set number of drops of a known concentration of oxytocin solution every minute. These pumps are reliable, easily adjusted, and have an alarm system to alert the midwife if problems should arise.

Oxytocin infusion to induce labor has the advantage that the obstetrician is not committed to delivery within a set time limit, as long as the membranes remain intact. It used to be the practice for infusions to run all day and be taken down at night if not effective, allowing the patient some sleep before they were begun again the following day. Disadvantages include the risk of amniotic fluid embolism, a sudden increase in the sensitivity of the uterus to oxytocin at rupture of the membranes leading to hypertonicity, and, very occasionally, antidiuretic effects of high-dose oxytocin leading to fluid retention and even water intoxication. Most commonly, however, the infusion is just not effective, leading to prolonged induction-delivery intervals, sometimes of several days, with a consequent increase in maternal and fetal morbidity. Because of this failure to induce labor effectively, oxytocin infusions before amniotomy have largely been abandoned.

Prostaglandins

The myometrium contains specific binding sites for prostaglandins (Kimbell et al., 1975). Activation of these sites causes uterine contraction. Intravenous

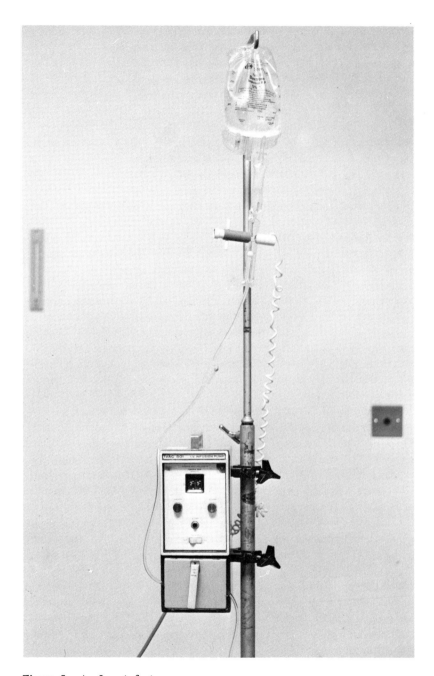

Figure 5. An Ivac infusion pump.

infusions of prostaglandin $F_{2\alpha}$ (Karim et al., 1968) and E_2 (Karim et al., 1970) have been used to induce labor and have been reported to lead to a short induction-delivery interval and cause very few unwanted effects. This has not been the experience of all obstetricians. Because prostaglandins are usually synthesized and released locally, leading to high local concentrations, they have to be given systemically in relatively large doses. A typical regime of 0.5-2.0 μg/min will cause adequate contractions even in the presence of intact membranes or early in pregnancy. Consequently, these drugs are useful for induction of abortion as well as labor. The problem, however, is that at these doses many patients suffer moderately severe gastrointestinal side effects, such as diarrhea, nausea, and vomiting. So, although these drugs are effective in inducing labor when given intravenously, their usefulness is limited by the unwanted effects.

Oral prostaglandins are effective in producing uterine contractions, and are given as tablets containing 0.5 mg prostaglandin E_2. The tablets are given hourly in increasing dose until adequate contractions are produced, up to a maximum dose of 2 mg/hr. With the higher doses, up to two-thirds of patients have labor induced successfully (Nelson and Bryans, 1978), but the incidence of diarrhea, vomiting, and, occasionally, uterine hypertonicity is also high. The dose of prostaglandin E_2 used, therefore, should rarely exceed 1.0-1.5 mg/hr, with a consequent reduction in efficiency. In term multigravidas with ripe cervices, oral prostaglandins may be used successfully to induce labor, with the advantage that the patient does not have an intravenous infusion and may be more comfortable.

Extra-amniotic infusions of prostaglandin E_2 are used for induction of second trimester abortion and are most successfully used to induce labor at a dose of 1 μg/min, increasing to 4 μg/min or until contractions are established (Calder et al., 1976). The solution of prostaglandin E_2 in 0.9% sodium chloride solution is infused through a number 12 Foley catheter placed in the extra-amniotic space. The method has a low incidence of unwanted effects, but is less acceptable to the patient because the catheter must be inserted through the cervical os. There is a risk of intrauterine infection and if contractions cease a vaginal examination must be performed to make sure that the catheter is still in place. These problems can be overcome by using a single dose of prostaglandin in Tylose gel. This technique is widely used to induce labor in cases of intrauterine fetal death, but because of the infection risk involved in pushing a catheter through the cervical os, it may be preferable to use prostaglandin gel in the vagina.

Prostaglandin E_2 given intravaginally is effective in inducing labor. The incidence of unwanted gastrointestinal effects is low and the technique is acceptable to the patient. The risk of intrauterine infection is not increased, and if a slow-release preparation is used it can be removed from the vagina if contractions become too strong or frequent. Using a glycine-based pessary, Mackenzie et al. (1981) found that labor became established in a significant proportion of patients. Primigravidas were given pessaries containing 5 mg of prostaglandin E_2 and multigravidas 2.5 mg prostaglandin E_2 pessaries. All of the patients had amniotomies after 3 hr; 66% of the primigravidas and 81% of the multigravidas established themselves in labor without oxytocin. As well as this efficiency in establishing labor, there is a marked reduction in the cesarean section rate when prostaglandin E_2 vaginal pessaries are used instead of ARM and oxytocin (Hefni and Lewis, 1980) and the length of labor is reduced. The only drawback is the relative inaccessibility of the fetus when the membranes are intact.

Prostaglandins can, therefore, be used to induce labor without ARM. The intravenous and oral routes have limitations, mainly because of unwanted gastrointestinal effects. Extra-amniotic delivery of the drug is very effective, but is more difficult and less acceptable to the patient than the use of vaginal pessaries. Whichever route is used, great care must be taken if oxytocin is subsequently given during labor, because prostaglandins and oxytocin act synergistically and a tonic contraction may result.

USE OF OXYTOCICS IN CONJUNCTION WITH AMNIOTOMY

At one time it was conventional to delay syntocinon infusion for 24 hr folowing ARM, because 70% of these patients would by then have delivered or be established in labor. This clearly added to the risks of infection and caused many patients to undergo a prolonged induction-delivery interval. Using amniotomy and simultaneous syntocinon infusion, Bradford and Gordon (1968) showed that 78% of their patients were delivered within 12 hours. Patterson (1971) compared amniotomy alone with amniotomy and simultaneous syntocinon infusion and showed 12-hr delivery rates of 38.5 and 85.5%, respectively. It has now become standard practice to commence the syntocinon infusion at amniotomy. A typical regime would begin at 1 mU/min and increase by 3mU/min every 15 min until adequate contractions became established. The dose of syntocinon would be titrated against the uterine response, either approximately, by reducing the dose of drug given once labor was established and progressing well (Beazley et al., 1975), or with an automated infusion system, regulated by the strength of the contractions, such as the Cardiff Infusion System (see Fig. 6).

The advantages of ARM and syntocinon used together are an acceptably short induction-delivery interval and access to the liquor and fetus so that meconium can be seen, a scalp electrode applied, and fetal blood sampled when necessary. The method has disadvantages. Great care has to be taken with the oxytocin infusion, to prevent overstimulation, leading to uterine hypertonicity

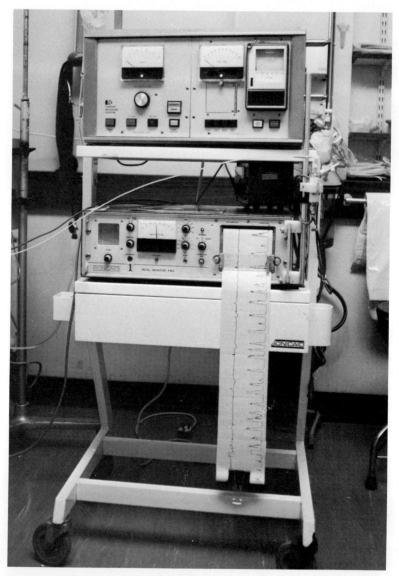

Figure 6. The Cardiff Infusion System.

and consequent fetal distress. If the patient has a relatively unripe cervix the induction-delivery interval may be very prolonged and there is a danger of intrauterine infection. The patient is relatively immobile during labor because of the intravenous infusion. Despite these problems, ARM and syntocinon are commonly used for induction of labor, being reasonably efficient and safe when used with care.

Prostaglandins may be used in conjunction with ARM and are particularly useful when the cervix is relatively unfavorable or the patient is not at term. Intravenous prostaglandins carry too great a penalty in side effects and still immobilize the patient. Oral prostaglandins are of limited use, only being effective in the multigravidas with a ripe cervix. Intravaginal prostaglandins are of value, if used shortly before ARM, in ripening the cervix, establishing contractions, and leading to rapid delivery with a low incidence of fetal problems. The patient does not necessarily need an intravenous infusion and may be more mobile and comfortable.

CHOICE OF METHOD OF INDUCTION OF LABOR (see Fig. 7)

The choice of method of induction depends upon the state of the cervix. If it is unripe ARM may be difficult, and if performed will lead to a high incidence of failed induction, prolonged labor, and a resulting increase in morbidity and mortality. The most convenient, safe, and effective methods of ripening the cervix are with vaginal prostaglandin E_2 or estrogen gel. Both will cause ripening, but both will cause uterine activity as well, although estrogens will do this rather less than prostaglandins. The patient may become

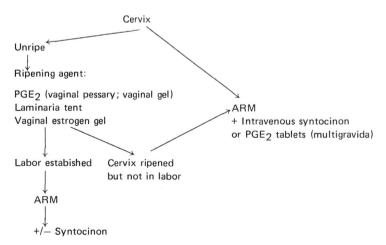

Figure 7. Choice of method of induction.

established in labor without further intervention, but, if not, amniotomy and syntocinon infusion may be instituted at a later stage. If the cervix is ripe, amniotomy may be performed and a syntocinon infusion begun; the dose is increased until contractions are established. Alternatively, a prostaglandin E_2 pessary can be put into the vagina to cause ripening and establish contractions. Amniotomy is then performed 3 hr later and labor augmented with syntocinon if necessary.

RISKS OF INDUCTION OF LABOR

The risks of this procedure are damage to mother or fetus or failure to induce labor at all. Failed induction is now relatively uncommon. Its avoidance depends on use of an appropriate method of induction, ripening the cervix where necessary. The consequence of a failed induction is a cesarean section and it must be stressed that induction of labor should not be entered into lightly.

Because individual response to oxytocics is very variable, hypertonicity, potentially leading to uterine rupture or fetal asphyxia, can only be avoided by using low doses of oxytocics and gradually increasing them until contractions are established. If the patient has true indications for induction she must be "at risk" and use of oxytocics in these patients is a form of "stress test" on the fetus. Consequently, the fetal heart rate should be monitored continuously throughout ripening and induction. This is inconvenient for the doctor and patient, but the procedure cannot be regarded as safe without this watch on fetal welfare.

The object of induction of labor is to effect delivery safely and rapidly with the minimum of inconvenience to the patient. It is clear that the key to this is the ripe cervix, but if cervical ripening techniques are as dangerous as induction itself, the patient is bound to be inconvenienced or the fetus put at risk. Development of cervical ripening agents that work solely by altering the ground substance of the cervix, without concurrent uterine activity or fetal stress, would clearly be a major advance.

REFERENCES

Agress, R. L., and Benedetti, T. J. (1981). Intrauterine fetal death during cervical ripening with laminaria. *Am. J. Obstet. Gynecol. 141*:587-588.

Anderson, M. M. (1965). The state of the cervix and surgical induction of labour. *J. Obstet. Gynaecol. Br. Commonw. 72*:711-716.

Beazley, J. M., Banovic, I., and Feld, M. S. (1975). Maintenance of Labour. *Br. Med. J. 2*:248-250.

Beazley, J. M., and Gillespie, A. (1971). Double-blind trial of prostaglandin E_2 and oxytocin in induction of labour. *Lancet i*:152-155.

Bradford, W. P., and Gordon, G. (1968). Induction of labour by amniotomy and simultaneous syntocinon infusion. *J. Obstet. Gynaecol. Br. Commonw.* 75:698-701.

Brant, H. A. (1970). Amniotomy. *Br. J. Hosp. Med.* 3:116-120.

Calder, A. A., Embrey, M. P., and Tait, T. (1977). Ripening of the cervix with extra-amniotic prostaglandin E_2 in viscous gel before induction of labour. *Br. J. Obstet. Gynaecol.* 84:264-268.

Calder, A. A., Mackenzie, I. Z., and Embrey, M. P. (1976). Intrauterine (extra-amniotic) prostaglandins in the management of unsuccessful pregnancy. *J. Reprod. Med.* 16:271-275.

Cocks, D. P. (1955). Significance of initial condition of cervix uteri to subsequent course of labour. *Br. Med. J.* 1:327-328.

Dillon, T. F., Douglas, R. G., Du Vigneaud, V., and Barber, M. L. (1960). Transbuccal administration of pitocin for induction and stimulation of labour. *Obstet. Gynaecol.* 15:587-592.

Drew-Smythe, H. J. (1931). Indications for the induction of premature labour. *Br. Med. J.* 1:1018-1020.

Ekman, G., Wingemp, L., and Ulmsten, U. (1980). Clinical experiences with a new gel for intracervical application of prostaglandin E_2 before therapeutic abortion or induction of term labour. *Acta Obstet. Gynaecol. Scand. [Suppl.]* 93:83.

Ellwood, D. A., Mitchell, M. D., Anderson, A. B. M., and Turnbull, A. C. (1980). The in vitro production of prostanoids by the human cervix during pregnancy: Preliminary observations. *Br. J. Obstet. Gynaecol.* 87:210-214.

Embrey, M. P. (1962). The effects of intravenous oxytocin on uterine contractility. *J. Obstet. Gynaecol. Br. Commonw.* 69:910-923.

Francis, J. C., Turnbull, A. C., and Thomas, T. F. (1970). Automated oxytocin infusion equipment for induction of labour. *J. Obstet. Gynaecol. Br. Commonw.* 77:594-602.

Friedman, E. A. (1962). Determinant role of initial cervical dilatation on the course of labour. *Am. J. Obstet. Gynecol.* 84:930-935.

Gordon, A. J., and Calder, A. A. (1977). Oestradiol applied locally to ripen the unfavourable cervix. *Lancet* 2:1319-1321.

Hefni, M. A., and Lewis, G. A. (1980). Induction of labour with vaginal prostaglandin E_2 pessaries. *Br. J. Obstet. Gynaecol.* 87:199-202.

Karim, S. M. M., Hillier, K., Trussell, R. R., Patel, R. C., and Tamusange, S. (1970). Induction of labour with prostaglandin E_2. *J. Obstet. Gynaecol. Br. Commonw.* 77:200-210.

Karim, S. M. M., Trussell, R. R., Patel, R. C., and Hillier, K. (1968). Response of pregnant human uterus to prostaglandin $F_{2\alpha}$ induction of labour. *Br. Med. J.* 4:621-623.

Kierse, M. J. N. C., and Turnbull, A. C. (1976). The fetal membranes as a possible source of amniotic fluid prostaglandins. *Br. J. Obstet. Gynaecol.* 83:146-151.

Kimball, F. A., Kirton, K. T., and Wyngarden, L. J. (1975). PGE$_1$-specific binding in rhesus myometrium. *Prostaglandins 10*:853-864.

Mackenzie, I. Z., Bradley, S., and Embrey, P. (1981). A simpler approach to labor induction using lipid-bound prostaglandin E$_2$ vaginal suppository. *Am. J. Obstet. Gynecol. 141*:158-162.

Mackenzie, I. Z., and Embrey, M. P. (1977). Cervical ripening with intra-vaginal prostaglandin E$_2$ gel. *Br. Med. J. 2*:1381-1384.

Mitchell, M. D., Kierse, M. J. N. C., Anderson, A. B. M., and Turnbull, A. C. (1976). Evidence for a local control of prostaglandins within the uterus. *Br. J. Obstet. Gynaecol. 84*:35-38.

Nelson, G. H., and Bryans, C. I. (1978). Induction of labour with oral prostaglandin E$_2$ in normal and high risk pregnancies. *Am. J. Obstet. Gynecol. 132*:642-648.

Nixon, W. C. W., and Smyth, C. N. (1959). Old and new methods of induction of labour and of premature labour. *Am. J. Obstet. Gynecol. 77*:393-405.

Patterson, W. M. (1971). Amniotomy with or without simultaneous oxytocin infusion. *J. Obstet. Gynaecol. Br. Commonw. 78*:310-316.

Quinn, M. A., Murphy, A. J., Kuhn, R. J. P., Robinson, H. P., and Brown, J. B. (1981). A double-blind trial of extra-amniotic oestriol and prostaglandin F$_{2\alpha}$ gels in cervical ripening. *Br. J. Obstet. Gynaecol. 88*: 644-649.

Sellers, S. M., Hodgson, H. T., Mitchell, M. D., Anderson, A. B. M., and Turnbull, A. C. (1980). Release of prostaglandins after amniotomy is not mediated by oxytocin. *Br. J. Obstet. Gynaecol. 87*:43-46.

Soloff, M. S. (1975). Uterine receptor for oxytocin: Effect of estrogen. *Biochem. Biophys. Res. Commun. 65*:205-212.

Stewart, P., Kennedy, J. H., Barlow, D. H., and Calder, A. A. (1981). A comparison of oestradiol and PGE$_2$ for ripening the cervix. *Br. J. Obstet. Gynaecol. 88*:236-239.

Tohan, N., Tejani, N., Vasanasi, M., and Robbins, J. (1979). Ripening of the term cervix with laminaria. *Obstet. Gynecol. 54*:588-590.

Turnbull, A. C., and Anderson, A. B. M. (1967). Induction of labour. Part 1: Amniotomy. *Gynaecol. Br. Commonw. 74*:849-854.

Valentine, B. H. (1977). Intravenous oxytocin and oral prostaglandin E$_2$ for ripening of the unfavourable cervix. *Br. J. Obstet. Gynaecol. 84*:846-854.

Wilson, P. D. (1978). A comparison of four methods of ripening of the un-favourable cervix. *Br. J. Obstet. Gynaecol. 85*:941-944.

11

Monitoring of Uterine Contractility

PHILIP J. STEER / St. Mary's Hospital Medical School, London, England

Early clinical investigators of uterine activity including Brown-Sequard, J. Y. Simpson, and Milne-Murray quoted in Bell (1952), simply observed uterine contractions without any attempt at recording or quantitating them objectively. It is generally agreed that the first successful attempt to record intrauterine pressure in labor in the human was made by Schatz in 1872 (Bourne and Burn, 1927; Bell, 1952). He used a rubber bag inserted into the uterus and connected by tubing to a pressure manometer. The resulting rise and fall of the water or mercury in the manometer was recorded on a revolving kymography drum.

This method remained in use for more than 60 years. It required nitrous oxide or chloroform anesthesia of the patient (Bourne and Burn, 1927) for insertion of the bag and for this reason never became widely used for routine clinical purposes.

Attempts were therefore made to record uterine contractions externally, from the mother's abdomen. Rubsamen in 1913 (quoted in Bell, 1952) used a complicated system of pulleys to rest a weight on the mother's abdomen. As the weight rose and fell with each uterine contraction, its movement was recorded by a writing lever. For successful results, it was necessary for the mother to be absolutely still at all times. This was clearly impractical.

Details of the 'tambour' recorder were first published by Lorand in 1913 (Reynolds et al., 1948; Bell 1952; Smyth 1957). An inverted cup covered with a flexible membrane (usually rubber) was strapped firmly onto the mother's abdomen by means of a belt. As the uterus contracted, it pressed firmly against the tambour and reduced the volume of the tambour chamber. This increased the pressure of the contained air. This increase was recorded on a water/float manometer and kymograph drum. Because air is easily compressed, and the increase in pressure rather small, a sensitive manometer is required to produce adequate amplitude of recording, and this makes the system very sensitive to vibrational artefact.

A comprehensive assessment of tambour transducers was made by Lacroix in 1968. He compared the pressure recorded by the gas-filled nonelectronic "parturiograph," with intrauterine pressure recorded by an intrauterine catheter connected to an external Statham strain gauge transducer in 22 patients. Identical pressures were only recorded in 25%. In the other 75%, the attenuation of the contraction amplitude measurement was very dependent on the pressure of the gas within the system, and errors of 2.7KPa (20 mmHg) were not uncommon.

Sensitivity to artefact was reduced somewhat by the development of the strain gauge dynamometer (Reynolds, 1948). When a thin metal strip is bent by an external force, its electrical resistance is changed. The external force is transduced from a contraction using a piston which indents the uterus. The piston is held in place by a brass ring attached to the patient's abdomen with double-sided adhesive tape. A contraction of the uterus pushes up the indenting piston, and deforms the thin metal strip. The change in electrical resistance of the strip is measured using a Wheatstone Bridge, and can be recorded using an amplifier and chart recorder.

This type of dynamometer is still widely used today in commercial fetal monitors. It can be calibrated accurately in grams of force on the central piston, but it cannot provide an accurate measure of true intrauterine pressure. This is because it is affected not only by intra-amniotic pressure, but also by local uterine muscle tension. Both of these are attenuated to a variable degree by the thickness of the abdominal wall. Intra-amniotic pressure is the same for all parts of the uterine cavity which are in fluid continuity (except for the hydrostatic effect of depth), because fluid, being almost incompressible, transmits pressure equally in all directions. The amniotic fluid pressure therefore represents the summation of muscle tension in various parts of the uterus. The reading of this component of recorded pressure will be the same wherever the transducer is placed (hydrostatic element apart). The component due to muscle tension will, however, depend largely on the contractile state of the uterus at the point at which the transducer is applied. There will also be a variable component of abdominal wall attenuation. It follows that, while the ability of the external tokodynamometer to register true intra-abdominal pressure is limited, a number of these devices can be used to provide information about the propogation of muscular activity through the uterus.

Physiological studies using such a multiple tokodynamometer technique (Hellman et al., 1950) showed that a normal contraction wave originates at the fundus of the uterus, and passes down towards the cervix. Contractions are also stronger and longer lasting at the fundus than lower down in the uterus. This is termed *fundal dominance*. It explains why the best external recordings of uterine activity (UA) with the external tokograph are obtained when it is placed over the upper third of the uterus.

A study of the relationship between external tokography and amniotic fluid pressure was published by Caldeyro (Barcia), Alvarez, and Reynolds in 1950. They used a combination of three Reynolds tokodynamometers, four uterine polygraph (tambour) transducers, and intra-amniotic fluid-pressure measurement. To record the intra-amniotic pressure, a 15-gauge stainless steel needle was used to puncture both the abdominal and uterine walls. The needle was then connected to a recording mercury manometer. The results of these studies confirmed that incoordinate uterine activity can be seen equally clearly with intrauterine pressure (IUP) recordings as with multiple external transducers. When the amniotic fluid pressure changes are smooth and regular and there is normal progress in labor, it can be assumed that there is normal uterine contraction polarity (fundal dominance).

Because of the clinical unacceptability of routine abdominal wall puncture, a further attempt was made by Smyth in 1957 to improve the accuracy of external transducers. He designed the guarding tokodynamometer, the principle of which is as follows.

If a small area of the abdominal wall and underlying uterine wall is turned into a flat diaphragm by pressing upon the external surface with a flat plate, the pressures on each side of the body wall will be equal. By measuring the force upon the plate, the internal pressure can be measured if the area of contact is known. To define the area of contact exactly, and also to eliminate any pressures arising from bending of the body wall at the edges of the flattened area, the pressure plate is surrounded by a guard plate which is held exactly level with the measuring area and flattens an additional "surround" of body tissues. The force on the "surround" or "guard" ring is not measured. The force on the central pressure plate is measured with the usual strain gauge and Wheatstone Bridge arrangement.

There are major clinical drawbacks to what is in theory a very effective system.

1. The instrument has to be applied over a fluid-filled part of the uterus. If it is applied over the fetal back, for example, its accuracy is severely reduced. This restriction in the site of application in turn restricts the patient's choice of posture (she cannot lie on the tokodynamometer). Considerable skill is needed to ensure correct application.

2. The instrument must be held in position by a stiff elastic belt passed around the patient. The belt must be very tight: a force of at least 1 kg must be applied to flatten the abdominal wall over the 40 cm^2 of application. Even at this pressure, contact may be lost at the peak of a very strong contraction. Smyth notes that this tight application becomes uncomfortable after a while and recommends that the belt be left loose for long term recordings. Accurate measurements can therefore only be obtained in the short term.
3. In order to acheive a sufficient central component of force, it is necessary to pass the retaining belt over a handle 5 cm high on the transducer. This produces a further impediment to patient mobility.
4. Excessive tension of the belt will itself raise the intrauterine pressure.

Smyth claimed that, provided the system is operated within the constraints described above, a true recording of intrauterine pressure can be obtained. However, although the traces shown in his paper confirm the correspondence of the two methods, he cites only one case in which simultaneous tocographic and amniotic fluid pressure recordings were made.

Wood et al. (1965) reported comparison of recordings made with the Smyth tocodynamometer and a direct recording of IUP in a further six cases. They found that the pressures recorded with the Smyth tokodynamometer varied between 70 and 100% of the true IUP. "In order to obtain satisfactory results with this instrument, care in the choice of site of its application, and the correct tension of its fastening are necessary."

For the reasons enumerated above, external methods of monitoring uterine activity have not continued to be used for scientific investigation (Csapo, 1970). The external tokodynamometer has, however, been widely used as an adjunct to continuous fetal heart rate monitoring (Steer, 1977). For this purpose, precise determination of contraction pressure is unnecessary, and a simplified form of the external tocograph is perfectly adequate and, equally important, acceptable to the patient.

However, for the investigation of abnormally slow labor, or the control of oxytocin infusion, a more accurate measurement of IUP is desirable. A clinically acceptable method for such measurement was described by Williams and Stallworthy in 1952. It involved the transcervical insertion of a flexible polythene catheter into the uterus via an introducer such as the Drewe-Smythe catheter. The catheter, filled with a sterile fluid, is connected to a pressure-recording device. In their original description this was a mercury manometer, but this has now been replaced by an electronic strain gauge.

MEASUREMENT USING A POLYTHENE CATHETER

Preparation of the Apparatus

The recorders used when measuring pressure using a fluid-filled catheter attached to an external pressure transducer will nearly always be fetal monitors. Recordings are made with a heated stylus on heat-sensitive waxed or chemical paper. The scale is generally from 0 to 100 mmHg (0-13.33KPa) over 4 cm (1mm chart amplitude $\equiv$ 2.5 mmHg $\equiv$ 0.3KPa), speed 1-3 cm/min. Simultaneous recordings of fetal heart rate are usually made on the same chart paper (60-210 bpm over 7 cm UK, 30-240 bpm over 7 cm, USA). The external transducers used are generally flat diaphragm strain gauge types, with a two-outlet dome (e.g., Statham or Bell and Howell) (see Fig. 1). Occasionally, single-outlet dome types are used (for example, Kulite) (see Fig. 2).

Calibration
The calibration of the pressure transducers can be checked easily (see Fig. 3):

1. Ensure an airtight fit of the dome to the transducer.
2. Fit one or more plastic disposable three-way taps to the outlets of the dome in the closed position.
3. Force the three-way tap(s) into the "incorrect" fourth position so that all the pathways are open (care must be exercised to prevent damage to the transducer dome (see Fig. 3).
4. Connect the mercury manometer of a sphygmomanometer to one of the vacant arms of the three-way tap.
5. Check that zero pressure is recorded on the monitor and on the manometer. Adjust as necessary.
6. Connect the arm cuff to the second vacant arm of the three-way tap.
7. Inflate the cuff and squeeze it with one hand until the mercury manometer reads 100 mmHg. Check that the monitor shows the correct full scale deflection. Adjust as necessary.

Sterilization of the Pressure Transducer
This is necessary to prevent bacterial invasion of the uterus. If the catheter is accidentally filled with an inappropriate fluid (e.g., 5% dextrose, or amniotic fluid) bacteria may grow down the catheter into the uterus (Roberts and Steer, 1977). Transfer of bacteria into the uterus can also occur if flushing of the catheter after insertion is performed incorrectly (see below).

The dome should be removed from the transducer, and the dome and diaphragm cleaned. Care should be used because the dome is expensive and nondisposable, and the pressure-sensitive diaphragm is easily damaged by excessive pressure or scratching. The dome and transducer should then be

(A) FLUSH IU CATHETER

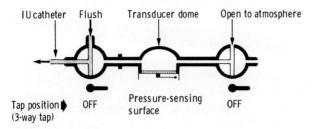

(B) FLUSH TRANSDUCER

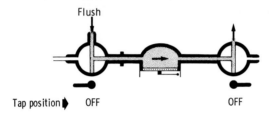

(C) RECORD IU PRESSURE

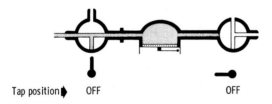

Figure 1. Tap positions in calibration of pressure transducers for monitoring intrauterine pressure.

reassembled by screwing the dome down firmly to prevent leaks and avoiding cross-threading. A three-way tap can then be fitted to the dome outlet(s). With each tap open to atmosphere (two-outlet type) or the dome loosened slightly (single outlet), the transducer should then be filled with a sterilizing solution, such as Cidex (2% aqueous activated glutaraldehyde, Cidex-Arbrook Ltd., Scotland), so as to exclude any air bubbles. Cidex-Arbrook Ltd. state that Cidex kills all vegetative organisms within 10 min, and spores (including tetanus) within 3 h. A minimum 3-h sterilization is therefore recommended. Cidex remains active for 14 days after preparation.

CLOSED

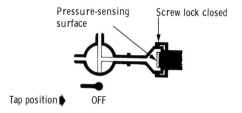

Figure 2.   Input to transducer: ensure airtight fit to dome.

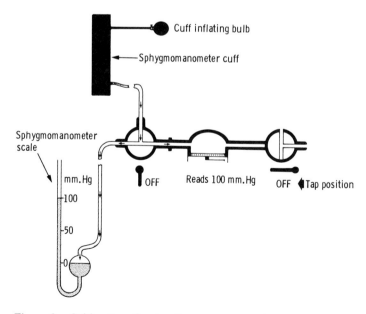

Figure 3.   Calibration, forcing three-way tap to incorrect position.

Preparation of the Intra-Uterine Catheter

Sterilized catheter packs are available from a number of manufacturers (e.g., Hewlett Packard or Portex Ltd.) Open the pack onto a sterile towel. Add syringes, a needle, and three-way tap(s), if not included in the pack. The operator should then "scrub up" in the normal way, wearing a mask, and should then don a sterile gown and gloves. The catheter is attached to the male connector of the three-way tap using the female adaptor fitted or supplied. (Note that the end of the catheter to be inserted into the patient has a number of holes cut in the side of the catheter; the other end is the one to be connected to the three-way tap.) The catheter is then filled with sterile fluid. Sterile water alone is probably sufficient (Roberts and Steer, 1977) but as an additional safeguard against infection it is widespread practice to add 1 g of a suitable antibiotic (such as ampicillin in nonsensitive patients, or cephaloridine) to 100 ml of sterile water of 1: 1,000 chlorhexidine solution. The solution is drawn up in the 20 ml syringe then used to fill the catheter via the three-way tap. If the syringe is left attached to the three-way tap, it acts as a weight to help prevent the end of the catheter being pulled off the towel-covered trolley onto the floor during insertion of the catheter. It also prevents the fluid running out when the catheter is handled.

Preparation of the Patient

Insertion of an intrauterine catheter should be performed as a sterile procedure, to prevent accidental contamination of the catheter on insertion. The procedure is explained to the patient, and she is then placed in the lithotomy position by two assistants. A wedge should be used to produce lateral tilt of the patient's trunk and prevent supine hypotension, particularly if the patient has received an active epidural anesthetic. With increasing skill and experience on the part of the operator, it is possible to insert the catheter with the patient in the left lateral position, if she or the fetus will not tolerate the supine position.

The perineum should be thoroughly cleansed with an antiseptic non-irritant solution such as Savlon. Sterile towels are used to cover the legs, with a "split-sheet" for the perineum. A vaginal and bimanual examination should be performed to establish the position of the fetal head and the state of the cervix.

Position of the Placenta

Insertion of a transcervical intra-uterine catheter is clearly contraindicated in abnormal cases, such as placenta previa. If a mid- or last-trimester ultrasound examination has been performed, and the position of the placenta recorded, this can provide a useful guide for the best direction to insert the catheter, both to facilitate introduction and avoid trauma to the placenta. For example, a low anterior placenta recorded on ultrasound suggests that the catheter should be passed posterior, or lateral to the fetal head, depending on other factors (see below).

The procedure now adopted depends upon the state of the cervix and membranes, and upon the position of the fetal head. The two commonest situations will be described in detail.

Induction of Labor

The cervix is usually 1-3 cm dilated, with intact membranes, and the head or breech is not fixed in the pelvis but can be dislodged upwards with gentle digital pressure. Two fingers of the examining hand are introduced into the vagina until they lie in contact with the cervix. The curved plastic introducer supplied with the sterile catheter set is then passed gently with the other hand down the groove between the two fingers in the vagina until the tip enters the cervix. The introducer can then be passed a few centimeters at a time, upwards and backwards between the fetal head or breech, and the posterior wall of the uterus. It is not necessary to rupture the membranes beforehand, as they will usually be ruptured during this procedure. As the introducer perforates the membranes, liquor will pour out of its external end. It can be inspected for meconium or blood. If, unexpectedly, (no clinical suggestion of placental abruption) the liquor is heavily blood-stained, the introducer should be withdrawn and reinserted in a different direction.

Under no circumstances should more than light pressure be used or be necessary when placing the introducer. Undue force carries with it the danger of perforation of the placenta or uterus.

Light upward pressure on the fetal head (or breech) by the fingers in the vagina will often assist in disimpacting the head sufficiently to allow the introducer to slip easily between the fetus and the uterine wall until the distal tip lies freely in the amniotic fluid above the presenting part (Fig. 4). Excessive disimpaction should not be used because of the risk of cord prolapse (Fig. 5).

Once the proximal end of the introducer is within 2-3 cm of the vulva, the intrauterine catheter may be inserted, open end first. Once 20 cm has been inserted (the length of the introducer), resistance to further insertion may be felt. In this case, force should not be used to push the catheter through. There is a risk of perforation of the uterus, or damage to fetus or placenta, because of the relative sharpness and stiffness of the catheter emerging from the end of the introducer. Instead, the fingers in the vagina (and if possible, through the cervix) should be used to move the introducer from side to side, maintaining steady pressure on the catheter, until it suddenly slides through easily. Once this easy movement has been obtained, a further 30 cm of

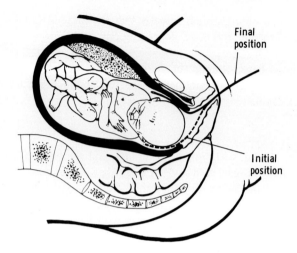

Figure 4. Preferred position of intrauterine catheter when the head is low and cervix is 4+ cm dilated.

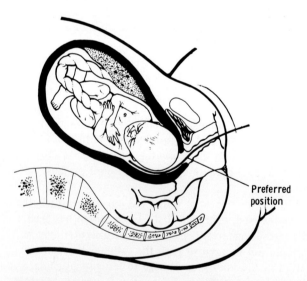

Figure 5. Preferred position of intrauterine catheter when the head is high and cervix is closed.

catheter should be inserted. More than this produces a risk of entanglement with the umbilical cord (Cave et al., 1979).

The catheter should then be held stationary, and the introducer withdrawn over it, leaving the catheter in situ.

With some types of catheter, the introducer must be left in place at the far end of the catheter; with others, the end fitting can be disconnected, allowing removal of the introducer. This allows a brief flow of liquor into the catheter, which should later be flushed out to minimize the risk of infection (Roberts and Steer, 1977). The brief flow of liquor serves to confirm the correct placement of the catheter. Slight blood-staining of the liquor is of no significance, being produced by minor trauma to the uterine wall. If it persists, or becomes heavy, fetal condition must be observed closely (usually by electrode placement and continuous fetal heart-rate monitoring) to exclude the risk of placental or fetal vessel damage. This would eventually be manifest as an abnormal fetal heart-rate pattern. The blood can also be tested by Singer's test (differential hemolysis with sodium hydroxide) or a simple tablet test to exclude fetal hemoglobin (Trudinger and Pryse-Davies, 1978).

The patient's legs can now be taken down, and she can be placed in any comfortable position. A small piece of suitable hypoallergenic tape (e.g., Micropore) can be used to attach the catheter to the patient's upper thigh to minimize the risk of accidental dislodgement.

The three-way tap at the end of the catheter can now be used to replace (one of) the three-way tap(s) on the transducer (Fig. 6). A water-tight connection must be ensured to prevent leakage, which will cause a flow of liquor down the catheter, resulting in probable blockage with vernix. The tap should be closed to the transducer and the 20-ml syringe used to flush through and clear the catheter of any liquor, vernix, or blood clot. The tap is then closed to the catheter, and the other three-way tap on the transducer is opened to atmosphere (two-tap transducer; on the one-tap transducer, the dome is loosened). The transducer is then flushed through to remove any trapped air bubbles. Note that (1) the catheter should never be flushed across the transducer and (2) the second tap must be open when the transducer is flushed, or severe damage will be inflicted on the pressure-sensitive membrane.

A final check of correct zero-pressure reading can be made with the tap open to atmosphere or the dome loosened, adjustment made as necessary, and then the tap or dome closed (Fig. 6). The three-way tap attached to the catheter is adjusted to connect the catheter to the transducer.

The transducer must now be positioned so that an appropriate intrauterine pressure is registered. This means attachment of the transducer to the fetal monitor level with the symphysis pubis of the patient (or to a special legplate

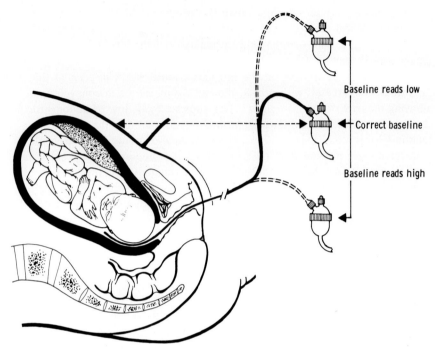

Figure 6. Calibration of intrauterine pressure.

on the patient's upper thigh). If the catheter is excessively long, it can be coiled up and taped to the patient's upper thigh.

The catheter can be checked for patency by asking the patient to cough. A 7.5-15-mmHg (1-2 KPa) positive deflection should be seen in the recorded pressure. Correct placement of the catheter can be checked by bimanual lateral compression of the uterus, when a 7.5-11-mmHg (1-1.5 KPa) positive deflection should be seen in the recorded pressure. A negative deflection in this situation indicates that the tip of the catheter is below the fetal head; lateral compression of the uterus tends to raise the fetus up and create a fall of pressure in the vagina and uterus below the presenting part. For this reason, pressure on the fundus should not be used, as this can be transmitted through the fetal trunk and recorded as a rise in pressure even when the catheter is incorrectly placed in the vagina or uterus below the presenting part.

Established Labor

This is defined as the cervix being 1 or more cm dilated, and fully effaced, and the head or breech well down into the pelvis. The pressure of the presenting part against the posterior wall of the uterus and sacrum usually prevents easy posterior insertion of the introducer.

The general preparation is as described above. The two fingers in the vagina are inserted into the cervix, and passed posteriorly behind the presenting part as far as possible (usually 4-5 cm) without causing undue maternal discomfort. The introducer is passed down the groove between the fingers until the tip lies level with the ends of the fingers. The fingers and introducer are then swept laterally around between the presenting part and the uterus until they lie anterior to the presenting part. They now lie between the presenting part and the uterus and pubic bone. In this direction, the distance to the pool of liquor behind the presenting part and above the pubic bone (often used for amniocentesis) is small. A very small advancement of the introducer beyond the tips of the fingers will normally enter this pool of liquor. Correct positioning is usually rewarded with a flow of liquor down the introducer. When the introducer seems to be correctly placed, gentle attempts should be made to feed the catheter through; once again excessive force should not be used or be necessary. If the catheter fails to advance, gentle deviation of the introducer towards one side or the other will generally be successful. Connection of the inserted catheter to the transducer is as previously described.

If these techniques are followed correctly, safe insertion of the intra-uterine catheter should be possible in the great majority of cases. Success improves with experience. The exceptional failures are usually in patients in whom there is no room to pass the catheter alongside the presenting part. Failure of catheter insertion in this situation may therefore represent relative disproportion.

COMPLICATIONS

Perforation of the Uterine Wall

Chan et al. (1973) reported three such cases. All were asymptomatic, and two were only found incidentally at cesarean section. There were no complications from these perforations. Tutera and Newman (1975) described a single case, also found at cesarean section. The perforation in the posterior lower uterine segment was closed easily with chromic catgut; the patient's postoperative course was uneventful.

Perforation of the Placenta

This may occur particularly if the placenta is low-lying. Personal experience shows that in approximately 2% of insertions, apparently pure maternal blood gushes back down the introducer and/or catheter as it is inserted. It is then necessary to withdraw the catheter and insert it in another direction. There have been no reports of serious sequelae following such a perforation unless hemorrhage at the time of insertion heralds rupture of a fetal vessel (see below).

Puncture of a Fetal Vessel

Fetal vessel puncture with subsequent demise of the fetus has been reported by Trudinger and Pryse-Davies (1978). A 41-year-old primigravida in spontaneous labor at 38 weeks had a polythene fluid-filled intrauterine catheter inserted. Although a fresh bright red blood loss was noted, the fetal heart was not monitored, and the patient delivered a fresh stillborn infant (weight 2.72 kg). Postmortem examination confirmed a ruptured fetal placental vein. The same authors report three further cases of fetal vessel puncture with fetal anemia in which the fetuses fortunately survived.

Compression of the Umbilical Cord

Cave et al. (1979) have reported a case of fetal demise, which they have attributed to compression of the umbilical cord by a kinked and entangled catheter. Their analysis can be disputed since there are late decelerations on the published fetal heart-rate tracing, before the acute deceleration which they claim was due to attempts to remove the catheter. The patient had received an epidural anesthetic, so postural hypotension associated with the dorsal position on attempting to remove the catheter may also have been contributory. The fetal heart rate recovered after the initial attempt to remove the catheter, but unfortunately a repeat attempt to remove the catheter vaginally was made while the patient was anesthetized for the cesarean section. It would be surprising if one or even two episodes of acute cord compression could have caused fetal hypoxia unless the fetus was already compromised. Trudinger and Pryse-Davies report a similar case of entanglement in which traction on the catheter resulted in variable decelerations, but in which the infant was born in good condition.

Blockage of the Catheter

The catheter may be blocked with vernix or blood (Csapo, 1970; Odendaal et al., 1976). This is most likely to occur on insertion of the catheter and it is therefore normal practice to flush the catheter through with a few milliliters of sterile water or saline following insertion. Most commercially supplied catheters have additional holes in the side of the catheter, near the tip. Further blockage is therefore only likely if there is a leakage of fluid at the connection of the catheter to the transducer, or from the transducer itself. This causes a flow of liquor into the catheter, carrying with it vernix and/or blood clot. Complete blockage is easy to recognize because a totally flat tracing is produced. A partial blockage will only attenuate the signal with the result that a variable underestimate of uterine activity may be made. This can lead the obstetrician into infusing an excessive amount of oxytocin in an attempt to "improve" uteirne activity. This danger could theoretically be minimized by using two separate catheters and transducers, and only accepting the resulting measurement when each system registers the same pressure. This is not normally a practical solution, on grounds both of expense and convenience. In addition, Knoke et al. (1976) have shown that the reliability of open-ended fluid-filled catheters in the measurement of intrauterine pressure is only ±5.2-9.7 mmHg (0.7-1.3 KPa). This represents the range of standard deviation of three simultaneous estimates of intra-uterine pressure, measured in nine patients, using fluid-filled open-ended intrauterine catheters (the mean value was not appropriate because the distribution of differences was heterogeneous). Because of this inherent unreliability of the measurement, comparison of pressures recorded with two catheters may still yield different results even when both are functioning correctly. It would therefore be necessary to allow a 10 mmHg differential before concluding that one of the catheters had become blocked. This would inevitably increase the chance that simultaneous blockage of the two catheters could remain undetected.

The Problem of Determining True "Baseline Tone"

Baseline tone, or *resting intrauterine pressure* is the pressure within the uterus when it is not contracting. There is a component of pressure due to the elastic recoil of the tissues of the uterus, and an additional hydrostatic component which varies with the depth below the upper fluid level of the uterus. The contribution to overall measured pressure of the hydrostatic component will vary from zero when measured level with the upper fluid level of the uterus, to approximately 30 cm of water (25 mmHg, 3.4 KPa), if measured at the lower fluid level of the upright uterus. Baseline tone is therefore not a single value but varies according to the position of the measuring transducer. A measuring external transducer is usually placed level with the symphysis pubis (Williams and Stallworthy, 1952). Using this fixed point for the transducer, the contribution of hydrostatic pressure to the registered baseline tone will vary with the posture of the mother, and the consequent degree of "uprightness" of the uterus. The exact value of the hydrostatic component is usually unknown, and therefore the measurement of baseline tone is usually arbitrary within ±10 mmHg (1.3 KPa). Arroyo and Mendez-Bauer (1975) and Mendez-Bauer et al., (1975) have suggested attaching the transducer to the maternal abdomen over the fundus of the uterus to minimize the effects of changes in posture, but this technique is rather cumbersome and has not found general clinical acceptance.

The Risk of Infection

A number of workers have reported an increase in the incidence of endometritis with the use of intrauterine catheters (Amato, 1977; Hagen, 1975) although some say that this is rare (Chan et al., 1973), others find no effect (Tutera and Newman, 1975) and yet others claim that any effect is due to artificial rupture of membranes (Gibbs et al., 1976). Two potential sources of infection exist: (1) infection may be carried in during placement of the catheter; or (2) the pressure transducer may be sterilized inadequately before use. If bacteria are present in the dome or on the diaphragm of the transducer, a direct fluid path exists between the bacteria and the uterine cavity. It has been shown that bacteria are unlikely to swim down a catheter filled with sterile water or saline within 24 hr, but if the catheter is filled with a nutritive medium (such as liquor), chemotactic growth down the catheter into the uterus is possible (Roberts and Steer, 1977). Effective sterilization of the transducer (e.g., with aqueous 2% activated glutaraldehyde) is therefore important, as is proper aseptic technique for placement of the catheter in the uterus. Catheters should be flushed through with sterile water, and not allowed to fill with liquor.

Miscellaneous

Fluid-filled catheters have a limited length, which restricts patient mobility. Movement of the catheter causes large artefactual variations in recorded pressure. Clinical use may be difficult because of the need for calibration, flushing, and asembly of parts.

MEASUREMENT USING A CATHETER-TIP PRESSURE TRANSDUCER

Because of the complications associated with fluid-filled catheters described above, a recent new approach has been the use of catheter-tip pressure transducers. These are produced in the United Kingdom for obstetric use by Gaeltec (Scotland) Ltd., and marketed by Sonicaid. A bridge strain gauge is deposited on a thin metal pressure-sensing surface. Initially, the transducer was mounted on the end of a 90 cm woven dacron catheter and situated so that it measured lateral and not head-on or impact pressure. The sensing surface is recessed, which minimizes the risk of accidental damage. The catheter and transducer were sealed with a silicone rubber sleeve, giving the catheter a diameter of 2.7 mm. Recent improvements have

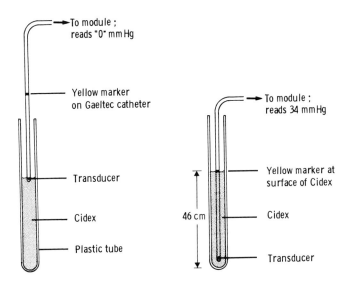

Figure 7. Calibration of the Sonicaid Gaeltec intrauterine catheter.

included the use of a more robust polyurethane sleeve and the incorporation of a thin stainless steel wire to within 2 cm of the catheter tip. this improves ease of insertion by increasing stiffness. The catheter tip itself is rounded and capped with a very soft silicone rubber tip to prevent trauma to the uterus or fetus.

The transducer is connected by a plug at the distal end of the catheter to a 2-m flexible extension cable which is in turn connected to the contraction socket of a fetal monitor. Full technical details have been reported by Steer et al. (1978).

Practical Details

Moisture is absorbed into the silicone rubber sleeve and will cause a positive pressure change of about 1.3 KPa (10 mmHg) unless the catheter is allowed to stabilize for at least 6 hr in a fluid.

The catheter is stored in a rigid lucite tube filled with Cidex and attached to the side of the fetal monitor. This means that the catheter is always sterile and ready to use provided at least 3 hr have elapsed since the last use. As storage is wet, there is no need for additional "stabilization" before use.

The electrical connector should never be allowed to become wet, as this causes a degree of "short circuit," producing baseline drift of the pressure recording.

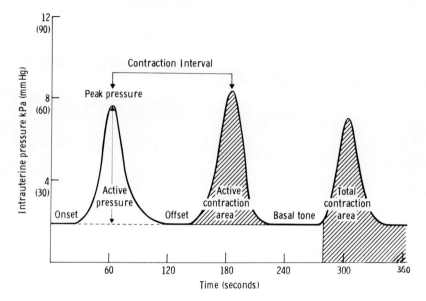

Figure 8. Active pressure = peak pressure minus basal tone. Active contraction area = integral of active pressure with time (over 15 min = 900 sec) = $\int_0^{900}$ active pressure $\times$ dt = kiloPascal sec/15 min (Système Internationale units). Active contraction area per 15 min is therefore the sum of the active contraction area of each contraction (or part of a contraction) within those 15 min.

Calibration is checked by connecting the catheter to the monitor input and observing the pressure readout (Fig. 7). The catheter is raised so that the lip is just below the surface of the Cidex (to avoid the surface-tension effects which occur if the transducer is exposed to air). The correct zero reading should then be observed, and can be corrected as necessary. The catheter is then reinserted into the Cidex and a check made that the deflection in mmHg corresponds to a depth of Cidex above the catheter tip (61 cm of Cidex is equivalent to 45 mmHg or 6 KPa). The span can then be adjusted as necessary.

The technique of insertion is essentially the same as for a fluid-filled catheter, except that an introducer is not needed.

Analysis of Intrauterine Pressure Readings (Fig. 8)

The classic parameters of uterine activity are frequency pressure and duration of contractions and baseline tonus. The first attempt to derive a single measure to represent all these variables was made by Bourne and Burn in 1927. They used a planimeter to measure the total area below a tracing which represented the intrauterine pressure varying with time. Unfortunately, they did not quantitate their units.

Caldeyro-Barcia introduced the Montevideo unit, a multiple of pressure of contractions with their frequency. (Caldeyro-Barcia et al., 1957). Finding the level of baseline tone difficult to measure accurately, and of apparently no significance in the majority of labors, these authors used for their unit the peak contraction pressure minus the baseline tone ("active" pressure) rather than the actual value of the maximum pressure. The Montevideo unit was therefore designed as mean active pressure per 10 min multiplied by frequency of contractions per 10 min.

El-Sahwi et al. (1967) preferred to include the duration of contractions in their measurement (the Alexandria unit) since this is an important variable in the interference of uterine activity with placental blood flow (Huch and Huch, 1977; Schneider et al., 1980). Their unit was otherwise identical to the Montevideo unit. Hon and Paul (1973) and Miller et al. (1976) described a unit which integrated the total intrauterine pressure (area) above zero pressure per 10 min (units: Torr min). They considered that since basal tone can have a profound influence on fetal oxygenation, through its effect on placental perfusion, integration of the total area under the pressure curve would be the ideal measurement. This technique has, however, serious practical drawbacks related to the difficulties in the measurement of "true" basal tone as described above. These difficulties can lead to errors in the measured basal tone which, when integrated, give rise to spurious values equal to those generated by the contractions themselves. Active contraction area measurement, however, (the area under the contraction curve, but above baseline tone) is almost independent of errors due to hydrostatic pressure and patient movement (Carter and Steer, 1976, 1978, 1980; Steer and Carter, 1977; Steer, 1977; Steer, 1979).

A number of different techniques for computing active contraction area have been described, using both computers (Henry et al., 1979), and dedicated on-line microcircuiting (Carter and Steer, 1980). The Système International unit of action contraction area is the kiloPascal second (kPas). The mean value of uterine activity in unselected spontaneous labour is 1100-1300 kPas (equivalent to 160-180 Montevideo units), standard deviation ±300 kPas (Steer, 1980).

REFERENCES

Amato, J. C. (1977). Fetal monitoring in a community hospital. *Obstet. Gynecol. 50*:269-274.

Arroyo, J., and Mendez-Bauer, C. (1975). The maintenance of a stable baseline in intrauterine pressure with varying maternal position—A practical approach. *J. Perinat. Med. 3*:129-131.

Bell, G. H. (1952). Abnormal uterine action in labour. *J. Obstet. Gynaecol. Br. Emp. 59*:617.

Bourne, A., and Burn, J. H. (1927). The dosage and action of pituitary extract and of the ergot alkaloids on the uterus in labour, with a note of the action of adrenalin. *J. Obstet. Gynaecol. Br. Emp. 34*:249-272.

Caldeyro (Barcia), R., Alvarez, H., and Reynolds, S. R. M. (1950). A better understanding of uterine contractility through simultaneous recording with an internal and a seven channel external method. *Surg. Gynecol. Obstet. 91*:641-650.

Caldeyro-Barcia, R., Sica-Blanco, Y., Poseiro, J. J., Gonzalez-Panizza, V., Mendez-Bauer, C., Fielitz, C., Alvarez, H., Pose, S. V., and Hendricks, C. H. (1957). A quantitative study of the action of synthetic oxytocin on the pregnant human uterus. *J. Pharmacol. 121*:18-31.

Carter, M. C., and Steer, P. J. (1976). An electronic method of controlling induced labour. In *Applications of Electronics in Medicine.* Institution of Electronic and Radio Engineers, London, pp. 293-300.

Carter, M. C., and Steer, P. J. (1978). A labour monitor for the measurement of uterine activity, and the control of oxytocin infusion. In *Biosigma 1978,* Comité du Colloque International sur les Signaux et les Images en Médicine et en Biologie, Imprimerie Emt, pp. 149-154.

Carter, M. C., and Steer, P. J. (1980). An automatic infusion system for the measurement and control of uterine activity. *Med. Instrum. 14*:169-173.

Cave, D. G., Swingler, G. R., and Skew, P. G. (1979). Hypoxic stillbirth due to entangled intrauterine catheter. *Br. Med. J. 1*:233.

Chan, W. H., Paul, R. H., and Toews, J. (1973). Intrapartum fetal monitoring— Maternal and fetal morbidity and perinatal mortality. *Obstet. Gynecol. 41*: 7-13.

Csapo, A. (1970). The diagnostic significance of intrauterine pressure. *Obstet. Gynecol. Surv. 25*:403-435.

El-Sahwi, S., Gaafar, P. A., and Toppozada, H. K. (1967). A new unit for evaluation of uterine activity. *Am. J. Obstet. Gynecol. 98*:900-903.

Gibbs, R. S., Listwa, H. M., and Read, J. A. (1976). The effect of internal fetal monitoring on maternal infection following daesarian section. *Obstet. Gynecol. 48*:653-658.

Hagen, D. (1975). Maternal febrile morbidity associated with fetal monitoring and caesarean section. *Obstet. Gynecol. 46*:260-262.

Hellman, L. M., Harris, J., and Reynolds, S. R. M. (1950). Characteristics of the gradients of uterine contractility during the first stage of true labor. *Bull. Johns Hopkins Hosp. 86*:234-248.

Henry, M. J., McColl, D. D. F., Crawford, J. W., and Patel, N. (1979). Computing techniques for intrapartum physiological data reduction—I. Uterine activity. *J. Perinat. Med. 7*:209-213.

Hon, E. H., and Paul, R. H. (1973). Quantitation of uterine activity. *Obstet. Gynecol. 42*:368-370.

Huch, R., and Huch, A. (1977). Continuous measurement of fetal pH and pO₂. In *The Current Status of Fetal Heart Rate Monitoring and Ultrasound in Obstetrics.* Eds. R. W. Beard and S. Campbell (Eds.), Royal College of Obstetricians and Gynaecologists, London.

Knoke, J. D., Tsao, L. L., Neuman, M. R., and Roux, J. F. (1976). The accuracy of measurements of intrauterine pressure during labour; a statistical analysis. *Comput. Biomed. Res. 9*:177.

Lacroix, G. (1968). Monitoring labor by an external tokodynamometer. *Am. J. Obstet. Gynecol. 101*:111.

Mendez-Bauer, C., Arroyo, J., Garcia-Ramos, C., Menendez, A., Lavilla, M., Izquierdo, F., Villa Elizaga, I., and Zamarriego, J. (1975). Effects of standing position on spontaneous uterine contractility and other aspects of labour. *J. Perinat. Med. 3*:89-100.

Miller, F. C., Yeh, S., Schifrin, B. S., Paul, R. H., and Hon, E. H. (1976). Quantitation of uterine activity in 100 primiparous patients. *Am. J. Obstet. Gynecol. 124*:398-405.

Odendaal, H. J., Neves De Santos, L. M., Henry, M. J., and Crawford, J. W. (1976). Experiments in the measurement of intrauterine pressure. *Br. J. Obstet. Gynaecol. 83*:221-224.

Reynolds, S. R. M., Heard, O. O., Bruns, P., and Hellman, L. M. (1948). A multichannel strain gauge tokodynamometer: An instrument for studying patterns of uterine contractions in pregnant women. *Bull. Johns Hopkins Hosp. 82*:446-469.

Roberts, A. M., and Steer, P. J. (1977). Bacterial motility and intrauterine catheter-borne infection. *Br. J. Obstet. Gynaecol. 84*:336-338.

Schneider, H., Strang, F., Huch, R., and Huch, A. (1980). Suppression of uterine contractions with fenoterol and its effect on fetal EcPO₂ in human term labour. *Br. J. Obstet. Gynaecol. 87*657-665.

Smyth, C. N. (1957). The guard ring tocodynamometer—Absolute measurement of intra-amniotic pressure by a new instrument. *J. Obstet. Gynaecol. Br. Commonw. 64*:59-66.

Steer, P. J. (1977). Monitoring in labour. *Br. J. Hosp. Med. 17*:219-225.

Steer, P. J. (1979). The clinical significance of uterine activity in labour. *J. Maternal Child Health 4*:271-275.

Steer, P. J. (1980). Unpublished data.

Steer, P. J., and Carter, M. C. (1977). Electronic assessment of uterine activity. In *Physical Science Techniques.* M. M. Black and M. J. English (Eds.), Pitman Medical, Tunbridge Wells, 1977, pp. 136-146.

Steer, P. J., Carter, M. C., Gordon, A. J., and Beard, R. W. (1978). The use of catheter-tip pressure transducers for the measurement of intra-uterine pressure in labour. *Br. J. Obstet. Gynaecol. 85*:561-566.

Trudinger, B. J., and Pryse-Davies, J. (1978). Fetal hazards of the intrauterine pressure catheter: Five case reports. *Br. J. Obstet. Gynaecol. 85*:567-572.

Tutera, G., and Newman, R. L. (1975). Fetal monitoring; its effect on the perinatal mortality and Cesarian section rates and its complications. *Am. J. Obstet. Gynecol. 122*:750-754.

Williams, E. A., and Stallworthy, J. A. (1952). A simple method of internal tocography. *Lancet 1*:330.

Wood, C., Bannerman, R. H. O., Booth, R. T., and Pinkerton, J. H. M. (1965). The prediction of premature labor by observation of the cervix and external tocography. *Am. J. Obstet. Gynecol. 91*:396-402.

12

Intrapartum Fetal Monitoring

BRIAN A. LIEBERMAN / Saint Mary's Hospital, Manchester, England

The last 50 years have witnessed a decrease in the perinatal mortality rate in the United Kingdom from 63.4:1000 total births in 1933 to 14.6 in 1979, a 76.7% improvement. Successive generations of obstetricians have responded by attempting to improve these results. At present the majority of perinatal deaths are associated with congenital abnormalities and preterm births. Mothers now embark on pregnancy knowing that the risk of maternal death is small and with the highest expectations of being delivered of a healthy infant. For the vast majority of women this will indeed be the case. Numerous factors have contributed to the decrease in the perinatal mortality rate. These include a general improvement in the mothers' state of health and nutrition, a reduction in maternal age and in the overall number of pregnancies per patient, easier access to legal abortion, improvement in the standard and availability of prenatal care, better understanding and prevention of intrapartum hypoxia, and improved standards of neonatal care. It is beyond the scope of this chapter to assess the contribution made by these and other factors to the decline in the perinatal mortality rate, but the death during labor or shortly after birth, or the permanent disability from severe perinatal asphyxia of an otherwise normally formed infant is a tragedy. Intrapartum stillbirths are to a large extent preventable since it is now possible to make the diagnosis and expedite delivery of the fetus. This chapter will discuss the assessment of fetal welfare during labor using standard clinical and electronic techniques of fetal heart-rate monitoring and fetal blood sampling.

Continuous fetal heart-rate monitoring is widely practiced throughout the United Kingdom and in the United States. Gillmer and Coombe (1979) reported that only 1 of 224 consultant obstetric units in the United Kingdom did not possess a fetal heart rate monitor, and Dilts (1976) stated that 278 of 279 obstetric services in the United States with residency programs had electronic fetal monitoring equipment. Gillmer and Coombe (1979) noted a bimodal distribution with respect to the percentage of patients being monitored with peaks at 20-30 and 80-90%, reflecting division of opinion about the need to monitor all or only high-risk patients.

The ability of the fetus to wishstand the stress of labor is to a large extent influenced by factors operative during pregnancy. Careful consideration of the mode of delivery and the need for intrapartum monitoring is essential in the presence of fetal growth retardation, an elevation in maternal blood pressure, proteinuria, chronic renal disease, rhesus isoimmunization, and diabetes. The incidence of intrapartum hypoxia is determined not only by these antenatal maternal and fetal complications but also may arise de novo during labor and, unfortunately, may be associated with avoidable factors. These include oxytocin- and prostaglandin-induced hyperstimulation of uterine activity; failure to diagnose cephalopelvic disproportion, resulting in prolonged labor with a difficult and prolonged second stage often requiring operative intervention; and unnecessary induction of labor with the possibility of cord prolapse or chorioamnionitis. The dangers associated with intrapartum hypoxia are well-recognized. These range from a stillbirth or neonatal death to severe birth asphyxia with the possibility of permanent brain damage, and milder forms of birth asphyxia associated with the meconium aspiration syndrome.

CLINICAL ASSESSMENT OF INTRAPARTUM FETAL WELFARE

Traditionally, during labor a Pinard's stethoscope has been used to auscultate the fetal heart. The value of this procedure has been enhanced by the knowledge gained from continuous intrapartum fetal-heart rate monitoring. Obstetricians and midwives are easily trained to detect decelerations in the heart rate during and immediately after a uterine contraction or the presence of a persistent fetal tachycardia or bradycardia. The reliability of this method of fetal monitoring is reduced by maternal obesity, the inability of the human ear to detect lack of baseline variability and reduction of beat-to-beat variation, and the need to auscultate during and after each contraction. In the event of a perinatal death due to intrapartum hypoxia the accuracy and reliability of this method of recording is open to criticism.

The presence of meconium in the amniotic fluid may indicate fetal hypoxia but a number of factors reduce the value of this observation. Preterm infants seldom pass meconium even when severely hypoxic although meconium is present in the ileum as early as 70-85 days' gestation. Meconium may not be observed if the fetal head is wedged tightly into the pelvis, in the presence of intact membranes, and may be a normal finding in breech presentations. It is well-recognized that in many instances of fetal distress and hypoxia, no meconium is passed and, conversely, that meconium is often present in the amniotic fluid without any evidence of fetal distress at birth. Abramovici et al. (1974) have postulated that the passage of meconium may indicate a state of temporary compensated fetal distress: well-oxygenated vital organs but with peripheral hypoxia or vasoconstriction. Fetal hypoxia is known to increase intestinal mobility (Desmond et al., 1957) and this may result in the passage of meconium. Lucas et al. (1979) have shown a fourfold increase in umbilical-cord plasma motilin levels in infants who experienced fetal distress during labor. They suggested that as motilin decreases small intestinal transit time, the high motilin levels associated with fetal distress and the rapid colonic time found in the neonate contribute to abnormal gut motility, resulting in the passage of meconium. The poor correlation between fetal hypoxia and the passage of meconium in preterm infants may be related to their substantially lower motilin levels. Krebs et al. (1980) analyzed the relationship between fetal heart-rate patterns and meconium staining of the amniotic fluid. They reported that the passage of meconium is associated with lower 1- and 5-min Apgar scores and higher neonatal mortality than a control group with clear amniotic fluid. Fetuses with meconium-stained amniotic fluid showed abnormal fetal heart rate patterns more often than the controls, and iatrogenically induced hypoxia and the direct effect of meconium on the pulmonary gas exchange at birth increased the number of low Apgar scores in those cases with normal fetal heart-rate patterns. The outcome of labor with abnormal fetal heart-rate patterns with meconium did not differ from that of abnormal fetal heart-rate patterns without meconium and heavy meconium was not associated with significantly low Apgar scores or more abnormal fetal heart-rate patterns than light meconium. They concluded that meconium should be used as a warning sign of fetal distress that warrants close intrapartum observation.

ELECTRONIC AND BIOCHEMICAL ASSESSMENT OF FETAL WELFARE DURING LABOR

Any decision regarding fetal welfare during labor should be based on a thorough assessment of the mother's health, the rate of progress of labor (by measurement of the rate of cervical dilatation and descent of the fetal presenting part), fetal maturity, and precise knowledge of the condition of the fetus. Although the risk of maternal death or serious morbidity following cesarean section is low, this should not be used to justify high cesarean section rates when the indication for the operation is fetal distress. The methods currently used to assess intrapartum fetal welfare can detect hypoxia but meticulous attention to detail and the commitment by those concerned with management to frequent determinations of the fetal pH is essential. Continuous intrapartum fetal heart rate monitoring is first and foremost a screening procedure to detect fetal hypoxia. The major drawback (from the obstetrician's point of view) to continuous fetal heart rate monitoring is the high percentage of false-positive results (the baby in good condition at birth following a suspicious or abnormal fetal heart rate pattern). On the other hand, false-negative results, that is, a normal fetal heart rate pattern but a baby in poor condition, are far less common providing that the second stage of labor is uncomplicated and in the absence of a placental abruption, cord prolapse, or surgical delivery. From the maternal point of view, continuous fetal heart rate monitoring does impose certain limitations on mobility; these are easily overcome by the use of telemetry or the provision of long leads between the mother and the monitor. Approximately 90% of mothers will be delivered within 12 hr of admission to a labor ward, provided that a policy of active management is pursued. Uncritical use of fetal heart rate monitoring will be associated with high cesarean section rates.

The Case for Continuous Monitoring

The vast majority of, if not all, intrapartum stillbirths or neonatal deaths due to severe intrapartum hypoxia are preceded by an abnormality in the continuous fetal heart-rate pattern. This abnormality is associated with increasing fetal hypoxia and lactic acidosis. At its simplest an electronic fetal heart rate monitor provides an accurate record of the fetal heart rate during labor. This is important for each individual pregnancy as it serves as an objective record of intrapartum welfare should the subsequent neonatal or infant development be abnormal. Even with the most meticulous prenatal care a number of fetuses will unexpectedly become hypoxic during labor. This unexpected hypoxia may be associated with existing but subclinical fetoplacental insufficiency or may be due to placental abruption, cord occlusion, uterine hyperstimulation, the supine hypotension syndrome, or hypotension associated with epidural analgesia. Parer (1979) analyzed 10 nonrandomized surveys that compared the results of monitored to unmonitored patients (Table 1). These studies varied widely in design, patient management, patient population, and the method of selection. Approximately half the studies compared the results of patients selected for monitoring with those whom it was elected not to monitor, generally within the same time period.

Table 1. Intrapartum Monitoring and Intrapartum Stillbirth (1958) and Neonatal Deaths (NND): Combined Results of Nonrandomized Trials[a]

Series	No. of patients		No. of IPSB		IPSB rate/1000		No. of NND		NND rate/1000	
	C	M	C	M	C	M	C	M	C	M
Paul and Hon, 1974	21,000	6,686	29	4	1.4	0.6	139	36	6.7	5.4
Tutera and Newman, 1975	6,179	608	37	1	6	2	49	0	8.0	0
Shenker et al., 1975	11,599	1,950	14	1	1.2	0.5	128	6	11.0	3.1
Koh et al., 1975	794	286	5	1	6.3	3.5	3	1	3.8	3.5
Edington et al., 1975	5,597	2,102	26	1	4.6	0.5	63	0	11.3	4.3
Lee and Baggish, 1976	4,323	3,529	16	1	3.7	0.3	56	21	13.0	6.0
Amato, 1977	2,981	4,226	9	1	3.0	0.2	24	4	5.7	0.9
Johnstone et al., 1978	9,099	7,312	11	3	1.2	0.4	..	..	..	..
Hughey et al., 1977	3,438	3,852	..	..	..	..	14	9	4.0	2.3
Neutra et al., 1978	8,664	7,182	..	..	..	..	48	23	5.5	3.2
Total	..	..	147	13	2.4	0.5	524	109	8.1	3.6
x^2	..	..	36.1($p < 0.0001$)		..	..	63.2($p < 0.0001$)		..	..

[a]Results of outcome of labor in 10 nonrandomized surveys comparing monitored (M) with unmonitored controls (C).
Source: Parer, 1979.

The other studies compared results of monitoring virtually all patients with results obtained either without or with limited monitoring in preceding years. The studies and sequential time periods may have introduced errors due to concomitant changes in patient care, such as improved neonatal care, which may give beneficial results incorrectly attributed to monitoring. Studies of patients selected for monitoring during the same time period contain errors because high-risk patients, with expected worse outcome, are usually in a monitored group. This would tend to dilute the apparent advantages of monitoring. The striking features in the combined analyses are the drop in the intrapartum stillbirth rate from 2.4 to 0.5:1000 and the halving of the neonatal death rate in association with monitoring; improved outcome with monitoring in every individual trial; the total number of patients (greater than 95,000) sufficient to demonstrate the differences statistically; incidences of intrapartum stillbirth and neonatal death rates less in randomized trials than in nonrandomized trials; neonatal death rates significantly less. In uncontrolled trials it is difficult to ascribe cause and effect to monitor use and decreased deaths, however it is equally difficult to refute such a relationship. Parer (1979) concluded that the intrapartum stillbirth rate will decrease by 1-2:1000 and neonatal deaths would halve if monitoring was widely used.

Continuous intrapartum fetal heart-rate monitoring has been used in virtually all patients delivering at St. Mary's Hospital, Manchester, in 1979 and 1980. Before this time most high-risk patients were monitored. The number of intrapartum stillbirths and first-day neonatal deaths classified by clinicopathological cause from 1976 to 1980 is shown in Table 2. Dr. A. J. Barson, perinatal pathologist at St. Mary's, performed the post mortem examinations and classified the results. The causes of death are largely self-explanatory. Hypoxia, uncomplicated, refers to those in which no other factor such as cord occlusion, birth trauma, or placental abruption was likely to have accounted for the perinatal death. The policy of total continuous intrapartum monitoring has been associated with a decrease in the number of perinatal deaths due to uncomplicated hypoxia; the results closely approximate the improvement forecast by Parer (1979). During this time span, the number of intrapartum and early neonatal deaths associated with hypoxia, decreased by three, and the number of neonates suffering from meconium aspiration syndrome decreased from 12 to 6 (Table 3).

The number of intrapartum stillbirths by weight for gestational age at St. Mary's from 1976 to 1980, excluding those with lethal congenital abnormalities and extreme prematurity, is shown in Table 4. A decrease in the number of growth-retarded fetuses dying in labor has been associated with an increase in the use of continuous fetal heart rate monitoring. In the Scottish Perinatal Survey (McIlwaine et al., 1979), 103 of the deaths

Table 2. Intrapartum and First-Day Deaths by Clinicopathological Cause, Saint Mary's Hospital, Manchester

	1976	1977	1978	1979	1980
Lethal malformation	17	12	10	7	11
Extreme prematurity (≤28 weeks)	3	3	3	5	8
Hyaline membraine disease/ intraventricular hemorrhage	3	2	0	3	2
Hypoxia, uncomplicated	4	4	3	0	1
Prepartum hemorrhage	1	4	2	1	7
Pre-eclampsia, hypertension	1	2	0	1	0
Other maternal disease	3	0	0	0	3
Cord occlusion	1	1	0	2	0
Birth trauma	3	2	2	3	0
Intrauterine infection	1	2	1	0	0
Total	37	32	21	22	32

Source: Courtesy of A. J. Barson, St. Mary's Hospital, Manchester, England.

occurred in growth-retarded but normally formed infants. Of these 103 deaths, 7 occurred in labor and 23 postpartum. It is likely that continuous fetal heart-rate monitoring will reduce the number of perinatal deaths in this group.

The number of live births by mode of delivery and gestational length at St. Mary's from 1975 to 1979 is shown in Table 3. The proportion of preterm deliveries by forceps decreased from 30.8% in 1975 to 17% in 1979; this resulted from a deliberate change in policy which precluded delivery by forceps in the preterm infant in the absence of fetal heart-rate or biochemical evidence of fetal distress. There has been no change in the rate of forceps deliveries from 1975 to 1979 in term pregnancies. The decreased number of deaths from intrapartum hypoxia has been associated with an increase in the proportion of women being delivered by emergency cesarean section. The indications for cesarean section are shown in Table 5. Although in 1975, 3.5% (142 of 4005) of women and in 1979 7.5% (319 of 4347) were delivered by emergency cesarean section, the proportion of emergency operations undertaken for fetal distress fell from 57.1% (81 of 142) in 1975 to 42.6% (136 of 319) in 1979 (Table 5). The results at St. Mary's Hospital, Manchester, show that (1) intrapartum fetal heart rate monitoring is associated with a decrease in the number of stillbirths and early neonatal deaths from intrapartum hypoxia and a decrease in the number of emergency cesarean sections for fetal distress, and (2) that the increased number of emergency cesarean sections

Table 3. Live Discharges by Mode of Delivery and Gestational Length, Saint Mary's Hospital, Manchester

		1975		1976		1977		1978		1979		Subtotal
		n	%	n	%	n	%	n	%	n	%	n	%
Preterm (≤ 36 weeks)	Spontaneous vaginal	153	54.4	129	47.9	166	50.9	126	40.3	198	52.6	772	49.3
	Forceps	87	30.8	89	33.2	87	26.7	101	32.3	64	17.0	428	27.3
	Elective cesarean	18	6.3	28	10.4	50	15.3	47	15.0	57	15.2	200	12.8
	Emergency cesarean	24	8.5	23	8.5	23	7.1	39	12.4	57	15.2	166	10.6
	Subtotal	282	100.0	269	100.0	326	100.0	313	100.0	376	100.0	1566	100.0
Term (≤ 37 weeks)	Spontaneous vaginal	2832	76.1	753	72.6	822	71.6	826	68.6	743	69.2	13976	71.5
	Forceps	608	16.3	673	17.7	651	16.5	721	17.4	643	16.1	3296	16.8
	Elective cesarean	165	4.4	210	5.5	231	5.8	303	7.4	323	8.1	1232	6.3
	Emergency cesarean	118	3.2	159	4.2	242	6.1	271	6.6	262	6.6	1052	5.4
	Subtotal	3723	100.0	3795	100.0	3946	100.0	4121	100.0	3971	100.0	19556	100.0
	Total	4005		4064		4272		4434		4347		21122	
Preterm	% of total	7.0		7.1		8.3		7.6		8.6		7.4	
Term	% of total	93.0		92.9		91.7		92.4		91.4		92.6	
Meconium aspiration syndrome		12	–	10	–	13	–	9	–	6	–	–	–

Table 4. Stillbirths (Excluding Lethal Malformations and Gross Prematurity), Saint Mary's Hospital, Manchester, by Weight for Gestational Age at Post Mortem 1976-1980

	1976	1977	1978	1979	1980
Birthweight for gestational age					
SD−2	8	5	2	1	2
SD−1	4	6	1	2	3
SD 0	6	2	3	2	5
SD + 1	−	−	−	−	1
SD + 2	−	1	−	−	1
Not ascertainable	1	−	−	−	1
	19	13	6	5	13[a]

[a]Seven of these 13 deaths in appropriately grown infants were associated with a placental abruption.
Source: Courtesy of A. J. Barson, St. Mary's Hospital, Manchester, England.

from 1975 to 1979 does not reflect an overdiagnosis of fetal distress but is associated with other changes in intrapartum management including greater recourse to cesarean section with fetal malpresentations or malposition, particularly when the fetus is immature, the desire to avoid prolonged labor, and early recourse to repeat cesarean section if labor is not progressing satisfactorily. These results are in keeping with two earlier studies, (Simmons and Lieberman, 1972; Beard et al., 1977), which reported a decrease in the cesarean section rate after introduction of electronic fetal heart-rate monitoring. These studies support the contention that the combined use of fetal heart-rate monitoring and fetal blood sampling enables the obsetetrician to determine the condition of the fetus more accurately than with the traditional methods (auscultation and meconium), thus not only avoiding unnecessary cesarean sections, but also indicating when the operation is required.

The Case Against Electronic Monitoring

The widespread acceptance of this technology by practicing obstetricians has been questioned. Banta and Thacker (1979) regard the evidence for benefit of electronic fetal heart rate monitoring as contradictory. Goodlin and Haesslein (1979) have concluded that in well-screened healthy populations, electronic fetal monitoring adds little except to increase the cesarean section rate. The results of three randomized trials have not shown a clear-cut advantage to electronic fetal heart rate monitoring (Havercamp et al., 1976, 1979;

Table 5. Indications for Emergency Cesarean Section, Saint Mary's Hospital, Manchester

	1975				1979				% Change 1975 to 1979
	Preterm	Term	Total	%	Preterm	Term	Total	%	
Fetal distress	13	68	81	57.1	23	113	136	42.6	− 14.5
Malpresentation or malposition	3	23	26	18.3	18	60	78	24.4	+ 6.1
Failure to progress in labor and maternal disorders	2	20	22	15.5	1	69	70	22.0	+ 6.5
Previous cesarean section	2	5	7	4.9	9	17	26	8.2	+ 3.3
Prepartum hemorrhage	4	2	6	4.2	6	3	9	2.8	− 1.4
Total	24	118	142	100.0	57	262	319	100.0	—

Table 6. Diagnostic Precision of Fetal Heart-Rate (FHR) Monitoring Using Apgar Score as the Measure of Outcome

Source		False positives (%)	False negatives (%)	Sensitivity	Specificity
FHR alone					
Bissonnette, 1975	714	20.3	5.7	57.3	82.3
1-min Apgar <7					
Gabert and Stenchever, 1973	749	33.8	8.6	84.2	79.5
1-min Apgar <6					
Schifrin and Dame, 1972					
1-min Apgar <7	307	57.1	7.0	53.8	89.6
5-min Apgar <7	307	79.6	0.7	83.3	87.2
Saldana et al., 1976	620	77.0	13.8	70.6	43.7
1-min Apgar <7					
Tipton and Shelley, 1971	100	18.5	6.8	81.5	93.2
1-min Apgar <7					
FHR + FSB					
Beard et al., 1971	270	43.6	19.9	32.4	91.6
1-min Apgar <7					

Source: Banta and Thacker (1979).

Kelso et al., 1978), while a fourth study by Renou et al. (1976) showed considerable benefit. Parer (1979) noted that the expected intrapartum stillbirth rate prior to the general use of intrapartum monitoring was approximately 2-3:1000 births (excluding deaths in infants less than 1000 g and with lethal congenital abnormalities) and the neonatal death rate with the same exclusions was approximately 10:1000 births. To show a decline in intrapartum stillbirth rate by 1-2:1000 births would require 14,000 patients and a control group of the same number. The total number of patients in the prospective studies is only 2027 (897 controls and 1130 monitored). There was only one intrapartum stillbirth (a control) and the difference between groups in the number of neonatal deaths was not significant (2.5:1000 compared with 3.5:1000).

The high false-positive rate (low sensitivity or extent to which abnormals are correctly classified) of fetal heart-rate monitoring as a measure of intrapartum hypoxia as assessed by the Apgar score at birth is well-recognized. The sensitivity ranges from 53.8 to 84.2% (Table 6), but the majority of reports confirmed the relatively high specificity of fetal heart rate monitoring (low false-negative rate or extent to which normals are correctly classified). With the single exception (43.7%) the majority of authors report specificity of fetal heart rate monitoring to range from 79.5 to 93.2%. These reports confirm

Table 7. Diagnostic Precision of Fetal Scalp Blood Sampling Using Apgar Score as the Measure of Outcome[a]

Source	n	False negatives (%)	False positives (%)	Sensitivity (%)	Specificity (%)
Beard et al., 1971					
1-min Apgar <7, pH < 7.25	279	19.1	42.1	32.4	92.4
Bowe et al., 1970					
1-min Apgar pH < 7.20	355	13.9	30.3	62.6	89.4
Coltart, 1969					
1-min Apgar <7, pH < 7.25	295	23.6	42.2	30.6	90.1
De la Rama and Merkatz, 1970					
1-min Apgar <7, pH < 7.20	208	9.0	56.7	44.8	90.5
Hon et al., 1969					
1-min Apgar <7, pH ≤ 7.2	214	15.4	69.2	39.0	79.2
5-min Apgar <7	214	5.6	84.6	47.1	77.7
Kubli, 1968					
1-min Apgar <7, pH < 7.20	78	10.2	55.6	57.1	84.1
Wood et al., 1967					
2-min Apgar <7, pH < 7.20	118	47.4	21.7	28.6	90.9

[a]Rates in many studies have been recalculated because of innaccurate estimates of false positives and false negatives.
Source: Banta and Thacker, 1979

what is widely accepted among practicing obstetricians: the heart in a healthy fetus can respond to a variety of stimuli by alterations in rate and rhythm and that a normal fetal heart-rate pattern is generally associated with the birth of a baby in good condition; but that the presence of an abnormal pattern does not necessarily reflect intrapartum hypoxia. The relationship between fetal pH determinations in labor and the Apgar score is shown in Table 7. The sensitivity ranges from 28.6 to 62.6% and the specificity from 77.7 to 92.4%. These findings are not unexpected and reflect inter alia differences in technique and terminology, the inconsistent timing of fetal blood sampling relative to delivery, and lack of appreciation of events in the second stage of labor that affect the outcome. Fetal pH determinations during labor measure the acid-base status at the time of sampling: what is required is a continuous pH or PO_2 measurement and an analysis of the outcome of labor not only by clinical events (e.g., Apgar score) but also by umbilical vein and artery acid-base determinations and careful analysis and control of the events in the second stage of labor that adversely affect the condition of the baby at birth.

The predictive value of fetal heart-rate monitoring and fetal blood sampling is the relationship between the sensitivity and specificity of these investigations

to the prevalence rate of intrapartum hypoxia. The predictive value of a
positive test is the percentage of time that it denotes a hypoxia; the predictive
value of a negative test is similarly the percentage of time that a negative test
detects an unaffected individual. Accepting that the sensitivity of fetal heart
rate monitoring is 80% and the specificity 90%, the predictive value of a negative or normal test is 99.5% assuming that the prevalence rate of intrapartum
hypoxia is 20:1000. According to Banta and Thacker (1979) these results
reflect the low prevalence of the disease rather than the diagnostic accuracy
of the test. The predictive value of a normal fetal heart-rate pattern would
remain 98% even if the sensitivity and specificity were as low as 50%. Assuming the same rates of sensitivity and specificity, the predictive value of a
positive abnormal fetal heart rate pattern is only 14%, thus the abnormal test
incorrectly predicts outcome 86% of the time. If the prevalence to rate of
the condition was 10:1000 the predictive value of the abnormal test would
also decline. These views are important because uncritical reliance on these
diagnostic tests will be associated with an increase in the cesarean section
rates. The cause of the fetal heart rate abnormality should be sought and the
condition of the fetus assessed by acid-base studies.

Intrapartum stillbirth and neonatal death due to hypoxia do still occur in
mature normally formed infants monitored during labor. Avoidable factors
are present in the majority of these unfortunate perinatal deaths. These include a failure of the attending staff to recognize or appreciate the significance of the abnormality, the gradual change from normal to abnormal over
the course of a prolonged labor, the inappropriate use of oxytocic drugs
(syntocinon and prostaglandin), and the use of forceps to deliver a baby in a
critical state, often after a prolonged labor. A major factor is the high false-
positive rate of fetal hypoxia detected by continuous fetal heart-rate monitoring; this tends to lull the obstetrician into the acceptance of a "minor
abnormality" as being of little importance, followed by delivery of a dead
or severely hypoxic fetus. Measurement of the fetal acid-base status is the
most precise method of assessing the condition of the baby during labor.
However, fetal blood samples only give an assessment of the fetal condition
at the time of sampling and continuing or deteriorating fetal heart-rate
patterns are an indication for repeated fetal blood samples.

COMPLICATIONS OF FETAL HEART-RATE MONITORING AND FETAL BLOOD SAMPLING

Fetal

Clinically significant hemorrhage from the scalp or buttock following an
intrapartum fetal blood sample is rare (0.3% according to Balfour et al.,
1970). The amount of bleeding is reduced by the operator applying direct

pressure to the puncture site following the sampling. If bleeding continues, the application of a fetal scalp clip electrode will staunch the loss. Equally important, however, is the rough removal of the electrode following delivery resulting in scalp lacerations, bleeding, and infection. The electrode should be unscrewed gently or the jaws of a scalp clip similarly eased apart.

Puncture of fetal vessels by intrauterine catheters has been reported by Trudinger and Pryse Davies (1978) and Nuttal (1978).

The reported incidence of neonatal scalp abscesses following intrapartum monitoring ranges from 03. to 4.5% (Balfour et al., 1970; Okoda et al., 1977; Plavidal and Werch, 1976). Other reported complications include septicemia, cranial osteomyelitis, and disseminated herpetic infection (Overturf and Balfour, 1975; Thadepalli et al., 1976; Turbeville et al., 1976).

No adverse affects have been reported following the use of ultrasound to record the fetal heart continuously during labor. While it is accepted that infants delivered abdominally develop respiratory distress syndrome (RDS) and hyaline membrane disease (HMD) more frequently than those delivered vaginally, even when gestational length is controlled, the indication for cesarean section itself may be causally related to the incidence of RDS and HMD. The majority of infants delivered by cesarean section do not in fact develop HMD but experience only transient tachypnea of the newborn (TTN).

Maternal

Physical
The risk of serious maternal morbidity or mortality already attributable to fetal heart-rate monitoring is low. Uterine perforation by intrauterine catheters has been reported by Chan et al. (1973) and Tutera and Newman (1975). The major risks are associated with cesarean section. However, although the cesarean section rate has steadily increased in the United Kingdom since 1952, there has been a significant decline in the number of deaths associated with this procedure.

The estimated fatality rate fell from 4:1000 operations in 1952 to 0.7:1000 in 1975; the cesarean section rate has risen from approximately 2.6% in 1952 to 5.8% in 1975 (Reports on Confidential Enquiries into Maternal Deaths, 1954-1975). The risk of maternal morbidity and mortality directly related to fetal heart rate monitoring is as yet undetermined.

Emotional
Precise data is lacking. Many women gain comfort from knowing that their baby's condition is constantly being recorded, while others find this technology unacceptable. General acceptance of monitoring with high-risk pregnancies is prevalent, although its value in apparently healthy women and fetuses is open to debate. The emotional trauma suffered by prospective

parents at the death during labor or permanent disability of a normally formed fetus from hypoxia persuades the author to continue advocating a policy of intrapartum fetal heart-rate monitoring provided that the indications for emergency cesarean sections are strictly controlled.

SCREENING FOR INTRAPARTUM HYPOXIA

Since 1979, the policy at St. Mary's Hospital, Manchester, has been to screen for fetal hypoxia during labor in all patients by continuous electronic fetal heart-rate monitoring and to assess the condition of the fetus by pH determination in the presence of a suspicious or abnormal pattern. During the first 2 years of operation this policy has been associated with a decrease in the number of fetal deaths from uncomplicated hypoxia. These results, 0.0:1000 births in 1979 and 0.2:1000 births in 1980 approximate closely those predicted by Parer (1979).

The fetal heart can respond to a variety of stimuli by alterations in both rate and rhythm. Under physiological conditions, the heart rate of a well-oxygenated fetus may not alter in response to the stress of uterine contraction but the transient hypoxia associated with a uterine contraction may provoke a temporary increase in the basal rate (an acceleration), while pressure on the fetal head by increasing vagal tone is often associated with a decrease in the basal rate (a deceleration). Sedative drugs such as pethidine hydrochloride or diazepam crossing the placenta may reduce the baseline variability of the fetal heart thereby mimicking one of the fetal heart rate patterns seen with intrapartum hypoxia (Scher et al., 1972). Beta-blocking agents such as propranolol impair the fetus' ability to respond to hypoxia by preventing an increase in the fetal heart rate (Lieberman et al., 1978).

The fetal heart responds to hypoxia by an increase in rate. This tachycardia commonly takes a form of an acceleration from the basal rate associated with a uterine contraction; the rate returns to normal at or just prior to the cessation of the contraction. Prolonged hypoxia associated with fetoplacental insufficiency, uterine hyperstimulation, or epidural anesthesia may manifest as a sustained tachycardia. With increasing hypoxia the fetal heart loses the ability to respond to vagal influences, which manifests as a loss of beat-to-beat variation. Sinusoidal patterns (a fetal heart rate pattern with 2-5 oscillations/min, each oscillation having an amplitude of at least five beats per minute), although uncommon, have been reported in cases of severe rhesus isoimmunization (Rochard et al., 1976), fetal hypoxia (Baskett and Koh, 1974), fetal anemia due to massive fetal maternal transfusion (Modanlou et al., 1977), and Kell incompatibility (Birkenveld et al., 1980).

Figures 1 to 10 show fetal heart rate patterns commonly seen during labor, which may, for clinical purposes, be subdivided into three groups:

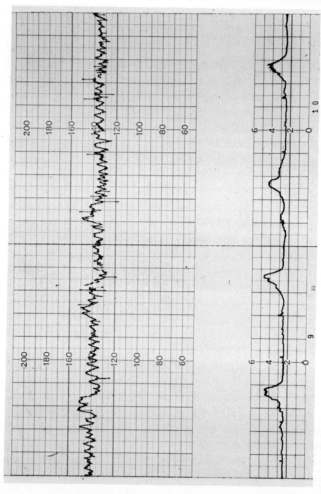

Figure 1. Normal fetal heart rate pattern, baseline rate 120-160 beats/min, baseline variability greater than five beats per minute. No decelerations. (Courtesy of R. Beard, St. Mary's Hospital, Manchester, England, and M. D. Gillmer, John Radcliffe Hospital, Oxford, England.)

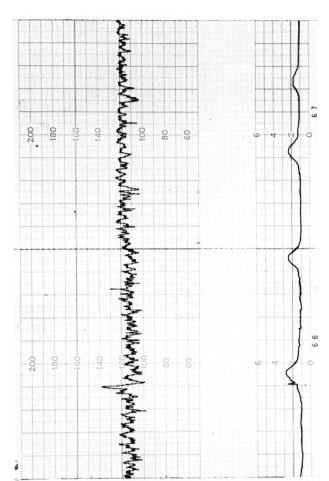

Figure 2. Normal fetal heart rate patterns with baseline bradycardia between 100 and 110 beats/min and baseline variability of greater than five beats/min. No decelerations. (Courtesy of R. Beard, St. Mary's Hospital, London, England, and M. D. Gillmer, John Radcliffe Hospital, Oxford, England.)

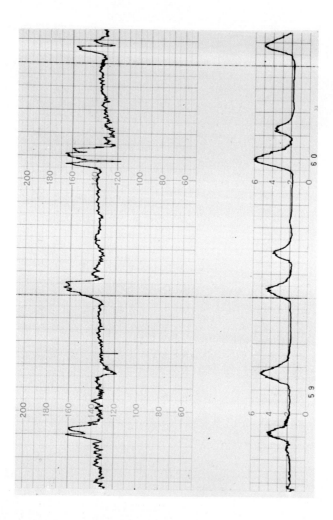

Figure 3. Normal fetal heart pattern with accelerations from baseline rate associated with contractions. Baseline rate and variability normal. (Courtesy of R. Beard, St. Mary's Hospital, London, England, and M. D. Gillmer, John Radcliffe Hospital, Oxford, England.)

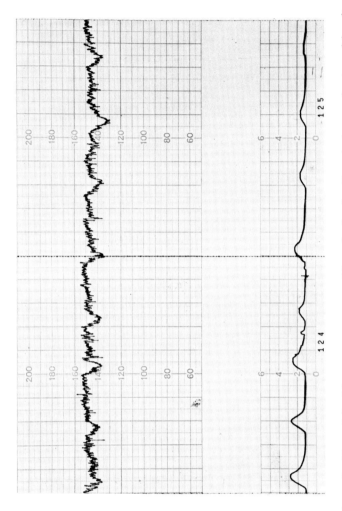

Figure 4. Normal fetal heart rate pattern with early decelerations but normal rate and baseline variability. (Courtesy of R. Beard, St. Mary's Hospital, Manchester, London, and M. D. Gillmer, John Radcliffe Hospital, Oxford, England.)

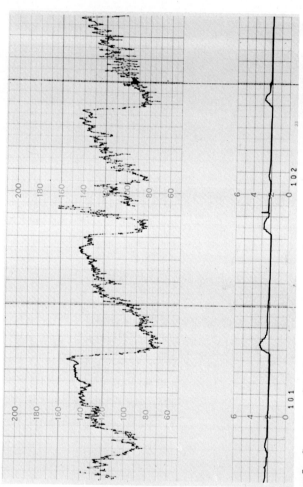

Figure 5. Suspicious fetal heart rate pattern with normal rate, baseline variability, and reactive accelerations but variable decelerations. (Courtesy of R. Beard, St. Mary's Hospital, London, England, and M. D. Gillmer, John Radcliffe Hospital, Oxford, England.)

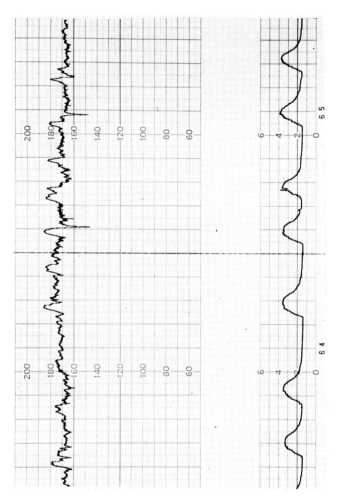

Figure 6. Suspicious fetal heart rate pattern with baseline tachycardia but normal baseline variability and reactive accelerations. (Courtesy of R. Beard, St. Mary's Hospital, London, England, and M. D. Gillmer, John Radcliffe Hospital, Oxford, England.)

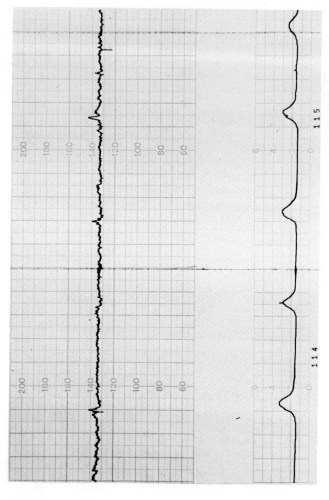

Figure 7. Suspicious fetal heart rate pattern with normal rate but lack of baseline variability and absence of reactive accelerations. (Courtesy of R. Beard, St. Mary's Hospital, London, England, and M. D. Gillmer, John Radcliffe Hospital, Oxford, England.)

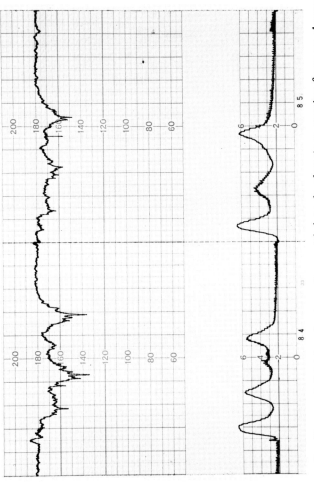

Figure 8. Abnormal fetal heart rate pattern with late decelerations starting from an abnormal baseline rate. (Courtesy of R. Beard, St. Mary's Hospital, London, England, and M. D. Gillmer, John Radcliffe Hospital, Oxford, England.)

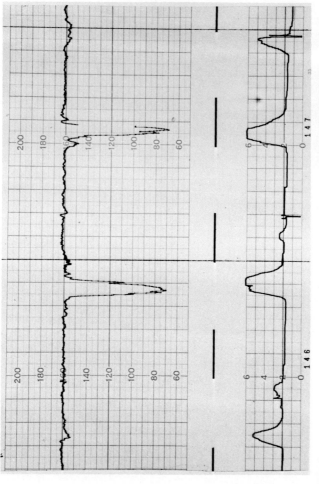

Figure 9. Abnormal fetal heart rate pattern with loss of baseline variability decelerations, tachycardia (>160 beats/min), and absence of reactive accelerations. (Courtesy of R. Beard, St. Mary's Hospital, London, England, and M. D. Gillmer, John Radcliffe Hospital, Oxford, England.)

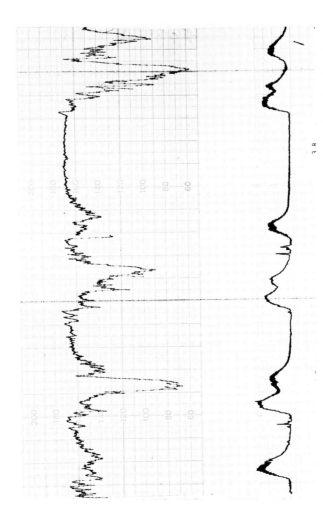

Figure 10. Abnormal fetal heart rate pattern with baseline tachycardia, late decelerations, and loss of baseline variability. (Courtesy of R. Beard, St. Mary's Hospital, London, England, and M. D. Gillmer, John Radcliffe Hospital, Oxford, England.)

(1) patterns likely to be associated with the birth of a baby in good condition (Apgar score equal to or grater than 7 at 1 and 5 min), hence referred to as normal fetal hart patterns; (2) suspicious patterns likely to procede to intrapartum hypoxia, and (3) abnormal patterns often associated with intrauterine hypoxia. This classification not only serves to screen for intrapartum hypoxia but is also useful as a teaching aid for both midwives and house officers. The principle of using the continuous fetal heart rate pattern as a *screening* test for intrapartum hypoxia is based on the observation that abnormal fetal heart-rate patterns are often associated with intrauterine hypoxia and that the fetal heart rate pattern is virtually *always abnormal* preceding an intrapartum stillbirth or the birth of a baby with severe perinatal hypoxia.

The relationship between these 10 fetal heart rate (FHR) patterns and intrapartum fetal blood pH values is shown in Figure 11. The proportion of FHR patterns associated with fetal blood pH values of <7.25 increases from approximately 1% with normal patterns to greater than 56.5% associated with variable decelerations and an abnormal baseline rate.

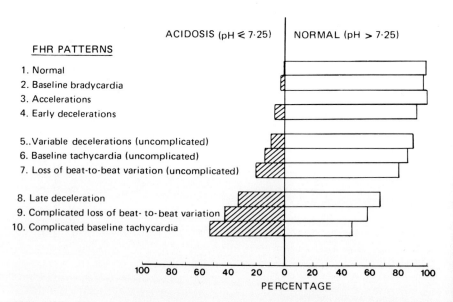

Figure 11. The relationship between fetal heart rate patterns and incidence of fetal acidosis during labor. (Courtesy of R. Beard, St. Mary's Hospital, London, England, and M. D. Gillmer, John Radcliffe Hospital, Oxford, England.)

Attention has already been drawn to the wide range in specificity and sensitivity of both intrapartum fetal heart rate patterns and fetal blood sampling in predicting the condition of the baby at birth. This lack of specificity and sensitivity has important clinical implications: uncritical use of this technology will result in unnecessarily high cesarean section rates. The cause of the fetal heart rate abnormality should be sought and the condition of the fetus assessed by fetal blood sampling. Management will obviously be influenced by the diagnosis, the condition of the fetus, and the stage of labor. Iatrogenic causes of fetal heart rate abnormalities are common. These include uterine hyperstimulation by intravenous oxytocin and prostaglandins, particularly in association with epidural anesthesia and supine hypotension. Maternal ketoacidosis, dehydration, and pyrexia are often associated with a fetal tachycardia, while fetoplacental insufficiency, fetal abnormalities, fetal anemia due to rhesus isoimmunization or a vasa previa, placental abruption, cord occlusion, and prolapse are well-recognized causes of fetal heart abnormalities.

In the second stage of labor the fetal heart rate shows an extremely wide range of response, making assessment of fetal welfare by heart rate monitoring virtually impossible. For practical purposes, the fetal heart rate should return to normal between contractions and a persistent fetal tachycardia or bradycardia should alert the clinician to the possibility of intrapartum hypoxia. A persistent fetal bradycardia between contractions or a delayed return to the normal rate following contraction is likely to be associated with intrapartum hypoxia and the delivery should be expedited.

Normal fetal heart rate patterns likely to be associated with the birth of the baby in a good condition are shown in Figures 1-4. The characteristics of these patterns include a baseline rate of 120-160 beats/min, the absence of decelerations with contractions, and a baseline variability of five beats per minute or more (Fig. 1). A baseline bradycardia with a rate of 100-199 beats/min, without decelerations and a normal baseline variability of five beats per minute or more *is also normal* and is often associated with a mature fetus with well-developed vagal tone (Fig. 2). Accelerations of fetal heart with the onset of a contraction, which return to the normal baseline rate before or shortly after the end of the contraction, indicate good reflex reactivity of the fetal circulation in response to the hypoxic stress of the contraction (Fig. 3). Early decelerations starting with the onset of the contraction that return to baseline rate by the end of the contraction, when the deceleration does not exceed 40 beats/min, are usually associated with a fetus in a good condition (Fig. 4). This pattern is due to head compression but may precede a suspicious or abnormal pattern and may thus reflect early hypoxia. Eight percent of these patterns are associated with fetal acidosis (intrapartum pH < 7.25) (Fig. 11).

Suspicious fetal heart patterns are shown in Figures 5-7. Uncomplicated variable decelerations are shown in Fig. 5; these consist of a normal baseline rate of 120-160 beats/min, a baseline variability of five beats per minute or more but with a decrease in the fetal heart at the onset of or early during the course of a contraction. The deceleration has an irregular shape that is variable from contraction to contraction, and the decrease in rate is usually more than 60 beats/min. This pattern may precede more abnormal patterns and is associated with fetal acidosis in approximately 10% of cases (Fig. 11).

An uncomplicated baseline fetal tachycardia is shown in Figure 6. The baseline fetal heart ranges from 160 to 180 beats/min, but the baseline variability is *normal* and there are no decelerations with contractions. This pattern is often secondary to maternal pyrexia, ketoacidosis, and dehydration and is associated with fetal acidosis in approximately 14% of patients (Fig. 11).

An uncomplicated loss of baseline variability is shown in Figure 7. The baseline fetal heart rate is normal but the baseline variability is less than five beats per minute. In the absence of decelerations, this pattern is often associated with the use of sedative or analgesic drugs but approximately 20% of these patterns will be associated with fetal acidosis. In general, the less baseline variability present, the greater the possibility of fetal hypoxia (Fig. 11).

Abnormal fetal heart rate patterns are shown in Figures 8-10. Late decelerations, when the nadir of the fetal heart rate occurs after the peak of the contraction, are shown in Figure 8. The interval between the nadir of the deceleration and the peak of the uterine contraction is referred to as lag time. In general the greater the lag time and the time taken for the deceleration to return to the normal baseline rate, the greater the possibility of fetal hypoxia. At least 30% of these patterns will be associated with fetal acidosis (Fig. 11). A complicated loss of baseline variability is shown in Figure 9. This pattern consists of an abnormal baseline rate (greater than 160 beats/min or bradycardia less than 120 beats/min) associated with a decreased baseline variability and or the presence of decelerations; 42% of these patterns are associated with fetal acidosis. A complicated tachycardia is shown in Figure 10. This consists of an abnormal baseline fetal heart rate (greater than 160 beats/min) associated with decelerations and a loss of baseline variability. More than 50% of these patterns will be associated with fetal acidosis (Fig. 11).

The management of labor in a patient with a suspicious or abnormal fetal heart rate pattern will be determined by the fetal pH value and the clinical features of the particular case. The patient should be put into the left lateral position and any obvious cause for the fetal heart rate abnormality, such as oxytocin hyperstimulation, maternal pyrexia, ketoacidosis or dehydration, treated and a vaginal examination performed to exclude full dilatation of the cervix and a cord prolapse. The fetal pH should be measured. No further action is required if the pH is equal to or greater than 7.26 and the fetal heart rate pattern returns to *normal*. Should the suspicious or *abnormal pattern persist* serial blood samples are indicated at 30-60 min intervals until delivery. A fetal pH of 7.20-7.25 is *abnormal*. A second sample should be taken and, if the acidosis is confirmed, delivery by the most appropriate means is indicated. This would be cesarean section if the cervix is not fully dilated or forceps should the cervix be fully dilated with vertex at or below the level of the ischial spines. A midcavity or rotational forceps delivery is contraindicated in the presence of fetal acidosis. A pH below 7.20 is *pathological;* the fetus should be delivered as expeditiously as possible.

FETAL HEART-RATE PATTERN IN PRETERM AND LOW-BIRTH-WEIGHT INFANTS

Martin et al. (1974) reported that in a group of 73 infants weighing less than 2000 g, the incidence of respiratory distress syndrome and the poroportion of neonatal deaths from RDS was increased in babies who had shown late severe variable decelerations during labor. A significant increase in deaths associated with RDS was apparent in infants who had shown a decreased baseline variability during labor (0-5 beats/min), and those with a marked tachycardia (>180 beats/min). They noted that this association between abnormal fetal heart rate patterns and death from RDS was limited to babies of less than 35 weeks' gestational age and was not apparent in more mature low-birth-weight infants. Bowes et al. (1980) analyzed the relationship between the continuous fetal heart rate patterns and the neonatal outcome in 61 infants weighing 1500 g or less. Normal patterns or good baseline variability correlated well with normal umbilical artery pH.

Although the value of intrapartum fetal heart rate monitoring in predicting the subsequent development of central nervous system hemorrhage, respiratory distress syndrome, and neonatal deaths was poor in these very low-birth-weight babies, the authors concluded that early intervention and operative delivery in infants with abnormal patterns may have influenced the outcome. Fetal heart rate patterns can therefore play an important role in the intrapartum assessment of these fetuses by identifying those who require prompt operative intervention and vigorous neonatal resuscitation.

PREDICTION OF THE BABY'S CONDITION AT BIRTH

Numerous classifications have been proposed for the prenatal assessment of fetal welfare by a scoring system dependent on the fetal heart rate and its response to fetal movement, Braxton Hicks contractions, and those stimulated by intravenous oxytocin (Kubli et al., 1977; Rochard et al., 1976; Pearson and Weaver, 1978; Earn, 1980).

The need for an intrapartum scoring classification is less important since the obstetrician has direct access to the fetus via fetal blood sampling and the wide range of response to intrapartum stimuli by the fetal heart reduces the validity of such a scoring system.

INTRAPARTUM FETAL ELECTROCARDIOGRAMS

The intrapartum fetal electrocardiogram (FECG) can be recorded continuously and stored on a computer. Marvell et al. (1980) have established the normal range of FECG values by passing these signals, after amplification and filtration, through an interface system to a digital computer. They noted changes in the FECG of normal babies that were previously thought to be characteristic of fetal distress. The PR interval was up to 10% shorter during contraction towards the end of labor and fell by 7% before delivery. The P wave amplitude fell by 30% in the hour before delivery. The QRS complex lengthened slightly toward the end of labor but the RR interval and ST segment displacement showed no significant change. They stressed the failure to diagnose fetal distress by simple changes in the fetal ECG and noted that the response of the FECG to the transient and long-term stresses of labor might provide the basis for understanding FECG in labor.

ACKNOWLEDGMENTS

I am extremely grateful to Dr. A. J. Barson, Perinatal Pathologist, St. Mary's Hospital, Manchester, for his invaluable and impartial analysis of the still-births and early neonatal deaths, and the Department of Medical Records at St. Mary's Hospital and North West Regional Statitician, Gateway House, Manchester for their help with Tables 4 and 5. I would like to thank Dr. M. D. Gillmer and Professor R. W. Beard for permission to reproduce Figures 1 to 11 from their Labour Wall Chart, printed by Hewlett Packard.

I am indebted to Mrs. V. E. Doney and Mrs. E. O. Stewart for typing the manuscript.

REFERENCES

Abramovici, H., Brandes, J. M., Fuchs, K., and Timor-Fritsch, I. (1974). Meconium during delivery: A sign of compensated fetal distress. *Am. J. Obstet. Gynecol. 118*:251.

Amato, J. C. (1977). Fetal monitoring in a community hospital: A statistical analysis. *Obstet. Gynecol. 50*:269-274.

Balfour, H. H., Bloc, S. H., Bowe, E. T., et al. (1970). Complications of fetal blood sampling. *Am. J. Obstet. Gynecol. 107*:288-294.

Banta, E. D., and Thacker, S. B. (1979). Assessing the costs and benefits of electronic fetal monitoring. *Obstet. Gynecol. Surv. 34*:8, 627-642.

Baskett, T. F., and Koh, K. S. (1974). Sinusoidal fetal heart rate pattern—A sign of fetal hypoxia. *Obstet. Gynecol. 44*:379-382.

Beard, R. W., Edington, P. T., and Sibanda, J. (1977). The effects of routine intrapartum monitoring in clinical practice. *Contrib. Gynecol. Obstet. 3*:14-21.

Birkenfield, A., Yaffe, E., and Sadovsky, E. (1980). Sinusoidal fetal heart rate pattern with severe fetal anaemia. *Br. J. Obstet. Gynaecol. 87*:916-919.

Bissonnette, J. M. (1975). Relationship between continuous fetal heart rate patterns and Apgar score in the newborn. *Br. J. Obstet. Gynaecol. 82*: 24-28.

Bowes, W. A., Gabbe, S. G., and Bowes, C. (1980). Fetal heart rate monitoring in premature infants weighing 1500 gms. or less. *Am. J. Obstet. Gynecol. 137*:7, 791-795.

Chan, W. E., Paul, R. E., and Toews, J. (1973). Intrapartum monitoring, maternal and fetal morbidity and perinatal mortality. *Obstet. Gynaecol. 41*: 7-13.

Desmond, M. M., Moore, J., Lindley, J. E., and Brown, C. A. (1957). Meconium staining of the amniotic fluid. *Obstet. Gynecol. 9*:91-203.

Dilts, P. V. (1976). Current practice in antepartum and intrapartum monitoring. *Am. J. Obstet. Gynecol. 126*:491-494.

Earn, A. A. (1980). A proposed international scoring system for predicting fetal status derived from fetal heart rate patterns. *Obstet. Gynecol. Surv. 35*:265-270.

Edington, P. T., Sibanda, J., and Beard, R. W. (1975). Influence on clinical practice of routine intrapartum fetal monitoring. *Br. Med. J. 3*:341-343.

Gabert, H. A., and Stenchever, M. A. (1973). Continuous electronic monitoring of fetal heart during labor. *Am. J. Obstet. Gynecol. 115*:919-923.

Gillmer, M. D. G., and Coombe, D. (1979). Intrapartum fetal monitoring practice in the United Kingdom. *Br. J. Obstet. Gynecol. 86*:10, 753-758.

Goodlin, R. C., and Haesslein, H. C. (1977). Where is it fetal distress? *Am. J. Obstet. Gynecol. 128*:440-447.

Haverkamp, A. D., Thompson, E. E., McFee, J. G., and Cetrulo, C. (1976). The evaluation of continuous fetal heart rate monitoring in high risk pregnancy. *Am. J. Obstet. Gynecol. 125*:310-320.

Haverkamp, A. D., Orleans, M. Langendoerfer, S., McFee, J., Murphy, J., and Thompson, E. E. (1979). A controlled trial of the differential effects of intrapartum fetal monitoring. *Am. J. Obstet. Gynecol. 134*:399-412.

Hughey, M. J., La Pata, R. E., McElin, T. W., et al. (1977). The effect of fetal monitoring on the incidence of Caesarean section. *Obstet. Gynecol. 49*: 513-518.

Johnstone, F. D., Campbell, D. M., Hughes, G. J. (1970). Has continuous intrapartum monitoring made any impact on fetal outcome? *Lancet 1*: 1298-1300.

Kelso, I. M., Parsons, R. J., Lawrence, G. F., Arora, S. S., Edmonds, K. D., and Cook, I. D. (1978). An assessment of continuous fetal heart rate—A randomized trial. *Am. J. Obstet. Gynecol. 131*:526-532.

Koh, K. S., Greves, D., Yung, S., et al. (1975). Experience with fetal monitoring in a University teaching hospital. *Can. Med. Assoc. J. 112*:455-460.

Krebs, H. B., Petes, R. E., Dunn, L. J., Jordan, E. V. F., and Segreti, A. (1980). Intrapartum fetal heart rate monitoring. Association of meconium with abnormal fetal heart rate patterns. *Am. J. Obstet. Gynecol. 137*:8, 936-943.

Kubli, F., Boos, R., Ruttgers, H., et al. (1977). Antepartum fetal heart rate monitoring. In *Proceedings of Scientific Meeting of the Royal College of Obstetricians and Gynecologists*. R. Beard and S. Campbell (Eds.), Royal College of Obstetricians and Gynecologists, London.

Lees, W. K., and Baggish, M. S. (1976). The effect of unselected intrapartum fetal monitoring. *Obstet. Gynecol. 47*:516-520.

Lieberman, B. A., Stirrat, G. M., Belsey, E., Cohen, S., Pinker, G. D., and Beard, R. W. (1978). The possible adverse effect of propranolol on the fetus in pregnancy complicated by severe hypertension. *Br. J. Obstet. Gynaecol. 85*:678.

Lucas, A., Christofides, N. D., Adrian, T. E., Bloom, S. R., and Aynsley-Green, A. (1979). Fetal distress, meconium and motilin. *Lancet, 718*.

McIlwaine, G. M., Howat, R. C. L., Dunn, F., and Macnaughton, M. C. (1979). The Scottish Perinatal Mortality Survey. *Br. Med. J., 2*:1103-1106.

Martin, C. B., Siassi, B., and Hon, E. H. (1974). Fetal heart rate patterns and neonatal death in low birthweight infants. *Obstet. Gynecol. 44*:4, 503-510.

Marvell, C. J., Kirk, D. L., Jenkins, H. M. L., and Symonds, E. M., (1980). The normal condition of the fetal electrocardiogram during labour. *Br. J. Obstet. Gynaecol., 87*:786-796.

Modanlou, D., Freeman, R. K., Oritiz, O., Hinkes, P., and Pillsbury, G. (1977). Sinusoidal fetal heart rate pattern with severe anaemia. *Obstet. Gynecol. 49*:537-541.

Neutra, R. R., Fienberg, S. E., Greenland, S., et al. (1978). Effect of fetal monitoring on neonatal death rate. *N. Engl. J. Med. 299*:324-326.

Nuttal, I. D. (1978). Perforation of a placental fetal vessel by an intrauterine pressure catheter. *Br. J. Obstet. Gynecol. 85*:573.

Okada, D. M., Chow, A. W., and Bruce, V. T. (1977). Neonatal scalp abscess and fetal monitoring, factors associated with infection. *Am. J. Obstet. Gynecol. 129*:185-189.

Overturf, G. D., and Balfour, G. (1975). Osteomyelitis and sepsis, severe complications of fetal monitoring. *Pediatrics 55*:244-247.

Paul, R. E., and Hon, E. H. (1974). Clinical fetal monitoring: Effect on perinatal outcome. *Am. J. Obstet. Gynecol. 118*:529-533.

Parer, J. T. (1979). Fetal heart rate monitoring. *Lancet 2*:632-633.

Pearson, J. F., and Weaver, J. B., (1978). A six point scoring system for antenatal cardiotocographs. *Br. J. Obstet. Gynaecol. 85*:321.

Plavidal, F. J., and Werch, A. (1976). Fetal scalp abscess secondary to intrauterine monitoring. *Am. J. Obstet. Gynecol. 125*:65-70.

Renou, P., Chang, A., Anderson, I., and Wood, E. C., (1976). A controlled trial of fetal intensive care. *Am. J. Obstet. Gynecol. 126*:470-476.

Rochard, F., Schrifin, B. S., Goupil, F., et al. (1976). Non stressed fetal heart rate monitoring in the antenatal period. *Am. J. Obstet. Gynecol. 126*:699.

Saldana, L. R., Schulman, H., and Yang, W. (1976). Electronic fetal monitoring during labour. *Obstet. Gynecol. 47*:706-710.

Shenker, L., Post, R. C., and Seiler, J. S. (1975). Routine electronic monitoring of fetal heart rate and uterine activity during labour. *Obstet. Gynecol. 46*:185-189.

Scher, J., Hailey, D. M., and Beard, R. W. (1972). The effects of diazepam on the fetus. *J. Obstet. Gynecol. Br. Commonw. 79*:635.

Schifrin, B. S., and Dame, L. (1972). Fetal heart rate patterns. Prediction of Apgar score. *JAMA 219*:1322-1325.

Simmons, S. C., and Lieberman, B. A. (1972). The combined use of cardiotocography and fetal blood sampling in monitoring the fetus in labour. *J. Obstet. Gynecol. Br. Commonw. 79*:816-820.

Thadepalli, H., Rambhatla, K., Maidman, J. E., et al. (1976). Gonococcal sepsis secondary to fetal monitoring. *Am. J. Obstet. Gynecol. 126*:510-512.

Tipton, R., and Shelley, T. (1971). An index of fetal welfare in labour. *J. Obstet. Gynecol. Br. Commonw. 78*:702-706.

Trudinger, B. J., and Pryse-Davies, J. (1978). Fetal hazards of the intrauterine pressure catheter. Five case reports. *Br. J. Obstet. Gynaecol. 85*:567.

Turbeville, D. F., Health, R. E., Bowen, F. W., et al. (1976). Complications of fetal scalp electrodes, a case report. *Am. J. Obstet. Gynecol. 122*:530-531.

Tutera, G., and Newman, R. L. (1975). Fetal monitoring, ets effect on the perinatal mortality and caesarean section rates and its complications. *Am. J. Obstet. Gynecol. 122*:750-754.

13

Predictors of Intrapartum Fetal Distress: The Role of Electronic Fetal Monitoring

FREDERICK P. ZUSPAN / The Ohio State University, Columbus, Ohio

E. J. QUILLIGAN / University of California at Irvine, Irvine, California

JAY D. IAMS / The Ohio State University College of Medicine, Columbus, Ohio

HERMAN P. van GEIJN / Academisch Ziekenhuis der Vrije Universiteit, Amsterdam, The Netherlands

National Institutes of Health (NIH) Consensus Development Conferences have been established to address in a broad manner recent developments in medical practice and research. The Task Force participants are chosen entirely from outside the NIH and are asked to provide a comprehensive review of the state of the art, including recommendations for current clinical practice and future research in a given area of medicine. The National Institute of Child Health and Human Development recently established three such Consensus Development Task Forces on antenatal diagnosis. This report summarizes the findings of the Task Force on Predictors of Intrapartum Fetal Distress. The other two concerned predictors of hereditary disease and congenital defects and predictors of fetal maturity; the findings in these two studies will be reported separately.

The format for such conferences calls for a broad and detailed examination of the topic at hand, by a task force composed of physicians, epidemiologists, sociologists, ethicists, economists, lawyers, and public (consumer) representatives.

The full text of this report was circulated to interested individuals, institutions, and organizations before being presented in summary form at a public forum on March 6, 1979, at the National Institutes of Health. Those interested in commenting on the draft report had an opportunity to do so at that time,

Report of the National Institute of Child Health and Human Development Consensus Development Task Force. Reproduced with permission from *Am. J. Obstet. Gynecol.* *135:*287-291, 1979. Copyrighted by The C. V. Mosby Company, St. Louis, Missouri.

either in writing or verbally, after which the Task Force reviewed the comments made and incorporated them into the report as necessary. The entire report may be obtained upon request from the Office of Research Reporting, NICHD, Room 2A 34, Bethesda, Maryland 20014.

Because of the complexity of the subject and length of the report, only the Summary and Conclusions and the Recommendations sections are reprinted here. This report is being concurrently published by *The Journal of Reproductive Medicine,* the *Journal of Pediatrics,* and the *American Journal of Obstetrics and Gynecology.*

SUMMARY AND CONCLUSIONS

The following conclusions reflect the consensus of the Task Force based upon currently available information.

Intrapartum events are currently estimated to account for 20% of still-births, 20-40% of cerebral palsy, and approximately 10% of severe mental retardation, less than estimates based upon earlier retrospective studies. Nevertheless, adverse intrapartum events continue to be an important source of potentially preventable death and damage. Neonatal morbidity and mortality secondary to intrapartum asphyxia are well-known, but the precise magnitude of these problems is not known. The possibility of subclinical neurological dysfunction has been suggested in animal studies, but current outcome measures are inadequate to assess the subclinical effects of intrapartum hypoxia in humans.

Intrapartum hypoxic events may occur in any pregnancy but are more common in pregnancies defined as high-risk during either the prepartum or intrapartum period. Unfortunately, current risk-assessment profiles do not predict all instances of intrapartum morbidity and mortality.

Intermittent methods of fetal surveillance during labor (auscultation of the fetal heart rate every 15 min in the first stage and every 5 min during the second stage, in both instances for a period of 30 sec immediately after a uterine contraction) provide an acceptable method for intrapartum monitoring in low-risk pregnancies. This intensive supervision requires adequate numbers of well-trained personnel at the patient's bedside.

A normal fetal heart-rate pattern on continuous electronic fetal monitoring indicates a greater than 95% probability of fetal well-being. Laboratory and clinical studies have demonstrated that fetal hypoxia reliably produces changes in fetal heart rate patterns; however, these abnormal patterns may also occur in the absence of fetal distress.

Fetal distress in labor cannot be assessed by considering a single measurement such as intermittent or continuous fetal heart rate. Because fetal heart-rate patterns suggestive of hypoxia may occur in the absence of fetal distress, intermittent and continuous fetal heart rate assessments are screening, rather than diagnostic, techniques. Failure to appreciate this limitation may lead to inappropriate clinical decisions.

Intervention in labor to alleviate fetal hypoxia requires careful consideration of all available information. Fetal heart rate data indicating fetal distress require support from other clinical and laboratory information, including fetal scalp blood pH determination, when indicated, before a firm basis for intervention can be established.

The weight of present evidence from prospective and retrospective analyses shows no apparent effect of electronic fetal monitoring on perinatal mortality and morbidity in low-risk pregnancies. As maternal and fetal risk increases, there is a trend suggesting a beneficial effect of electronic fetal monitoring on intrapartum and neonatal morbidity and mortality. Specific obstetric risk factors especially amenable to intervention via electronic fetal monitoring have not yet been completely enumerated.

Maternal and fetal complications of electronic fetal monitoring have been reported. The most frequently reported fetal complication of internal monitoring is scalp abscess at the site of electrode application. Internal fetal monitoring by itself does not appear to be an important factor in the incidence of maternal postpartum infection. Other complications less frequently reported relate predominantly to errors in application of the fetal scalp electrode or intrauterine pressure catheter. The known risks of the external mode of fetal monitoring at present are minimal. There are no conclusive data on the long-term effects of continuous ultrasound application.

The effect of electronic fetal monitoring on the incidence of cesarean section may vary with the manner in which monitoring data are interpreted. In two of four randomized clinical trials in teaching hospital settings statistically significant increased rates of primary cesarean section have been demonstrated in monitored women. Several large retrospective studies in teaching hospitals have found this increase to be independent of the use of electronic fetal monitoring. The effect of electronic fetal monitoring on the cesarean delivery rate in any particular hospital may depend on the clinical use and norms of practice in that hospital. There is evidence that the simultaneous use of fetal scalp blood sampling provides additional information and may reduce the incidence of monitoring-associated cesarean section. The ideal use of electronic fetal monitoring in influencing more appropriate cesarean delivery has yet to be determined.

A number of additional promising fetal assessment techniques are currently under investigation. These include the use of computer microprocessors in combination with heart-rate monitors, telemetry systems, continuous monitoring of scalp pH, transcutaneous monitoring of oxygen tension, evaluation of fetal movements, and electroencephalography. None of these has been sufficiently evaluated to merit introduction into obstetric practice.

Techniques introduced into obstetric practice in the last decade may conflict with the concept of family-centered childbirth. Although limited research in this area has been done, currently available data suggest that electronic fetal monitoring need not diminish the human experience of childbirth when properly employed and explained by knowledgeable and supportive medical personnel. This early research also suggests that pregnant women who have an opportunity to discuss the potential uses and limitation of electronic fetal monitoring are less likely to have a negative reaction to its use.

Many of the ethical issues presented by electronic fetal monitoring are related to uncertainties about its risk and benefits and to the unique psychological situation of a woman in labor. Both increase the difficulties of achieving truly informated decision-making. Other such issues arise from the current concern about medical malpractice litigation, the increasing use of technology in childbirth, and questions of social justice and allocation of scarce resources. Future research to define proper use of electronic fetal monitoring may disclose additional issues.

Under present methods of application, electronic fetal monitoring increases the cost of obstetric services, although not by a large amount. These costs must be considered against the economic savings and benefits generated by electronic fetal monitoring. The development of more reliable estimates of these benefits must await definitive studies of the impact of electronic monitoring on perinatal morbidity and mortality.

Courts of law should recognize that intrapartum hypoxia is only one of many potential factors involved in the development of handicaps and perinatal death and that current research and clinical data do not allow comprehensive definition of prepartum and intrapartum risk or of means to reduce risk of adverse outcome.

RECOMMENDATIONS FOR CURRENT CLINICAL PRACTICE

The Task Force recognizes that pregnant women and those who attend them are now confronted with decisions regarding optimum intrapartum care which must necessarily be based on incomplete information. The conclusions reached by the Task Force do, however, provide a basis for the following recommendations for current obstetric practice.

The electronic fetal monitor or any other technology should never be a substitute for clinical judgment. Electronic fetal monitoring is only one method of fetal assessment.

Proper use of both intermittent auscultation and continuous electronic fetal monitoring in both high- and low-risk pregnancies, should, at the outset, include a discussion with the patient of her wishes, concerns, and questions concerning benefits, limitations, and risks of fetal monitoring. Women should have the opportunity to discuss the use of all forms of monitoring during the course of prenatal care and again on admission to the labor suite.

The use of all forms of monitoring should be accompanied by supportive and knowledgeable personnel who are attentive to the patient's expectations regarding the conduct of her labor. Hospital personnel should be cognizant of the potential impact of electronic fetal monitoring on family-centered childbirth.

Periodic auscultation of the fetal heart rate is an acceptable method of assessing fetal condition in pregnancies at low risk of intrapartum fetal distress. Interpretation of auscultated fetal heart rate data should include an understanding of the relationship of fetal heart rate changes to uterine contractions. Although the Task Force finds no evidence that electronic fetal monitoring reduces morbidity and mortality in low-risk pregnancies, it recognizes that under certain circumstances mothers or physicians may choose to use electronic fetal monitoring even in low-risk situations.

The use of electronic fetal monitoring should be strongly considered in high-risk pregnancies. Some of the high-risk situations may include: (1) low birth weight, prematurity, postmaturity, and intrauterine growth retardation; (2) medical complications of pregnancy; (3) meconium staining of the amniotic fluid; (4) intrapartum obstetric complications; (5) use of oxytocin in labor; and (6) the presence of abnormal auscultatory findings.

The medical record should reflect careful consideration of the benefits and risks to each individual, including a discussion of the indications for electronic fetal monitoring with the patient.

Since unexpected risk factors may arise during labor in patients without prior evidence of risk, all hospitals and birthing centers providing maternity care should have the necessary trained staff and equipment to assess carefully the status of each fetus in labor and to take appropriate action.

In order that electronic fetal monitoring be used appropriately, the medical profession and others should encourage, through their various educational modalities, a thorough understanding of the principles and procedures of intrapartum fetal heart rate assessment, by all personnel responsible for the care of pregnant women. Special attention should be given to the benefits, limitations, and risks of each mode of assessment. Acquisition of expertise in the use of continuous fetal heart rate and intrauterine pressure data requires the opportunity for supervised practical training in the interpretation of monitoring tracings, use of scalp blood sampling, and the integration of such data into the clinical setting.

The use of fetal scalp blood pH determination is strongly encouraged as an adjunct to electronic fetal heart rate monitoring.

Attention to the known potential hazards of electronic fetal monitoring should accompany its use. Placement of the fetal scalp electrode and intrauterine pressure catheter should be performed with attention to aseptic and atraumatic technique. Prolonged supine position of the mother should be avoided, and her mobility should not be unnecessarily limited.

Hospital personnel should be cognizant of the potential impact of electronic fetal monitoring on family-centered childbirth. Family-centered care and indicated intrapartum fetal monitoring are not mutually exclusive. Maternity services should be encouraged to integrate concepts of family-centered care with care of women who are electronically monitored.

RECOMMENDATIONS FOR FUTURE RESEARCH

Research into the effect of hypoxia on the developing fetus and neonate should be encouraged. The long-term neurologic sequelae of intrapartum hypoxia are of particular importance. Specific attention should be directed to the prognostic value of various modes of fetal assessment during labor.

Identification of risk factors for intrapartum fetal distress that may be successfully managed with electronic fetal monitoring is of critical importance. Additional epidemiologic research should be encouraged to develop clinically useful measurements of risk which would assit in early identification of patients who might benefit from electronic fetal monitoring.

Additional carefully designed and executed randomized clinical trials of electronic fetal monitoring in various categories of high-risk pateints should be conducted. Such trials should be based on risk factors identified in studies such as those suggested in the preceding recommendation and should be coordinated at the national level to provide optimum benefit from the data acquired. Low birth weight has already been identified as one such risk factor. Fetal scalp pH assessment should be included in these studies.

The development of noninvasive methods and equipment to assess fetal well-being accurately, both prepartum and intrapartum, is essential.

Investigation of additional techniques of intrapartum fetal assessment, such as fetal electroencephalography and behavioral states, fetal respiration, and continuous assessment of fetal acid-base values and oxygenation, should be encouraged. No technologic innovation to assess fetal health and distress should be introduced into clinical practice without carefully designed and executed clinical evaluations which include randomized trials of the potential risks, benefits, and limitations.

Further studies of the variables affecting the relationship between electronic monitoring and cesarean section and its complications are necessary and should be encouraged.

COMMENT

Many changes in obstetric practice and in society's attitude toward child-birth have occurred during the past decade. Rising interest in family-centered childbirth, concern about health care costs, increased participation of patients in medical decisions, and a national and individual desire for maximum fetal safety have all contributed to the current medical and public dialogue about electronic fetal monitoring. The Task Force report represents an effort to provide a consensus basis for current use of intrapartum monitoring and to suggest future research areas.

Several of the conclusions and recommendations warrant emphasis. The electronic fetal monitor is clearly a screening and not a diagnostic tool. The usefulness of electronic fetal monitoring, like any screening procedure, will depend on the population to which it is applied and on any risks inherent in its use. It is apparent from the report that both the appropriate population and the magnitude of any inherent risks have not yet been fully identified. Specifically, should monitoring be applied to all or only selected laboring patients? Which risk factors are especially likely to lead to intrapartum distress? Conversely, what is the risk that an "inappropriate" cesarean section will be done because of data generated by continuous monitoring? There are no clear answers to any of these questions, and this becomes obvious in the Task Force report. Until better answers are available, the Task Force conclusions and recommendations for current clinical practice provide a reasonable basis for individual patient management.

14

Fetal Capillary Blood Sampling

EBERHARD MUELLER-HEUBACH / University of Pittsburgh School of
Medicine, Magee-Womens Hospital, Pittsburgh, Pennsylvania

The technique of obtaining samples of capillary blood from the presenting part
of the fetus during labor and delivery was first described by Saling in 1962.
This approach permits the determination of fetal acid-base state, glucose,
hemoglobin, hematocrit, platelet count, and serologic titers. Clinically, the
intermittent assessment of fetal acid-base state to diagnose fetal asphyxia
during labor and delivery has become the most important use of fetal capillary
blood sampling. The diagnosis of fetal asphyxia and subsequent obstetrical
intervention have become increasingly frequent during the last decade. Often
the diagnosis of fetal asphyxia or *fetal distress* is based on fetal heart rate abnormalities observed during continuous electronic monitoring of fetal heart
rate. Although a normal fetal heart pattern during electronic monitoring is
highly reliable in predicting a normal fetus (Kubli et al., 1969; Tejani et al.,
1975), the relationship between abnormal fetal heart rate patterns and the
presence of fetal asphyxia is far less reliable. Tejani et al. (1975) found a
fetal capillary blood pH $\leq$ 7.25 in only 23-34% of cases with various abnormal
fetal heart rate patterns. Similarly, abnormal fetal heart rate patterns were
associated with a depressed Apgar score at 1 min only in 37% of cases
whereas neonatal depression was present in 88% of patients when the last
fetal capillary blood pH was $\leq$ 7.20 (Tejani et al., 1976). In other studies,
fetal capillary blood sampling has also been shown to clarify the diagnosis of
fetal distress during fetal heart rate monitoring and, as a result, to prevent
unnecessary cesarean sections (Zalar and Quilligan, 1979; Ayromlooi and

Garfinkel, 1980, Young et al., 1980). Furthermore, fetal capillary blood sampling permits immediate assessment of fetal status when a patient with clinical evidence suggestive of fetal asphyxia arrives in the labor suite in active labor. In such instances, recording of fetal heart rate for long enough to permit evaluation of fetal heart rate patterns may produce delays in the diagnosis of fetal status which may make the difference between intact survival and fetal death or permanent damage.

The above considerations indicate the importance of fetal capillary blood sampling during labor and delivery. Nevertheless, this technique is presently used only in a limited number of larger obstetrical services. The usual argument advanced by obstetricians who do not use fetal capillary blood sampling is the technical difficulty of the procedure. This chapter will describe the details of the technique and provide guidance in the interpretation of obtained results.

THEORETICAL BASIS

During labor and delivery, perfusion of the intervillous space is intermittently impaired during uterine contractions. This results in transient decrease or interruption of oxygen transfer from mother to fetus. Under normal conditions, intervillous space perfusion between uterine contractions is sufficient to ensure a maternal-fetal oxygen transfer that meets fetal oxygen requirements. The factors that determine adequate oxygen supply to the fetus are oxygen content of maternal arterial blood, intervillous space blood flow, placental exchange surface, placental permeability for oxygen, and fetal circulatory performance. With adequate oxygen supply of fetal tissues (i.e., fetal arterial oxygen content of 2 mM or more) the fetus is able to meet its energy requirements by aerobic metabolism of carbohydrates (Meschia, 1979). When fetal tissue oxygenation is reduced, anaerobic glycolytic metabolism will occur with accumulation of lactic acid. This lactic acid is buffered by the buffer base of whole blood which consists mainly of bicarbonate and hemoglobin, but a very small amount of buffer is represented by plasma protein and plasma and red cell phosphate. Anaerobic breakdown of glucose is very inefficient, producing only 2 high-energy ATP molecules compared with 38 ATP molecules per molecule of glucose during aerobic breakdown. Lactic acid causes an increase in hydrogen ion concentration with a corresponding decrease in buffer base. Hydrogen ion concentration $[H^+]$ is frequently expressed as pH, which is the negative logarithm to the base of 10 of $[H^+]$. A pH of 7.4 represents a hydrogen ion concentration of 40 nmol and when pH falls to 7.0, $[H^+]$ is 100 nmol. pH can decrease as a result of an increase in PCO_2 in the fetus (respiratory acidosis) or as a result of lactic acid accumulation (metabolic acidosis). Measurement of pH in fetal body fluids is a good indicator of fetal hypoxia. It permits the identification of those fetuses experiencing intrauterine asphyxia (i.e., hypoxia having led to acidosis) before fetal cells have suffered irreparable asphyxial damage.

INDICATIONS

The most frequent indication for fetal blood sampling is an abnormality of fetal heart rate observed during electronic fetal heart rate monitoring. The fetal heart rate patterns that are indications for fetal blood sampling are listed in Table 1. Decreased beat-to-beat variability of fetal heart rate may be a sign of fetal acidemia and requires fetal blood sampling. Frequently it is uncertain whether decreased variability is a result of fetal asphyxia or a result of maternal drug administration and placental drug transfer. Fetal blood sampling can clarify this. Variable deceleration of fetal heart rate is the most frequently observed decelerative fetal heart rate pattern. Usually there is no fetal compromise unless the pattern persists for more than 30 min and fetal heart rate falls to 80 beats/min or below. In this case, fetal blood sampling is indicated. Late decelerations of fetal heart rate are an indication of fetal hypoxia (Myers et al., 1973) and fetal blood sampling is necessary to assess the degree of fetal acidosis and to decide about the timing of delivery. Prolonged deceleration, in contrast with persistent bradycardia, presents usually as a sudden decrease in fetal heart rate to 80 beats/min or below. In this instance the patient must be prepared as quickly as possible for emergency cesarean section because this is usually a sign of umbilical cord compression and it is uncertain if and when fetal heart rate will return to normal. When fetal heart rate has returned to normal after preparations for cesarean section are completed, fetal blood sampling should be done and repeated 15 min later to determine fetal acidosis and, whether the fetus is recovering from it. If fetal

Table 1. Indications for Fetal Blood Sampling
Based on Fetal Heart Rate Abnormalities

Persistent tachycardia > 160 beats/min
Persistent bradycardia < 120 beats/min
Decreased beat-to-beat variability
Persistent variable decelerations
Late decelerations
Prolonged deceleration
Fetal arrhythmia
Sinusoidal pattern
Any unusual or unexplained pattern

heart rate is still low, cesarean section must be performed. In patients with fetal arrhythmias, an electronic recording of fetal heart rate can often not be obtained because the electronic instrument rejects the irregular fetal heart rate signals as artifacts. In these instances fetal blood sampling has to be done serially during labor. In some instances the fetal arrhythmia turns out to be the result of a congenital cardiac malformation. The causes of a sinusoidal pattern of fetal heart rate are unknown; however, it is often found in cases of fetal anemia due to isoimmunization or fetomaternal hemorrhage. Prolonged periods of sinusoidal fetal heart rate (30 min or more) may be an indication of fetal compromise and require fetal blood sampling. Patients with unusual patterns of fetal heart rate that are difficult to interpret also should undergo fetal blood sampling to be sure about the condition of the fetus. Any pH value of fetal capillary blood < 7.25 as well as a persistent abnormal fetal heart rate pattern require repeat fetal blood sampling in 15 min to determine whether progressive fetal acidosis is present.

The presence of meconium on admission of a patient in active labor to the labor room is an indication for immediate fetal blood sampling. The fetus may be acidotic. While a tracing of fetal heart rate sufficient for interpretation is obtained, valuable time may be lost in an already acidotic fetus until fetal compromise is suspected based on abnormalities of the fetal heart rate tracing.

Fetal blood has also been sampled for a variety of indications other than pH determination, although far less frequently. Oxygen and carbon dioxide tension and base deficit have been measured. Hematocrit of fetal blood can be determined in cases with likely fetal anemia, such as fetal erythroblastosis (Hobel, 1970) or sinusoidal fetal heart rate pattern. Fetal blood glucose concentrations have been measured in capillary blood sampled from the presenting fetal part (Paterson et al., 1967). In mothers with immunologic thrombocytopenic purpura, Scott et al. (1980) have suggested fetal blood sampling to obtain fetal platelet counts for the diagnosis of fetal thrombocytopenia.

CONTRAINDICATIONS

Fetal capillary blood sampling can only be performed after rupture of membranes. General obstetrical contraindications to artificial rupture of membranes (such as a high presenting fetal part) have to be considered when capillary blood sampling is contemplated in women with intact membranes. In patients with placenta previa or umbilical cord prolapse, attempts to sample fetal capillary blood are obviously contraindicated. Brow and especially face presentations represent contraindications because of the risk of fetal injury. Maternal infectious complications such as clinically apparent chorioamnionitis, active herpes simplex type II infection, or known infection with gonorrhea, syphilis, or beta-hemolytic streptococci preclude the use of fetal blood sampling because of the increased risk of fetal infection via the scalp incision. In cases where a fetal hematologic disorder such as hemophilia or von Willebrand's disease is suspected fetal blood sampling is contraindicated because it may lead to fetal exsanguination. Increased intracranial pressure in the fetus with gaping sutures of the skull as found in hydrocephalic babies may cause leakage of cerebrospinal fluid from a scalp incision for fetal blood sampling and carry the risk of subsequent meningitis. Malformations of the presenting part such as bony defects of the fetal skull as seen in anencephaly or encephalocele are contraindications to fetal blood sampling. In breech presentations fetal blood sampling from fetal genital organs which may be edematous from repeated maternal vaginal examinations has to be avoided. The number of fetal blood samples taken from a single fetus should not exceed six because of the increasing risk of infection and damage to fetal scalp tissue.

TECHNIQUE

Equipment

The equipment necessary for fetal capillary blood sampling can be assembled and packaged in each obstetrical unit or a ready made kit (Sherwood Medical Industries, St. Louis, Missouri) can be used. The components of the disposable sterile kit are illustrated in Figure 1. The conical endoscope is made of plastic and requires a cervical dilation of at least 2.5 cm before it can be introduced. Several cotton swabs are necessary to wipe the presenting part clean and to apply a film of silicone which aids in drop formation. The small blade protrudes 2 mm from the blade holder. The capillary tubes are 30 cm long coated with heparin and have a volume of 100 $\mu l/11.3$ cm of tube length. Either a plastic cover or clay is used to seal the capillary tubes. Small metal rods 7 mm long are inserted into the capillary tube. A 1-cm magnet with a central opening of 3 mm is used to move the metal rod in the tube. Not shown in the figure is the light source used to illuminate the field consisting of a rechargable handle with a switch of the same type as used for ophthalmoscopes or otoscopes. A flexible cable is attached to the tip of the handle with a small bulb at the other end.

Capillary Blood Sampling

Proper positioning of the patient is essential to facilitate the sampling procedure. An inverted bedpan is placed under the sacrum of the patient with the higher part pointing toward the patient's feet. The legs are flexed in the hip and knee joints and spread wide apart. In this position the examiner has easy access to the vagina while the patient is able to steady herself on

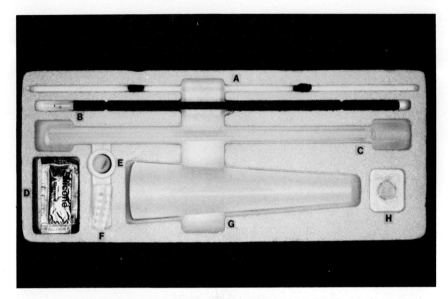

Figure 1. Equipment kit for fetal blood sampling. A: Heparinized capillary tubes; B: Blade holder with blade on left; C: Cotton swabs; D: Silicone; E: Magnet and small metal rods in small plastic box; F: Plastic covers to seal ends of heparinized capillary tubes; G: Conical endoscope (20.3 cm long, outer diameter 2.4 cm at narrow end, 5.2 cm at wide end.); H: Small container with clay.

the bedpan with her legs. Fetal blood sampling can also be done with the patient in stirrups on the delivery table or in a lateral or Sims's position. The vulvar area is cleansed with an antiseptic solution, and some centers also suggest draping with sterile drapes. The examiner wears cap, mask, and sterile gloves. Pelvic examination is carried out to determine cervical dilation and station of the presenting fetal part. If the membranes are intact, artificial rupture of membranes has to be done. In patients in whom the presenting fetal part is high, an assistant should apply fundal pressure to fix the presenting part in the pelvis and prevent it from being pushed cranially by the pressure of the endoscope as it is held against the fetal scalp or buttock. During the vaginal examination the conical plastic endoscope is introduced along the palm and index and/or middle finger of the right hand into the vagina. The index finger which has been placed into the cervical canal is removed and replaced by the endoscope (Saling, 1964a). When the cervix is posterior in patients in early labor, the endoscope has to be directed posteriorly to introduce it into the cervical canal. Then, for visualization of

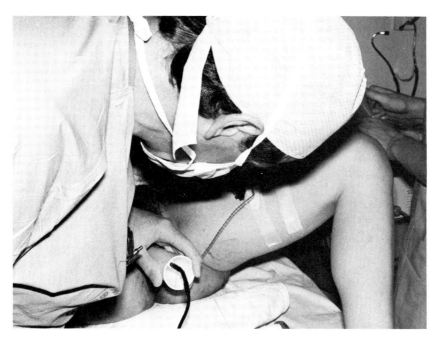

Figure 2. Conical endoscope in vagina with light source attached. Operator holds endoscope in place. Draping has not been done to allow better demonstration.

the presenting fetal part, the cervical canal has to be brought more anterior by pressing the outer end of the endoscope downwards using the perineum as a fulcrum. When the endoscope has been introduced, an assistant places the bulb end of the cable from the light source into the appropriate slot of the endoscope. The endoscope should be rotated so that the attached light is either lateral or at the upper part of the endoscope (towards the ceiling). If the light and the cable are attached to the lower part of the endoscope (towards the floor), they will act as an obstruction for the maneuverability of the blade-holder and the capillary tubes. Although it has been suggested that the light source be handled in an aseptic manner (James, 1974) we have found that contamination is easily avoided with some experience when a nonsterile light source is attached properly by an assistant. This saves storage of the light source in a sterilizing solution and handling of the light source with sterile forceps. Figure 2 illustrates the position of the patient and the endoscope being held in place by the examiner. The use of plastic endoscopes is easier than the metal endoscopes with removable obturator originally described by Saling (1964a).

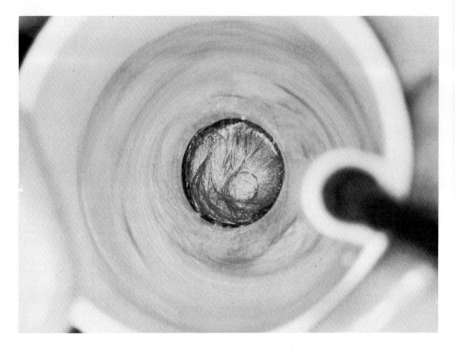

Figure 3. Endoscope held in place against hairy fetal scalp. Light source attached to endoscope on the right side.

At this point the presenting fetal part is in view (Fig. 3) and the hairy fetal scalp can be seen. It is essential to hold the endoscope with light pressure against the presenting fetal part to prevent the entry of amniotic fluid or mucus into the area within the endoscope; at the same time, excessive pressure has to be avoided so as not to interfere with capillary blood flow. The endoscope must be angled so that it rests evenly against the presenting fetal part. The higher the fetal presenting part, the lower the outside end of the endoscope. Upon initial inspection there is usually some mucus or amniotic fluid on the surface of the presenting fetal part. Figure 4 illustrates how the presenting fetal part is wiped clean with a long cotton swab. During the manipulation an assessment of the peripheral circulation of the fetus can be made. In a healthy fetus the skin appears pink whereas in a severely asphyxiated fetus the skin is pale as a result of peripheral vasoconstriction. This evaluation is more difficult or impossible when the fetus has a lot of hair or a dark skin color. Saling (1964a) originally suggested spraying the presenting fetal part with ethyl chloride to produce hyperemia of the skin. We have not found the ethyl chloride application to be necessary for good

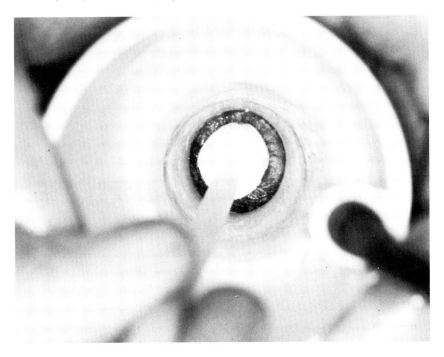

Figure 4. Wiping of fetal scalp with cotton swab to clean of mucus and amniotic fluid. Silicone is applied to fetal scalp is done in a similar fashion with a separate cotton swab.

blood flow from the skin incision. Lumley et al. (1971) have shown that omission of ethyl chloride does not make the blood sample more venous as a result of less effective hyperemia. Thus, the next step is the application of a small film of silicone to the presenting fetal part by means of a cotton swab which has been dabbed in silicone. The silicone aids in drop-formation of the blood. The area of the presenting fetal part closest to the examiner (usually the center of the field) has to be inspected again to ascertain whether there is a clean field for incision and drop formation. If the fetus has a great deal of hair, it may be necessary gently to stroke some hair aside with the butt end of the blade holder before incision to expose an area of fetal skin large enough for incision and blood drop formation.

The incision into the presenting fetal part is not illustrated because it must be done at a right angle to the surface of the presenting fetal part. The blade in the blade holder is rested gently against the area of the intended incision under direct vision. The blade holder is then turned at a right angle to the surface which means that the view of intended incision site will be obscured

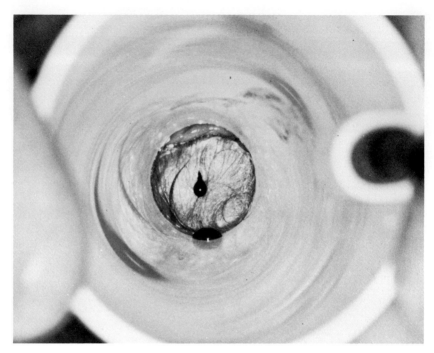

Figure 5. Fetal blood coming from scalp at site of incision. A drop of blood has collected on the lower surface of the endoscope. A second drop is on the surface of the scalp at the lower angle of the scalp incision.

by the examiner's hand holding the blade holder. A quick jab is made for the incision. It is essential not to rotate the blade while it is within the fetal tissue. Incisions should not be made over suture lines or fontanelles but in scalp areas overlying bony skull. Sufficient experience in applying the correct pressure to the blade for an incision which extrudes drops of fetal blood is quickly acquired. It is preferable to make the incision early during a uterine contraction because the presenting fetal part is pushed towards the examiner and relatively fixed. Furthermore, the presenting part may rotate during a uterine contraction, occasionally away from the field within the endoscope. With experience, a second incision is necessary in less than 10% of procedures. No more than three incisions should ever be made to obtain a single blood sample, particularly when serial blood sampling during labor is anticipated. Figure 5 illustrates a drop of blood which is extruded from the incision and, due to gravity, collects just below the incision. After the incision has been made a heparinized capillary tube should be held quickly into the globule of blood formed just below the incision (Fig. 6). Collection of fetal blood into

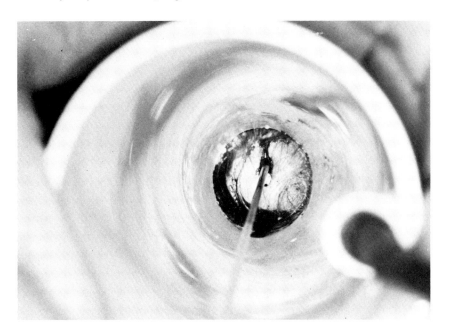

Figure 6. Heparinized capillary tube collecting blood from fetal scalp. The capillary tube is partially filled with fetal blood.

the capillary tube is not possible without some degree of air exposure. Kubli et al. (1966), Zernickow (1966), and Saling (1968) have shown that changes in blood gas composition during 5 sec of air exposure are negligible. Originally Saling (1964a) used tubes made of polyvinylchloride, but Kubli et al. (1966) found tubes of this material to be gas-permeable and recommended glass tubes, which are impermeable. Glass capillary tubes are now generally used. In the original technique of Saling (1964), the tube was filled by sucking blood through a mouthpiece into the capillary tube. Aspiration of air into the tube is a problem with this approach. Lumley et al. (1971) have shown in blood gas analyses of a column of fetal blood in a capillary tube that blood in the segment of tubing closest to the operator's mouth has a lower pH and higher PO_2 and PCO_2. For these reasons the original technique of Saling (1964a) has generally been abandoned and glass capillary tubes are filled by capillary action and gravity. The principle of filling the heparinized capillary tubes is illustrated in the schematic drawing in Figure 7. The capillary tube is rested gently against the skin of the presenting fetal part in the area just below the incision where extruded blood is collecting in drops. Although it has been suggested to place the tip of the capillary tube in contact with the globule of blood rather than the skin (James, 1974), we have found it difficult to keep

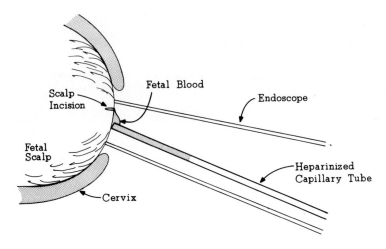

Figure 7. Schematic drawing of fetal blood collection into heparinized capillary tube. See text for details.

the tip of a 30-cm-long glass tube steady within a small drop of blood while holding the tube at the opposite end. As seen in Figure 7, the lower part of the tip of the tube is rested against the fetal skin and a small opening is created at the upper part of the tube tip by holding the outside end of the tube towards the floor. This permits entry of blood from the incision into the tube, which fills by capillary action and gravity. With experience the speed of filling of the capillary tube versus the amount of blood coming from the incision can be matched by changing the angle of the capillary tube and, thus, changing the opening at the tip of the tube and the force of gravity. This will prevent air bubbles from entering the tube and provide an un-interrupted column of fetal blood. Air bubbles in the blood column within the capillary tube do not change pH, PO_2, or PCO_2 of fetal blood (Lumley et al., 1971). During uterine contractions blood flow from the incision in-creases and filling of the capillary tubes is easier. Fetal blood collected dur-ing uterine contractions does not differ in blood gas composition from that collected between contractions (Lumley et al., 1971). The capillary tube should be filled with at least 100 μl of fetal blood to permit duplicate de-termination. Thus, the tube has to be filled at least slightly more than one-third of its length (100 μl = 11.3 cm). The capillary tube is then sealed with clay or plastic covers after one of the small metal rods has been introduced. This is best done by an assistant because the examiner still has to hold the endoscope in place to observe the incision site for bleeding. The incision site is compressed with a cotton swab through the next uterine contraction.

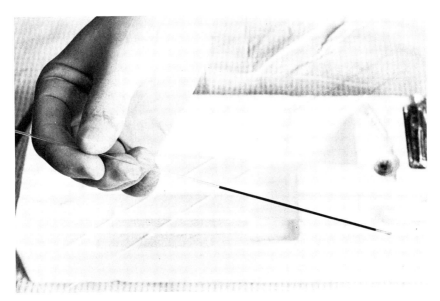

Figure 8. Heparinized capillary tube partially filled with fetal blood. The capillary tube is sealed with clay.

When there is no more bleeding from the incision on visual inspection after the next contraction, the endoscope is removed. Otherwise, compression of the incision site and intermittent inspection for bleeding have to be continued until the bleeding has stopped. The patient is then taken off the bedpan and placed into a lateral position. If electronic fetal heart rate monitoring is done during the fetal blood sampling procedure, transient fetal bradycardia may be observed which represents a vagal reflex due to pressure against the fetal head.

Fetal capillary blood sampling as described above can also be done in patients with breech presentation (Eliot and Hill, 1972; Liu, 1973). We would consider such sampling only in patients with frank breech presentation as it is our policy to deliver patients with footling breech presentations by cesarean section. Sampling of fetal blood from the buttocks can be done in the same manner as described above. The external genitalia have to be avoided when the incision is made. Incision of the buttocks requires slightly more pressure than incision of the scalp. There is less resistance to pressure and an incision tends to be more superficial with inadequate bleeding when pressure on the blade during incision is not greater than that exerted during a scalp incision.

Maternal arterial or venous blood samples may have to be taken after fetal capillary blood sampling as discussed in the section on Interpretation.

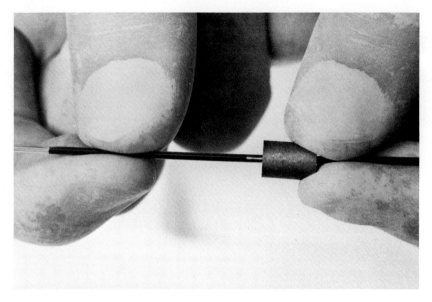

Figure 9. Mixing of fetal blood in the heparinized capillary tube. To the left of the external magnet a small metal rod is seen in the capillary tube.

Handling of Blood Samples

Figure 8 shows a heparinized capillary tube partially filled with fetal blood. Admixture of heparin to blood does not alter the pH value and only high heparin concentrations in blood will change PO_2, PCO_2, and base excess (Cissik et al., 1977a). The mixing of fetal blood with the heparin coating the glass capillaries is accomplished using a small metal rod introduced into the capillary tube. A magnet with a central hole is slipped over the tube and moved along the tube, thus moving the metal rod in the tube. Figure 9 demonstrates the magnet with the capillary tube through its central hole; the small metal rod within the tube can be seen to the left of the magnet. Mixing of fetal blood in the capillary tube should be done while the sampling is being carried to the acid-base instrument. Since fetal capillary blood sampling is done when there is a suspicion of fetal distress, measurements on fetal blood should be done immediately to ascertain fetal condition. Never-the less, blood samples stored in capillary tubes at room temperature have stable pH values for up to 25 min (Sato and Saling, 1975).

Acid-Base Determination

Depending on the acid-base instrument, 50-250 μl of fetal blood are necessary to obtain fetal blood pH measurements. Recently, instruments have become available that allow pH measurement with as little as 15 μl of fetal blood. It is preferable to use an instrument that requires no more than 50 μl for a single determination. In some instruments this can be achieved by switching to a micromethod. Many problems arise from inexperience of physicians in proper handling of acid-base instruments. The instrument's thermoregulatory mechanism has to be turned on at all times to ensure that measurements are made at $37°C$. Proper calibration with two standard buffers should be done daily by a laboratory technician. Then the obstetrician has to make only one calibration with a standard buffer before reading a fetal blood sample. It is essential that the system be flushed between buffers and fetal blood as well as at the end of sample measurement. The glass electrode used for pH measurement is unstable or nonfunctioning most frequently because of inadequate flushing out of fetal blood after a previous measurement.

The acid-base instrument should be in the labor room area and in good working order at all times. In some institutions arterial blood samples from the entire hospital are sent to the labor room for determination because this ensures continuous use and proper calibration by an experienced technician. Using acid-base instruments, standards of accuracy of duplicate pH measurements with various instruments under optimal conditions are at best $\pm$ 0.02 pH units (Hill and Tilsley, 1973; Vinet, 1976; Cissik et al., 1977b). It is unlikely that blood pH measurements in clinical routine are more accurate than $\pm$ 0.03-$\pm$ 0.05 pH units (Kater et al., 1968). A difference of 0.07 pH units or more in duplicate determinations of the same sample points to a technical error. The result should be disregarded and another sample should be obtained (Saling, 1968).

COMPLICATIONS

Three types of complications may occur with fetal capillary blood sampling, all of which are very rare.

Hemorrhage

Hemorrhage from the scalp incision has been reported by several authors. In a series of 1200 samples from 678 infants, three cases with substantial hemorrhage from scalp incisions were reported (Balfour et al., 1970). One of these patients was thought to have hemorrhagic disease. Hull (1972) and Hull and Wilson (1972) have pointed out the possibility of blood clotting defects requiring urgent management when bleeding from a fetal scalp incision is observed. More recently a case of congenital syphilis with disseminated intravascular coagulation and massive hemorrhage from the fetal scalp has been reported (Modanlou and Linzey, 1978). In one of the two reported lethal cases of fetal hemorrhage from a scalp incision, evidence for a coagulation defect was found. In the other case the scalp incision was too deep and a tributary vein into the longitudinal sinus had been opened (Beard et al., 1967). The latter problem has disappeared since blades of no more than 2-mm length have been introduced. Compression of the incision site with a cotton swab is necessary through at least one uterine contraction after the end of fetal blood sampling with subsequent observation of the fetal scalp for bleeding (Coltart et al., 1969). Wood (1978b) has attributed one of the two cases with fetal hemorrhage in his experience of more than 2000 scalp blood collections to the use of the vacuum extractor, but Lee (1970) has observed no bleeding from the site of scalp incisions in 63 cases of vacuum extraction subsequent to fetal blood sampling. In patients with vaginal bleeding after fetal blood sampling the source of blood can be determined by assessing the presence of fetal hemoglobin with the Singer (Singer et al., 1951) or Apt (Apt and Downey, 1955) test.

Following delivery observation of the scalp incision sites in the newborn is necessary because slight hemorrhage may occasionally occur which is usually controlled by compression (Kubli et al., 1966). This is particularly important when peripheral vasoconstriction has taken place in the fetus during labor and delivery as a result of asphyxia. Occasionally it may be necessary to close the scalp incision with a suture or a skin clip.

Blade Breakage

Breaking of the blade during fetal blood sampling has occurred as a result of faulty technique or faulty blades. This complication is very rare with the current quality of blades, provided certain caveats in technique are observed. Incision of the scalp at a right angle to the surface (Roberts and Whitehouse, 1969) and avoidance of rotation of the blade once inserted into the scalp (Nelson et al., 1971) are the most important steps to prevent blade breakage. After each scalp incision the blade has to be inspected to rule out breakage. If breakage has occurred, the incision should be probed and the blade removed by means of a surgical clamp or forceps with an attached magnet. Localizing a broken blade can be difficult even using x-rays.

Scalp Abscess

This is generally a localized problem that responds to local therapy. There is a relationship between the risk of scalp abscess formation and the number of scalp incisions; therefore, the number of incisions should be limited to no more than six. Fetal scalp abscess formation has been reported by Kubli et al., (1966) as well as in three cases in the series of 678 patients with 1200 fetal blood samples of Balfour et al. (1970). Strict aseptic technique during fetal blood sampling may decrease the incidence of scalp abscess formation although it will not eliminate this problem because of the normally contaminated vagina. The pediatrician caring for a newborn who had fetal capillary blood sampling has to be informed about this procedure so as to be alert to the possibility of abscess formation.

Fetal capillary blood sampling does not lead to increased puerperal morbidity as a result of increased vaginal manipulation during the procedure (Kubli et al., 1966). The overall risk of fetal blood sampling is less than 1% (Balfour et al., 1970) and most of the observed complications are not serious. Thus, the information gained from fetal blood sampling about the condition of the fetus far outweighs the small risk inherent in this procedure.

RELIABILITY

The clinical value of capillary blood sampling depends on the relationship between pH values of fetal capillary blood and in blood in the central circulation of the fetus. A direct comparison by simultaneous sampling of fetal capillary blood and blood from the cephalic circulation can only be made in experimental studies in animals. Such studies have been done in the fetal lamb (Gare et al., 1967) and, more importantly, in the fetal rhesus monkey (Adamsons et al., 1970). A close relationship between pH values of fetal capillary blood and blood from carotid artery or jugular vein was found. Studies of the reliability of fetal blood sampling in the human have compared pH values of fetal capillary blood sampled shortly before delivery and in umbilical venous and arterial blood after delivery. These studies have demonstrated that pH values of fetal capillary blood are between those of umbilical venous and arterial blood (Saling, 1964; Kubli et al,, 1966; Teramo, 1969; Bowe et al., 1970; Pontonneri et al., 1978; Fusi and Beard, 1980). Thus, pH values of fetal capillary blood are of reliable clinical value in determining the presence of fetal acidosis. The presence of caput succedaneum seems to have only minimal effect on the pH of capillary blood obtained from the presenting fetal part (Lumley et al., 1971; Boenisch and Saling, 1976).

The reliability of fetal capillary blood sampling depends on a variety of conditions detailed in the Technique section. Measurement of oxygen and carbon dioxide tension in fetal blood is less reliable than pH for assessment of fetal condition because these gas tensions may change rapidly. A poor relationship between fetal condition and oxygen tension of fetal capillary blood has been noted in studies by Kerenyi et al. (1970) and Lumley and Wood (1973). We have recently noticed in animal experiments in our laboratory that transcutaneous PO_2 measured continuously will return much more slowly to normal than PO_2 of carotid arterial blood after a transient decrease in fetal oxygen supply (Mueller-Heubach and Battelli, 1981). Thus, the most reliable indicator of fetal condition which can be measured quickly in a small fetal capillary blood sample remains its pH.

INTERPRETATION

The result from fetal capillary blood sampling should be available within 5 min from the moment the decision for blood sampling is made (including calibration of the acid-base instrument). With experience this can be easily accomplished.

Fetal blood pH values of 7.25 or more are considered normal (Bretscher and Saling, 1967). These authors have also shown that the role of respiratory acidosis is negligible when actual pH of fetal blood is compared with pH measured after equilibration with carbon dioxide at a tension of 40 mmHg. pH values in the range of 7.24-7.20 are considered preacidotic and values of 7.19 and below as acidotic. When interpreting pH values, it has to be remembered that they are a logarithmic function of hydrogen ion concentration $[H^+]$. Therefore, a pH decrease from 7.4 to 7.3 represents a $[H^+]$ increase of 10 nmol/liter whereas a pH decrease from 7.1 to 7.0 equals a $[H^+]$ increase of 21 nmol/liter.

During labor and delivery some degree of fetal and maternal metabolic acidosis is normal (Berg et al., 1966; Wulf et al., 1967; Bretscher and Schmid, 1970; Modanlou et al., 1973). The relationship between maternal and fetal metabolic acidosis developing during labor is normally stable, that is, the differences in pH, base excess, or lactate remain the same and fetal pH does not decline below 7.25. The pH value of fetal blood is normally 0.1 pH units below that of maternal venous blood (Khazin and Hon, 1971; Rooth et al., 1973). This gradient appears necessary for elimination of hydrogen ions from the fetus via the umbilical circulation to the mother. Transplacental exchange of hydrogen ions or lactate and change in bicarbonate are slow processes (Blechner et al., 1967; Schmid and Bretscher, 1970). Thus, pH changes in fetal blood due to asphyxia will become apparent before hydrogen ions are transferred into the maternal circulation. Fetal asphyxia will produce an increase in pH difference (Δ pH) between mother and fetus. Rooth et al. (1973) have suggested considering a Δ pH of 0.15-0.19 pH units as pre-acidosis and Δ pH $\geqslant$ 0.20 pH units as acidosis. Similarly Beard (1968) has considered a base deficit difference between mother and fetus of more than 3.0 meq/liter as indicative of fetal acidosis. When maternal acidosis develops, fetal pH will be influenced by maternal hydrogen ion concentration because fetal hydrogen ions need a sufficient transplacental gradient to be eliminated.

Therefore, in a small number of fetuses with pH values < 7.20. the acidosis is not a result of fetal asphyxia but derives from excessive maternal acidosis. This was the case in 7.6% of 355 newborns in the series of Bowe et al. (1970). When interpreting low fetal pH values, this possibility of an "infusion acidosis" of maternal origin over a prolonged period of time has to be considered since babies born with acidosis of this origin are not depressed. Therefore, it has been suggested that a maternal venous blood sample should be taken for acid-base determination and the maternal-fetal differences in pH and/or base deficit should be determined (Beard, 1968; Rooth et al., 1973).

   In clinical practice, the finding of a fetal pH > 7.25 is reassuring in terms of fetal condition and labor can be allowed to continue. In patients in whom a suspicious fetal heart rate pattern persists and/or the initial pH values was between 7.20 and 7.24, fetal capillary blood sampling should be repeated in 15 min to ascertain whether progressive acidosis is present. In serial fetal blood pH determinations a change can only be considered relevant when it is more than 0.05 pH units (Wood, 1978a) due to problems inherent in the procedure (see Technique). When the initial fetal blood pH is < 7.20, the pH determination should be repeated immediately. Therapeutic action should never be taken based on a single determination (Lumley et al., 1971). If a repeat determination again yields a pH value < 7.20 and the indication for fetal blood sampling has been an abnormal fetal heart rate tracing, it is advisable to proceed with delivery. It is very unlikely in this circumstance that the low fetal pH value is due to maternal acidosis. In cases in which a fetal pH value < 7.20 is obtained without an accompanying abnormal fetal heart rate tracing, a maternal venous blood sample should be obtained to exclude maternal acidosis as a cause of the low fetal pH. Fetal acidosis of maternal origin can be treated with intravenous glucose administration to the mother, which results in a return to normality of the fetal acid-base balance (Beard 1968). This recommendation holds true only when no remediable cause of fetal asphyxia can be identified (e.g., maternal hypotension, uterine hyperactivity). If therapeutic avenues other than delivery are available it is essential to verify improvement of fetal condition as a result of therapy by serial pH determinations. When newborns are evaluated by Apgar score after delivery it must be recognized that low Apgar scores may not necessarily reflect fetal asphyxia. A newborn with a normal capillary blood pH shortly before delivery may have a low Apgar score due to drug depression (Bowe et al., 1970). In those rare instances where fetal blood pH is < 6.90 it is questionable whether an emergency cesarean section should be done because the fetus will almost always die before or shortly after delivery (Bretscher and Saling, 1969).

   The use of fetal capillary blood sampling as described in this chapter, with proper recognition of the limitations of the technique and necessary considerations concerning interpretation of results, represents a major advance in obstetrics. This technique permits considerable refinement in the diagnosis of fetal asphyxia in patients with abnormal fetal heart rate tracings. As a result, fetal capillary blood sampling will help to lower perinatal mortality and morbidity while preventing unnecessary obstetrical intervention. Training of physicians in the specialty of obstetrics is incomplete without instruction in fetal capillary blood sampling.

REFERENCES

Adamsons, K., Beard, R. W., and Myers, R. E. (1970). Comparison of the composition of arterial, venous and capillary blood of the fetal monkey during labor. *Am. J. Obstet. Gynecol. 107*:435-440.

Apt, L., and Downey, W. S. (1955). "Melena" neonatorum—Swallowed blood syndrome; simple test for differentiation of adult and fetal hemoglobin in bloody stools. *J. Pediatr. 47*:6-12.

Ayromlooi, J., and Garfinkel, R. (1980). Impact of fetal scalp blood pH on the incidence of cesarean section performed for fetal distress. *Int. J. Gynaecol. Obstet. 17*:391-392.

Balfour, H. H., Block, S. H., Bowe, E. T., and James, L. S. (1970). Complications of fetal blood sampling. *Am. J. Obstet. Gynecol. 107*:288-294.

Beard, R. W. (1968). Maternal-fetal acid base relationships. In *Diagnosis and Treatment of Fetal Disorders*. K. Adamson (Ed.), Springer-Verlag, New York, p. 151-162.

Beard, R. W., Morris, E. D., and Clayton, S. G. (1967). pH of fetal capillary blood as an indicator of the condition of the fetus. *J. Obstet. Gynaecol. Br. Commonw. 74*:812-822.

Berg, D., Hüter, J., Köhnlein, G., and Kubli, F. (1966). Die Mikroblutuntersuchung am Fetus. Die physiologische fetale Azidose. *Arch. Gynaekol. 203*:287.

Blechner, J. N., Stenger, V. G., Eitzman, D. V., and Prystowsky, H. (1967). Effects of maternal metabolic acidosis on the human fetus and newborn infant. *Am. J. Obstet. Gynecol. 99*:46-54.

Boenisch, H., and Saling, E. (1976). The reliability of pH values in fetal blood samples. A study of the second stage. *J. Perinat. Med. 4*:45-50.

Bowe, E. T., Beard, R. W., Finster, M., Poppers, P. J., Adamsons, K., and James, L. S. (1970). Reliability of fetal blood sampling. *Am. J. Obstet. Gynecol. 107*:279-287.

Bretscher, J., and Saling, E. (1967). pH values in the human fetus during labor. *Am. J. Obstet. Gynecol. 97*:906-911.

Bretscher, J., and Saling, E. (1969). Azidotische Extremwerte beim menschlichen Fetus. *Zentralbl. Gynaekol. 91*:31-34.

Bretscher, J., and Schmid, J. (1970). Untersuchungen über die metabolische Komponente des Säure-Basenhaushaltes beim menschlichen Feten. I. Lactat-und Pyruvatparameter beim ungestörten Geburtsablauf. *Arch. Gynaekol. 208*:283-316.

Cissik, J. H., Salustro, J., Patton, O. L., and Louden, J. A. (1977a). The effects of sodium heparin on arterial blood-gas analysis. *J. Cardiovasc. Pulmon. Technol. 5*:17-20.

Cissik, J. H., Salustro, J., and Patton, O. L. (1977b). Confidence limits of duplication in arterial blood-gas analysis. *J. Cardiovasc. Pulmon. Technol. 5*:40-42.

Coltart, T. M., Trickey, N. R., and Beard, R. W. (1969). Fetal blood sampling. Practical approach to management of fetal distress. *Br. Med. J. 1*:342-346.

Eliot, B. W., and Hill, J. G. (1972). Method of breech management incorporating use of fetal blood sampling. *Br. Med. J. 4*:703-706.

Fusi, L., and Beard, R. W. (1980). Capillaries in the fetal scalp. *Lancet 8166*:483.

Gare, D. J., Whetham, J. C. G., and Henry, J. D. (1967). The validity of scalp sampling. *Am. J. Obstet. Gynecol. 99*:722.

Hill, D. W., and Tilsley, C. (1973). A comparative study of the performance of five commercial blood-gas and pH electrode analysers. *Br. J. Anaesth. 45*:647.

Hobel, C. J. (1970). The value of fetal scalp blood hemoglobin determination in Rh erythroblastosis fetalis. *J. Pediatr. 77*:460.

Hull, M. G. R. (1972). Perinatal coagulopathies complicating fetal blood sampling. *Br. Med. J. 4*:319.

Hull, M. G. R., and Wilson, J. A. (1972). Massive scalp hemorrhage after fetal blood sampling due to hemorrhagic disease. *Br. Med. J. 4*:321.

James, L. S. (1974). Fetal blood sampling. *Clin. Perinatol. 1*:141.

Kater, J. A. R., Leonard, J. E., and Matsuyama, G. (1968). Junction potential variations in blood pH measurements. *Ann. N.Y. Acad. Sci. 148*:54.

Kerenyi, T. D., Falk, S., Mettel, R. D., and Walker, B. (1970). Acid-base balance and oxygen saturation of fetal scalp blood during normal and abnormal labors. *Obstet. Gynecol. 36*:398.

Khazin, A. F., and Hon, E. H. (1971). Observations on fetal heart rate and fetal biochemistry. II. Fetal-maternal pH differences. *Am. J. Obstet. Gynecol. 109*:432.

Kubli, F., Berg, D., Köhnlein, G., Hüter, J., and Bretz, D. (1966). Die Mikroblutuntersuchung am Fetus: I. Kritik der Methode. *Geburtschilfe Frauenheilkd. 26*:1537.

Kubli, F. W., Hon, E. H., Khazin, A. F., and Takemura, H. (1969). Observations on heart rate and pH in the human fetus during labor. *Am. J. Obstet. Gynecol. 104*:1190.

Lee, K. H. (1970). Vacuum extraction after fetal blood sampling. *Aust. N.Z. J. Obstet. Gynaecol. 10*:205.

Liu, D. T. Y. (1973). Breech management with fetal blood sampling. *Br. Med. J. 1*:613.

Lumley, J., Potter, M., Newman, W., Talbot, J. M., Wakefield, E., and Wood, C. (1971). The unreliability of a single estimation of fetal scalp blood pH. *J. Clin. Lab. Med. 77*:535.

Lumley, J., and Wood, C. (1973). Unexpected oxygen tensions in fetal acidosis. *J. Perinat. Med. 1*:166-173.

Meschia, G. (1979). Supply of oxygen to the fetus. *J. Reprod. Med. 23*:160-165.

Modanlou, H., Yeh, S.-Y., Hon, E. H., and Forsythe, A. (1973). Fetal and neonatal biochemistry and Apgar scores. *Am. J. Obstet. Gynecol. 117*: 942-951.

Modanlou, H. D., and Linzey, E. M. (1978). An unusual complication of fetal blood sampling during labor. *Obstet. Gynecol. 51*:7s-8s.

Mueller-Heubach, E., and Battelli, A. F. (1981). Unpublished observations.

Myers, R. E., Mueller-Heubach, E., and Adamsons, K. (1973). Predictability of the state of fetal oxygenation from quantitative analysis of components of late decelerations. *Am. J. Obstet. Gynecol. 115*:1083-1094.

Nelson, G. H., Wages, H. S., Hahn, D. A., Aziz, E. M., and Freedman, D. S. (1971). A complication of fetal scalp blood sampling. *Am. J. Obstet. Gynecol. 110*:737-738.

Paterson, P., Phillips, L., and Wood, C. (1967). Relationship between maternal and fetal blood glucose during labor. *Am. J. Obstet. Gynecol. 98*:938-945.

Pontonnier, G., Grandjean, H., Derache, P., Reme, J. M., Boulogne, M., and de Mouzon, J. (1978). Intérêt de la mésure du pH sanguin dans la surveillance foetale pendant l'accouchement. *J. Gynecol. Obstet. Biol. Reprod. 7*: 1065-1077.

Roberts, H. R. N., and Whitehouse, W. L. (1969). Broken blade in fetal scalp sampling. *Br. Med. J. 2*:510.

Rooth, G., McBride, R., and Ivy, B. J. (1973). Fetal and maternal pH measurements. *Acta Obstet. Gynecol. Scand. 52*:47.

Saling, E. (1962). Neues Vorgehen zur Untersuchung des Kindes unter der Geburt. Einführung, Technik und Grundlagen. *Arch. Gynaekol. 197*:108.

Saling, E. (1964a). Technik der endoskopischen Mikroblutentnahme am Feten. *Geburtshilfe Frauenheilkd 24*:464-469.

Saling, E. (1964b). Mikroblutuntersuchungen am Feten: Klinischer Einsatz und erste Ergebnisse. *Z. Geburtshilfe Gynaekol. 162*:56-76.

Saling, E. (1968). *Foetal and Neonatal Hypoxia in Relation to Clinical Obstetric Practice.* Williams & Wilkins, Baltimore.

Sato, I., and Saling, E. (1975). Changes of pH values during storage of fetal blood samples. *J. Perinat. Med. 3*:211.

Schmid, J., and Bretscher, J.: Untersuchungen über die metabolische Komponente des Säure-Basenhaushaltes beim menschlichen Feten. II. Lactat-und Pyruvatparameter beim pathologischen Geburtsablauf. *Arch. Gynaekol. 208*:317-352.

Scott, J. R., Cruikshank, D. P., Kochenour, N. K., Pitkin, R. M., and Warenski, J. C. (1980). Fetal platelet counts in the obstetric management of immunologic thrombocytopenic purpura. *Am. J. Obstet. Gynecol. 136*:495-499.

Singer, K., Chernoff, A. I., and Singer, L. (1951). Studies on abnormal hemoglobins. I. Their demonstration in sickle cell anemia and other hematologic disorders by means of alkali denaturation. *Blood 6*:413-428.

Tejani, N., Mann, L. I., Bhakthavathsalan, A., and Weiss, R. R. (1975). Correlation of fetal heart rate-uterine contraction patterns with fetal scalp blood pH. *Obstet. Gynecol. 46*:392-396.

Tejani, N., Mann, L. I., and Bhakthavathsalan, A. (1976). Correlation of fetal heart rate patterns and fetal pH with neonatal outcome. *Obstet. Gynecol. 48*:460-463.

Teramo, K. (1969). The validity of foetal capillary blood samples during labor. *Gynaecologia 167*:511-522.

Vinet, B. (1976). An evaluation of three new blood-gas analyzer systems. *Can. Anaesth. Soc. J. 23*:85-91.

Wood, C. (1978a). Diagnostic and therapeutic implications of intrapartum fetal pH measurement. *Acta Obstet. Gynecol. Scand. 57*:13-18.

Wood, C. (1978b). Fetal scalp sampling: Its place in management. *Semin. Perinatal. 2*:169-179.

Wulf, H., Künzel, W., and Lehmann, V. (1967). Vergleichende Untersuchugen der aktuellen Blutgase und des Säure-Base-Status in fetalen und maternen Kapillarblut wahrend der Geburt. *Z. Geburtshilfe Gynaekol. 167*:113-155.

Young, D. C., Gray, J. H., Luther, E. R., and Peddle, L. J. (1980). Fetal scalp blood pH sampling: Its value in an active obstetrical unit. *Am. J. Obstet. Gynecol. 136*:276-281.

Zalar, R. W., and Quilligan, E. J. (1979). The influence of scalp sampling on the cesarean section rate for fetal distress. *Am. J. Obstet. Gynecol. 135*: 239-246.

Zernickow, K. (1966). Der Luftkontakteinfluss auf Mikroblutproben des Feten. *Gynaecologia 161*:277-287.

15

Epidural Analgesia in Obstetrics

J. SELWYN CRAWFORD / Birmingham Maternity Hospital, Birmingham,
England

ANATOMICAL CONSIDERATIONS

The epidural space is contained within the entire extent of the vertebral canal
from the foramen magnum to the sacral hiatus. Its bony and cartilaginous
external boundary is punctured by the paired series of paravertebral foramina,
through which pass the emergent spinal nerve roots (see Figs. 1 and 2). The
dural sac provides an internal boundary but this, in the adult, extends usually
only as far as the level of the second sacral vertebra; below this is the cauda
equina and the filum terminale. In the lumbar region, the cross-sectional profile of the epidural space is roughly triangular, the apex of the triangle being
dorsomedial. Recently reported observations (Husemeyer and White, 1980)
suggest that the triangulation can, in some subjects, be so pronounced as to
lead to compartmentalization of the space into two dorsolateral and one vertical
component having virtually no communication between them at various spinal
levels.

The epidural space contains predominantly loose fatty tissue and blood
vessels, mainly veins. In pregnancy the distention of the veins, and possibly
the volume of fat, increases, resulting in a reduction in the capacity of the
space to accept injected fluid. For this reason, in order to achieve a desired
segmental spread of nerve block in a pregnant patient, only two-thirds of the
volume used to produce a block of similar extent in a nonpregnant person of
the same age and height is required (Bromage, 1967). This opinion has, however, been contradicted by Grundy et al. (1978). It is also worthy of note that

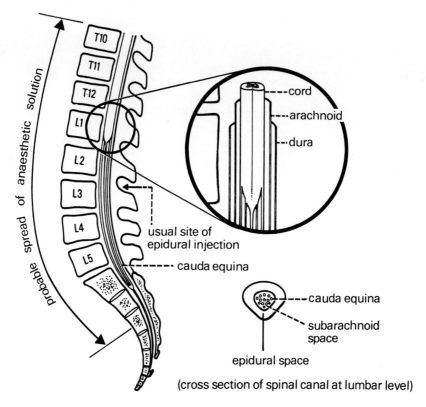

Figure 1. Lateral longitudinal view of the anatomical features related to the lower end of the epidural space. Sensation from the uterus is transmitted via nerves entering the spinal cord, root values T11 and T12 (with possibly some overlap from T10 and L1), and from the lower birth canal via S2, S3, and S4.

the extent of spread of local anesthetic injected into the epidural space of an obese patient is comparatively wide (Hodgkinson and Husain, 1980), presumably because of an abnormally large mass of fat within the space. The potential capacity of the space is further reduced if the mother is exposed to inferior vena caval compression, during a painful uterine contraction, during a painfree uterine contraction if the anterior abdominal wall muscles contract, or during a period of bearing-down (Messih, 1981). For these reasons, contrary to previously held opinion, the pressure within the epidural space in pregnancy is slightly above atmospheric (Messih, 1981).

The spinal nerve roots traverse the epidural space, each carrying with it a tunic of dura mater, which merges into the more easily penetrable nerve sheath at about the level of the intervertebral foramen (Bromage, 1978).

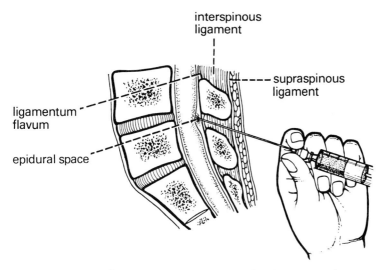

Figure 2. View of the epidural space in the lumbar region showing site of epidural injection.

The sensory nerve supply of the entire uterus is by sympathetic fibers contained within the emergent spinal roots T11 and T12, although the T10 and L1 segments are usually also involved. Thus the pain of a uterine contraction and of cervical dilatation is referred specifically to the sensory distribution of these roots. The low-back pain which is a frequent accompaniment of labor is probably due to pressure on structures in the posterior wall of the pelvis (lumbosacral plexus). Distention of the lower birth canal, which is the additional component of pain in the second stage of labour, stimulates impulses that travel via the S2, 3, and 4 nerve roots. Fibers in these roots also provide the afferent arc of the bearing-down reflex, and have their origin in the fibromuscular elements of the pelvic floor.

TECHNIQUE OF CANNULA PLACEMENT

The objective of lumbar epidural analgesia is to introduce local anesthetic into the epidural space so that it will block the passage of impulses that subserve the pain associated with labor. There are secondary objectives, such as abolition of the bearing-down reflex, and reduction of maternal blood pressure, which will be referred to subsequently. In obstetric practice entry into the epidural space is now predominantly via a lumbar vertebral interspace. The caudal route, via the sacral hiatus, was very popular until recently, and is still used by many practitioners, but will not be discussed here.

The patient is usually placed in the flexed lateral position, although some anesthetists prefer her to be sitting, especially if obesity makes identification of landmarks difficult. A lumbar vertebral interspace (usually L2/3 or L3/4) is approached in the precise midline (a lateral approach has been advocated by Carrie, [1971]) with a thin-walled (16-gauge internal, 18-gauge external) needle, either a Tuohy or a straight short-bevelled. The needle pierces, successively skin, subcutaneous tissue, supraspinous ligament, interspinous ligament, and ligamentum flavum to enter the epidural space. Entry is usually assessed by diminished resistance to pressure applied via the needle, either intermittently ("loss of resistance" technique) or continuously (inflated Macintosh balloon). Local anesthetic solution can be injected into the space through the needle, either in a "single-shot" technique or as the first dose of a continuous epidural block, but we advise against this lest the needle's point inadvertently pierce the dura during injection. It is preferable to thread an epidural cannula into the space (2-4 cm beyond the needle tip), withdraw the needle over it, then begin the series of intraepidural injections. We also advise the invariable use of a bacterial filter through which to inject solutions into the cannula, to avoid injecting either contaminated material or particulate matter (James et al., 1976; Seltzer et al., 1977) although the necessity for this has been questioned. (Abouleish et al., 1977).

Although a variety of clinical factors influence the decision to administer an epidural to a pregnant patient, several essential requirements common to all situations must be satisfied before a block is initiated:

1. The patient must be told in reasonable detail (without gloss and without alarmist suggestions) how an epidural is performed and what are the anticipated results of the treatment. In an efficiently organized obstetric department this information will be provided in the course of prenatal instruction.
2. Having been so informed, the patient must give assurance that she consents to the procedure. In the United Kingdom, written consent is not required and should not be sought.
3. The blood pressure should be recorded before the start of the procedure.
4. An intravenous infusion of crystalloid solution must be initiated before the start of the procedure. Preferably a liter of such fluid should have been administered before the first injection of local anesthetic into the epidural space. This is particularly important in patients who have been starved (as overnight) or who have been in labor for a considerable time.
5. A fetal heart rate monitor must be in operation (applied either externally or internally) from before the start of the procedure. Even in the most accomplished hands the time elapsing from positioning the patient to taping the epidural cannula in place can be 20-30 min. This is too long to be

unaware of the fetal status. For somewhat similar reasons, intermittent conversation with the mother should be maintained. Acute flexion even in the lateral position can cause aortocaval compression, and the silent mother might be experiencing cerebral hypoxemia.

Complications

Pain
There is no excuse for failing to warn the patient that the procedure might be painful. Sometimes it is painfree, often it is uncomfortable, sometimes it is painful. Pain can be caused by trauma to a tough supraspinous ligament, from periosteum as a passage is sought between the vertebrae, or from a nerve root impinged upon during threading of the cannula.

Failure
The incidence of failure is correlated with experience, but probably never reaches zero. The failure rate is higher in relation to maternal obesity, the active phase of labor ("moving target"), and the presence of bony abnormalities. There can also be failure to thread the cannula into the space, usually due to a posteriorly bulging dura. Compassion dictates that, except under very unusual circumstances, the epiduralist should not persist longer than 30 min in attempting to place the cannula within the space.

Hemorrhage
Our experience suggests that blood is shed within the space, during insertion of either the needle or the cannula, in approximately 10% of cases. No harm befalls the patient because of this, but if the blood tracks back through the needle or the cannula it should be withdrawn and reinserted through an adjoining interspace.

Dural Tap
Dural puncture is most commonly effected with the needle, but, occasionally, penetration of the membrane is with the cannula. The incidence of the complication diminishes with increasing experience of the practitioner, but has probably never reached zero in any reasonably large series. The incidence in a well-run obstetric unit is unlikely to exceed 2% annually.

The complication is a matter for regret but not for panic or distress. The procedure to be followed consequent upon a dural tap is straightforward, although varying in detail between obstetric units. The cannula is inserted into the epidural space via an adjoining intervertebral space, and analgesia is provided in the customary manner. Subsequent to completion of the third stage of labor (or of cesarean section), crystalloid solution is infused through the filter and cannula, at a rate such that approximately 1.5 l is given within 24-30 hr. During this period the patient can sit at will. At a convenient time thereafter, the infusion is stopped and the cannula withdrawn. Postural headache will subsequently be experienced by 25-30% of patients so treated, compared with 70% who will experience such a headache if no measure other than "forced fluids" is adopted (Crawford, 1972). If a postural headache does develop, the patient is offered an epidural blood patch. This consists of injecting up to 20ml of the patient's blood into the epidural space to form a firm clot over the dural puncture. It cannot be administered if the patient is receiving anticoagulant therapy, or has clinical evidence of systemic infection. We have administered a blood patch to 150 patients (after inadvertant tap or spinal analgesia) with no complications, and since adopting the dose of "up to 20ml" the incidence of total success has been 98% (Crawford, 1980a). The patient should be assured that her headache will clear spontaneously on the sixth day following the dural puncture, and allowed to decide for herself whether or not she will accept the provision of a blood patch. The blood injected will not lead to difficulties with subsequent epidurals. We have successfully administered an epidural to five patients who had a patch following a previous labor and a similar experience has been reported by Abouleish et al. (1975).

Broken Cannula
The terminal portion of a cannula breaking and lying within the epidural space occurs less frequently than used to be the case, for two reasons. It is now more widely appreciated that the cannula must never be withdrawn through the needle, lest the end be sheared off. Secondly, the characteristics of the cannulas produced commercially have greatly improved. We have records of nine such incidents in our service. No harm has subsequently befallen the patients. The advised routine to be adopted has been detailed elsewhere (Crawford, 1978). Here it is sufficient to emphasize that it is unwise to attempt surgical retrieval of the broken piece.

Serious Neurological Complications
Although reports of serious neurological complications are occasionally rumored, and sometimes appear in print, close investigation usually reveals that if such a complication did occur, it was the result of inattention to elementary details of procedure. The international incidence is impossible to estimate, and I can refer here only to our own experience. Two of our 18,000 patients have had a complication of this order. In one case an epidural abscess developed within blood which had been shed during initiation of the block. The infection was caused by blood-borne spread from the genital tract (Crawford, 1975). In the other case a minute specule of particulate matter was deposited in the epidural space, forming the nidus of a granulomatous reaction which pressed upon an emergent nerve root (Crawford et al., 1975). Both patients required a laminectomy and nerve function recovered completely in both.

DRUGS

The local anesthetics in predominant use are bupivacaine (available commonly in concentrations of 0.25 and 0.5% and, in some centers, 0.75%), lignocaine (available in a range of concentrations), etidocaine (0.5 and 1.0%), and chloroprocaine (2 and 3%). The latter has never been commercially available in the United Kingdom, despite requests from many anesthetists. Its advantages lie in its rapidity of onset and brief duration of action, and that because it is metabolized by serum cholinesterase, its systemic toxicity is low and the extent of placental transfer inconsiderable. However, recent reports (Covino et al., 1980; Ravindran et al., 1980; Reisner et al., 1980) have referred to serious neurological damage resulting from the inadvertent intrathecal injection of a considerable volume of chloroprocaine (both 2 and 3% solutions were implicated). The reason for these incidents is not yet clear. The drug has been widely used apparently without these complications for 25 years. It may reflect the low pH of the solutions (3.126 and 3.167). The invariable avoidance of an inadvertent injection intrathecally cannot be guaranteed in a busy clinical department, and it is therefore unlikely that chloroprocaine will be accepted into routine clinical practice in the United Kingdon.

Lignocaine is infrequently used to provide continuous epidural analgesia in labor, probably because of its relative brevity of action, but also because the dose required throughout a labor of average or longer than average duration leads to a level of concentration in maternal blood uncomfortably close to that associated with toxic responses.

Etidocaine favors the production of motor loss over sensory loss (Lofstrom, 1980) and it is thus better suited to operative procedures than labor. However, when bupivacaine fails to provide total relief from pain, etidocaine may sometimes rectify the deficiency.

Bupivacaine is the standard drug used internationally for epidural analgesia. Its effects are, to an extent dependent, on its concentration. At higher concentrations the onset of action is more rapid (but this is only a matter of a few minutes), its duration of activity longer, its effectiveness in producing sensory block more assured, and its induction of motor loss more pronounced (Scott et al., 1980). Abolition of the bearing-down reflex is more likely to occur if, for example, the 0.5% solution has been administered towards the end of labor than if the 0.25% solution has been used. In our own earlier series, 48.5% of the 4387 patients whose final top-up was with 0.25% bupivacaine did not have the urge to beardown, whereas the incidence was 55.9% among the 3365 patients whose final dose was with 0.5% solution. The time between receipt of the final dose and delivery was little consistent influence. Some clinicians have observed consistently good analgesia using 0.125% bupivacine (Bleyaert et al., 1979), whereas others have been unable to confirm this finding (Stainthorpe et al., 1978). The use of this very dilute solution has not become generally popular.

Bupivacaine is obtainable in solutions with adrenaline. I find little virtue in using this in obstetric practice. The presence of adrenaline extends the duration of perceived activity of bupivacaine by approximately 10 min, which is inconsequential for a continuous block for labor. The peaks of levels of blood concentration of bupivacaine are lower if adrenaline is included in the injected solution, but the levels reached under clinical circumstance using a plain solution are nowhere near that associated with toxic responses in either mother or infant, mainly because bupivacaine is so highly bound to serum protein (Mather and Thomas, 1978). On the other hand inadvertent injection of solution into an epidural vein does occur on occasion, and if the solution contains adrenaline the potential threat to maternal well-being will be considerable. The pH of the adrenaline-containing solution is 3.1 whereas that of the plain solution is 5.6, and the patient with pre-eclampsia is particularly susceptible to the hypertension engendering effects of catecholamine, (Zuspan et al., 1962; Talledo et al., 1968).

TECHNIQUE OF ADMINISTRATION

Three types of application of an epidural block may be distinguished in clinical practice on an international scale: continuous infusion, segmental block, and extensive block.

Continuous Infusion

Continuous infusion of the drug into the epidural space, either as a gravity-compelled drip, or, preferably, from a pump-driven syringe, has been reported (Zador and Nilsson, 1974; Glover, 1977; Hunton, 1979; Matouskova, 1979). There appears to be general agreement that although the results, in terms of adequacy of analgesia and freedom from complications, are reasonably good, the technique affords no outstanding advantages in routine clinical practice. After a loading dose of local anesthetic has been administered, and the infusion set at an appropriate rate (which can be determined only by observation of the patient's responses), there should be no further requirements for top-up doses. However, repetitive surveillance of the extensiveness of spread of the block, maternal blood pressure, and the state of her urinary bladder is obviously mandatory, so application of this technique does not reduce the demands made upon the staff in a delivery suite. Our own experience in trials of this technique has shown that roughly twice the amount of bupivacaine per hour is administered compared with that given when the intermittent technique is used. This finding reflects that of others reported informally.

Segmental or Selective Block

The technique of segmental or selective block has received considerable support (Hollmen et al., 1977; Jouppila et al., 1977; Willdeck-Lund et al., 1979, 1979b; Gal et al., 1979; Jouppila et al., 1979). The objective is initially to block only those spinal nerves that provide a pathway for sensory impulses from the uterus. The associated advantages are that the mother retains full sensation and power in her legs during the first stage and has no loss of bladder sensation. There can be no advantage in a limitation of vasomotor block, as the sympathetic outflow extends caudally only to L2, and the selective block technique is directed to the T10-L1 segments. The mass of drug to be injected at each top-up will probably be smaller than that used for a more extensive block, but this is of little consequence to either mother or fetus when bupivacaine or chloroprocaine is employed. The disadvantages are that, as has been detailed, the pain associated with the first stage is frequently not limited to that of a uterine contraction per se and, secondly, in a reasonably busy clinical practice the time of entry of each patient into the second stage of labor cannot be anticipated with precision, so that failure to prevent pain arising from the lower birth canal is likely to be common when selective block is used.

Extensive Block

For these reasons we greatly prefer to provide an extensive block, from T10 to S5 as early as possible in the procedure. Further discussion will be limited to consideration of this technique. The choice of volume of solution to be injected varies from one department to another, with seemingly little related variability in the incidence of either successful analgesia or complications. Our own practice is to inject 10 ml initially unless the patient is extremely small or very obese, in which case a smaller volume would be administered. Thereafter each top-up dose will consist of 10 ml unless the response to the previous dose had been an unnecessarily extensive block. The mother is placed in the lateral tilt position, with her head and shoulders comfortably raised on one or two pillows, and 2-3 min after the injection she is helped to turn onto her other side. The only exceptions to this procedure are: if the epidural is being started before surgical induction of labor, and, if, during labor, there is low-back pain or other evidence of failure to block to lower lumbar and sacral roots. Under these circumstances the injection is made while the mother is reclining against a backrest. It is mandatory that blood pressure be measured immediately before each top-up, and at 5-min intervals for at least 15 min after the injection.

EFFECTS

Primary

There is general consensus that approximately 85% of patients who receive an epidural for labor will be completely satisfied with the extent of analgesia. In our experience, which mirrors that of many other departments, in 3-4% of cases there is total failure to provide pain relief. In roughly half of such cases in our unit this is due to an attempt to initiate an epidural being made too late in labor. In the hands of most competent anesthetists the time elapsing between placing the mother into the appropriate position, and securing the catheter in place, is at least 20 min. If the mother is in strong labor it will be longer because of the need to halt advancement of the needle while a contraction is in progress. The latency period before the bupivacaine begins to provide effective analgesia might be another 10 min. For these reasons we are increasingly reluctant to start an epidural on a primigravida whose cervical dilatation has reached 9 cm or a multigravid at 8-cm dilatation, unless compelling reasons dictate otherwise. Other reasons for total failure include difficulty in entering or identifying the epidural space, and a mysterious, and fortunately very small, group in whom there is no apparent explanation.

Among the remaining group of "partial successes" the deficiency may have a variety of causes. Some are related to inappropriate positioning of the catheter, which might have traversed an intervertebral foramen (leading to the production of a profound, often markedly protracted, block of a single nerve root), or have advanced too far anteriorly around the dura so that a unilateral block is obtained. Intense low-back pain associated with a "flat sacrum" and a persistent occipitoposterior position of the fetal head can be extremely difficult to obliterate fully. Possibly the most frequently occurring reason for partial failure is the "missed segment." In this condition the pain of each uterine contraction is successfully abolished except for an area supplied by one nerve root or even, apparently, by a tributary peripheral nerve. In our own experience, as first reported by Ducrow (1971) and continued since then, this most frequently presents as pain in one or other groin, and appears to reflect involvement of the iliohypogastric and ilioinguinal nerves. Ducrow (1971) reported an incidence of 6.7% and the syndrome was persistent throughout labour in 1.5% of pateints. A similar incidence was reported by Bromage (1972) and Moir et al. (1976). Although it is reasonable to assume that a missed segment occurs because of failure of the local anesthetic to penetrate neural sheath and reach nerve axons, the roots of T12/L1, which are most often involved in our experience, are relatively thinly enveloped, whereas those of S1/2 have the thickest roots (De Campo et al., 1980). The latter authors suggest that the inguinal pain is of the referred type due to failure to block S1, but this is difficult to understand. No convincingly successful treatment of this partial failure has been reported. We inject a top-up of 0.5% bupivacaine, with the mother lying on the affected side, as a first line of therapy, and more recently have used 2.0% lignocaine, but the effectiveness of these manoeuvers is open to doubt. The incidence of missed segment, in our experience, is not related to a previous epidural, an observation which has been confirmed by Bray and Carrie (1978).

Loss of bladder sensation undoubtedly occurs as a result of an 'extended block.' This should not lead to the requirement of increased catheterization during labor. Our advocacy, and usual practice, is to encourage the mother to empty her bladder spontaneously before each alterante top-up, when sensation is returning.

Some degree of motor loss is virtually unavoidable. To an extent, the incidence and severity is directly correlated with the strength of the local anesthetic solution used for the final one or two top-up doses, but no discriminatory measurements have been reported from clinical practice. The duration of the epidural block appears also to be a contributory factor. Only infrequently does a patient have a total inability to move her legs voluntarily. It is important that mothers be warned in advance that neither the loss of sensation nor the weakness will disappear at the moment of birth. In our practice these two features persist for an average of 4-5 hr after delivery, rarely for longer than 8 hr, and, significantly, the return of sensation precedes by about 1 hr the return of power.

Pelvic and lower abdominal muscles are involved in the diminution of power. This attribute contributes to the characteristic association of a prolongation of the second-stage with epidural block, because of the diminished ability of the mother to bear down. Of much greater importance in this context however, is the abolition of the bearing-down reflex which will be experienced by roughly half the patients, rather more among those whose final dose consisted of 0.5% bupivacaine than among those who received the 0.25% solution. The result is due to depression of the sensory side of the reflex arc (root value S2-4). Abolition of the bearing-down reflex, and diminution of the ability to push, do not of themselves indicate that the mother will not be able to deliver spontaneously, although in clinical practice, they certainly increase the incidence of advised instrumental delivery. This will be further discussed later. One other noteworthy feature associated with the loss of bearing-down sensation is that it increases slightly the likelihood that the mother will experience a feeling of 'deprivation'. She will report that she feels she did not contribute satisfactorily to the delivery of her infant. However, the possibility of this response must be balanced against the possibility that in trying to avoid obtunding the bearing-down reflex there will be a failure to provide satisfactory analgesia. An analysis of data from our first 10,000 records demonstrated the following:

Urge to bear down	% Pain relief	% "Deprivation"
	Primigravid	
Absent	87.5	2.2
Present	80.0	1.3
	Multigravid	
Absent	80.8	2.9
Present	75.0	1.4

That mothers can certainly deliver spontaneously despite their diminished ability to bear down is due to the fact that uterine performance is not depressed by the epidural block. This holds equally as true for the first stage as for the second stage, and it can therefore be categorically stated that, all other things being equal, a continuous lumbar epidural has no significant influence on the duration of the first stage of labor. This is so whether labor is of spontaneous onset, or has been induced, or is augmented with an oxytocic (Table 1). There are only two ways in which an epidural can affect progress in the first stage. One is in the case of the mother whose pain has previously been poorly relieved, who is becoming exhausted, and whose progress has become desultory. The initiation of a successful epidural will tend to encourage a return to a satisfactory pattern of progress. The second instance is if the patient is permitted to become hypotensive, in which case uterine activity will be depressed.

Hypotension due to the vasomotor blockade induced by the epidural should not occur if the two essential precautions are observed: the avoidance of aortocaval compression and the correction, before initiation of the epidural, of any appreciable degree of hypovolemia. For purposes of documentation we define hypotension as a reduction of systolic blood pressure by at least 20 mmHg. Although some authorities prefer to extend the definition to include a fall of pressure to below 100 mmHg, I do not believe that to be sensible, because many of our patients (especially from the Indian subcontinent) sustain a baseline pressure at this level.

An analysis of our data carried out some years ago revealed a slightly higher incidence of hypotension associated with the administration of 0.5% bupivacaine (3.4% of 14,480 top-ups) than with the 0.25% solution (2.4% of 18,741 top-ups). Analysis of more recent data has yet to be undertaken, but the strong impression is that the current incidence is even lower than those first quoted. Fetal harm has not resulted from hypotension induced by any one of our epidurals. A vasopressor (the drug of outstanding choice in this situation being ephedrine) has been required in only 4 of the 17,000 laboring mothers who have, since 1969, received an epidural.

Table 1. Mean Duration of Labor (hours)[a]

		Epidural	P	No epidural
Spontaneous labor, no augmentation	Primigravid	7.25 (80)	<0.001	5.72 (503)
	Multigravid	3.93 (46)	<0.01	3.54 (899)
Spontaneous labor, with augmentation	Primigravid	12.44 (103)	N.S.	11.90 (147)
	Multigravid	9.18 (53)	N.S.	10.04 (124)
Induced	Primigravid	10.00 (292)	N.S.	9.95 (288)
	Multigravid	8.37 (204)	<0.01	7.45 (441)

[a]In groups of patients defined in respect to parity, presence of absence of oxytocic stimulation, and whether or not an epidural was administered. Patients with breech presentation, multiple pregnancy, significant prepartum hemorrhage, severe pre-eclampsia, abnormal fetus, or low birth weight baby (less than 2.5 kg) were excluded from the study.
Source: Data from Studd et al., 1980, and unpublished data.

The major concern regarding the potential hazard of maternal hypotension is the integrity of the intervillous blood flow. Until recently, this was presumed to be unimpaired because of the absence of any evidence of fetal distress resulting from the initiation and maintenance of an epidural. Reports of reliable comparative measurements of intervillous blood flow using the [133]Xenon clearance technique (Jouppila et al., 1978; Husemeyer and Crawley, 1979; Huovinen et al., 1979) have revealed that initiation and maintenance of an epidural does not diminish intervillous blood flow in the normotensive patient. Its effect in the hypertensive mother will be discussed later.

Secondary

It is now well-established that the abolition of pain, the reduction of anxiety, and the avoidance of fatigue conferred upon the mother are of considerable benefit to the fetus. The stress of poorly relieved labor results in an increased concentration of cortisol and reduced concentration of estriol in maternal plasma; these responses are not seen when an effective epidural has been provided (Jouppila et al., 1976; Maltau et al., 1978). This is similar to the process by which an epidural block extending from T10 to S5 inhibits the cortisol response and hyperglycemia which otherwise, are provoked by surgical procedures, (Engquist et al., 1977). As Morishima et al., (1978) observed, maternal anxiety alone can lead to fetal acidosis. These findings complement those reported by Pearson and Davis (1973, 1974) who observed that during poorly relieved labor there was a time-dependent increase in maternal acidosis and, presumably, by infusion, in fetal acidosis, which did not occur among patients receiving an epidural.

Because of the vasomotor blockade, and despite the diminution of lower-limb motor power, vascular perfusion of the pelvis and legs is enhanced during epidural block (Modwig et al., 1980). We have reason to suppose, on the basis of our own unpublished observations, that this is of benefit in reducing the incidence of postnatally developing deep-vein thrombosis.

As stated previously, a relatively prolonged second stage is undoubtedly an associated factor of the well-managed epidural. The reduction in tone of the pelvic floor musculature leads to some delay of rotation of the presenting fetal part. These features of epidural analgesia have provided the major focus of criticism of the technique. No doubt a considerable increase in the incidence of in-strumental deliveries has resulted, and an appreciable proportion of these have been rotational, or midforceps, with attendant birth trauma. Such trauma so caused has usually been relatively minor, and unassociated with long-term sequelae: cephalhematoma, facial nerve palsy, fractured clavicle, cerebral irritation, bruising of face. However, these do not reflect an unavoidable hazard of epidural analgesia, but a lack of obstetric discipline. The temptation to expedite delivery has proved irresistable to many obstetricians. Although an unfortunate tendency, it is understandable. The contributing factors include: the mother lies at ease with a relaxed perineum; other calls of a professional or social nature upon the obstetrician's time; and the well-ingrained concept that delay in the second stage poses an increasing hazard to the infant. A revision of obstetric understanding is required. There is no evidence to suggest that prolongation of the second stage is of itself inimical to fetal well-being, provided that the following criteria are satisfied: continuous monitoring of the fetal heart rate reflects no evidence of distress, the mother is not becoming exhausted, and aortocaval compression is avoided. Emphasis of these points in our own hospital practice has served to reduce the incidence of instrumented deliveries (Table 2), and to eliminate almost completely the incidence of avoid-able midforceps deliveries among patients receiving an epidural. The result has been a welcome reduction in the incidence of associated birth trauma. As a corollary, however, the features which led to an increase in the forceps rate are precisely those of advantage in the management of certain complications of delivery, as will be detailed later.

Table 2. Method of Delivery[a]

	Primigravidas				Multigravidas			
	n	Spontaneous (%)	Forceps/ventouse % (% of vaginal deliveries)	Emergency section (%)	n	Spontaneous (%)	Forceps/ventouse % (% of vaginal deliveries)	Emergency section (%)
1971	509	38.7	56.2 (59.2)	5.1	373	72.1	25.2 (25.9)	2.7
1972	611	40.4	50.4 (55.5)	9.2	414	75.8	21.3 (21.9)	2.9
1973	715	35.8	57.3 (61.6)	6.9	628	73.1	23.6 (24.4)	3.3
1974	751	29.2	61.5 (67.8)	9.3	738	62.7	32.2 (34.0)	5.0
1975	896	26.0	63.7 (71.3)	10.3	895	57.5	33.9 (37.0)	8.6
1976	887	20.0	64.0 (76.2)	16.0	830	55.1	37.2 (40.3)	7.7
1977	910	23.2	59.1 (71.8)	17.7	798	56.8	34.8 (38.0)	8.4
1978	902	22.9	60.9 (72.7)	16.3	798	50.8	39.3 (43.7)	9.9
1979	763	27.3	56.0 (67.2)	16.8	619	59.0	34.1 (36.6)	6.9
1980	826	33.5	46.9 (58.3)	19.6	643	66.7	29.7 (29.8)	3.3

[a]Among mothers with a singleton fetus presenting by the vertex, who received an epidural for labor.
Source: J. S. Crawford, Brimingham Maternity Hospital Report, Birmingham, England, 1980.

OUTCOME

Uncomplicated Pregnancy and Labor

Reference has already been made to maternal responses to an epidural. The infant of an uncomplicated pregnancy and labor will exhibit less birth asphyxia than will one whose mother received either no analgesia or centrally acting analgesia, and will not be subjected to drug-induced depression. However, the difference is marginal and, unless an unacceptably large dose of systemically administered drugs has been used in the "nonepidural" labor, is inconsequential to the immediate and long-term condition of the child. It is ethically unjustifiable to suggest to a healthy mother with a healthy fetus—with no reasonable prospect of difficulties to be encountered during labor and delivery—that by declining the offer of an epidural she is placing her infant at risk.

Nonobstetric Pathology

Mothers with various categories of nonobstetric pathology benefit from a continuous epidural for labor and delivery. The main advantage is the avoidance of maternal exertion and the reduction of fatigue, which result from total pain relief and abolition of the bearing-down reflex. Such categories include the following:

1. *Symptomatic cardiac and respiratory disease.* The specific cardiac lesion may be congenital (Gleicher et al., 1979) or acquired. The absolute contraindication to an epidural in these circumstances is if the mother is on sustained anticoagulant prophylaxis. If anticoagulants are to be withdrawn for the period of labor and delivery, an epidural may be administered, provided that the full "coagulation screen" has returned to normal.
2. *Musculoskeletal disease.* Specifically, abnormalities of the dorsolumbar spine, pelvis (including sacrum), or legs.
3. *Intracranial lesions.* (Tumor or cerebrovascular).
4. *Heterozygous sickle-cell disease or thalassemia.* The advantage here is twofold; maternal acidosis is avoided and the potential of venous stasis in the legs and pelvis is greatly reduced.
5. *Myesthenia gravis and myotonias.*
6. *Chronic neurological disease.*

An epidural can be of great benefit to mothers in each of these categories. However, it would be most unwise to embark on such a practice until all involved senior medical and nursing staff in the delivery suite have considerable experience of the management of unafflicted patients undergoing labor and delivery with epidural analgesia. Extreme vigilance is required to such matters as the avoidance of hypotension, the moving and positioning of mothers during labor, and into and out of lithotomy. The overenthusiastic acceptance of patients in these categories by relative novices is likely to lead to disaster.

Obstetric Pathology

This may be considered in two classes; diminished placental efficiency and potential hazards at vaginal delivery.

Placental Insufficiency

An epidural is beneficial to a poorly nourished fetus, whether the condition is related to pre-eclampsia, diabetes, Rh incompatibility, or intrauterine growth retardation of indeterminate origin. The avoidance of maternal and consequent fetal stress endowed by the epidural markedly reduces the hazard to which the rigors of poorly relieved labor would have exposed the fetus. Furthermore, a specific advantage is attributable to an epidural administered to the pre-eclamptic or diabetic mother. The block facilitates a significant improvement of intervillous blood flow (Kaar et al., 1980). Interestingly, this response can be observed when an extensive block, as previously described, is provided (Jouppila et al., 1980), but does not achieve a level of significance when a segmental block is given (Jouppila et al., 1979). Confusion exists about the influence of the hypotensive effect of an epidural given to a preeclamptic patient. In patients with pre-eclampsia, placental perfusion is flow-dependent rather than, as in the normotensive subject, pressure-dependent. The hypertension of pre-eclampsia is a manifestation of generalized vasoconstriction, in which the vessels supplying the placental site are involved. Vasodilatation thus facilitates uteroplacental perfusion despite an accompanying modest fall of blood pressure. However, an abrupt and severe epidose of hypotension would be as damaging in the pre-eclamptic as in the healthy mother. In this respect it is essential that the outstanding camouflaged characteristic of pre-eclampsia be borne in mind: hypovolemia (Gallery et al., 1979). The pre-eclamptic patient is maintaining a reduced circulating blood volume within a restrictive circulatory capacity. Vasodilatation without preparatory preloading is an invitation to profound hypotension. It is mandatory that initiation of an epidural in these patients be preceded by the intravenous infusion of at least 1, preferably 2, liters of crystalloid solution. The proposed use of human plasma protein fraction to increase circulatory volume by raising the oncotic pressure is interesting but beyond the scope of this chapter.

   An epidural will assist in the maintenance of a more stable level of blood pressure in the laboring pre-eclamptic patient but it is, in my opinion, unwise to use it as a specific antihypertensive measure. If antihypertensive drugs, such as hydrallazine are administered, it is advisable to reduce their rate of infusion for 10-15 min before each epidural top-up, to avoid the production of dangerously deep troughs of blood pressure. Further benefits accruing from an epidural given to a moderately or severely pre-eclamptic patient are likely to include improved renal perfusion and a reduction in catecholamine secretion. An epidural is contraindicated in pre-eclampsia only when there is an associated coagulation defect.

Hazardous Vaginal Delivery

Perinatal trauma associated with a difficult or precipitous delivery is a well-known complication of three situations: breech presentation, multiple pregnancy, and immaturity. A wealth of testimony now substantiates earlier claims that an epidural is highly advantageous in the vaginal delivery of a singleton breech (Breeson et al., 1978; De Crespigny and Pepperell, 1979) and of multiple births (Jaschevatzky et al., 1977; Weekes et al., 1977; Gullestad and Sagan, 1977). It is however, most unlikely that such benefit will accrue unless the mother is free from aortocaval compression throughout the second-stage, and unless the bearing-down reflex is totally abolished. The objective is to attain a gentle, unhurried delivery during which the painfree mother bears down with contractions at the request of the obstetrician. The advantage is especially marked in cases of prematurity, in which trauma, specifically intracranial hemorrhage, is a constant threat. Our own experience (Tables 3 and 4) testifies to this. The data in the tables do not distinguish between epidural and spinal but here there is no difference between the two. Although the information in the tables is somewhat unselective, the presence of accompanying pathology would be unlikely to influence the incidence of intracranial trauma.

A hint as to why a well-managed epidural is associated with reduced likelihood of evidence of cerebral trauma has recently been provided by Maltau and Egge (1980). They showed that in mature infants vaginally delivered by the

Table 3. Epidural Analgesia and Breech Delivery[a]

	Epidural or spinal (n = 56)	Other (n = 149)
1-min Apgar <5 (%)	35.7	48.3
5-min Apgar <7 (%)	28.6	25.5
Cerebral hemorrhage	0	6
Intrapartum stillbirth (%)	5.4	8.1
Neonatal death (%)	7.1	10.7

[a]Data from Birmingham Maternity Hospital (1968-1980) on vaginally delivered singleton breech of birth weight more than 0.99 kg and less than 2.5 kg., excluding cases of lethal congenital abnormality and prepartum death.

Table 4. Delivery of Twins and Epidural Analgesia[a]

	Vertex		Breech	
	Epidural or spinal	Other	Epidural or spinal	Other
First Twin				
n	58	134	22	40
1-min Apgar <5 (%)	5.2	10.4	27.3	20.0
5-min Apgar <7 (%)	1.7	6.0	13.6	10.0
Cerebral hemorrhage	0	2	1	1
Intrapartum stillbirth (%)	1.8	1.5	0	2.5
Neonatal death (%)	0	3.7	9.1	2.5
Second Twin				
n	43	86	39	85
1-min Apgar <5 (%)	4.7	16.3	20.5	29.4
5-min Apgar <7 (%)	0	3.5	2.6	9.4
Cerebral hemorrhage	0	3	0	1
Intrapartum stillbirth (%)	0	0	0	1.2
Neonatal death (%)	2.4	4.7	0	10.6

[a]Vaginally delivered first twins with birth weight between 0.99 and 2.5 kg, excluding cases of lethal congenital abnormality and prepartum death.

vertex, there was a significantly higher incidence of retinal hemorrhages (and the size of these was markedly greater) among infants of mothers who had delivered spontaneously without an epidural than among those whose mothers had had an epidural, had no urge to bear down, and had been delivered with forceps, despite the more protracted second stage in the latter group.

There is indeed a temptation to assert that if a reliable and efficient epidural service is available, failure to employ its services for the management of laboring patients in these three categories constitutes neglect.

Uterine Scar

An additional obstetric complication which does not fit into either of the above categories is scarred uterus. The provision of an epidural for a patient who has previously been delivered by cesarean section, or who has had a myomectomy, is beneficial, provided that monitoring is of an acceptably high standard. The signs of impending rupture are a change in the pattern of uterine activity, evidence of fetal distress, fresh vaginal bleeding, scar tenderness, and pain at the site of the scar. Of these, the latter two occur least frequently, but they will penetrate the otherwise effective pain-relief of an epidural (Crawford, 1976; Carlsson et al., 1980). Thus the requirement to distinguish between the pain of labor and pain due to impending scar rupture is avoided if an epidural is given. To date we have given an epidural to more than 400 laboring patients previously delivered by cesarean section, and are confirmed in our confidence in the safety and advisability of the measure.

COMPLICATIONS

There is an almost embarrassing freedom from maternal and neonatal complications of note associated with lumbar epidural block, with the exception of dural puncture. The mother is not more likely to develop headache or backache postnatally than is the 'nonepidural' patient, although some soreness at the site of puncture might be experienced for a day or two. Bladder disturbance (usually characterised as loss of bladder sensation, rarely as difficulty with micturition) occurs with equal frequency among epidural and nonepidural groups of mothers, if these groups are matched according to mode of delivery. Perineal pain may be appreciated more acutely by patients who had a painfree labor, but this is rarely bothersome for longer than 72 hr.

The only related complications among the neonates are those resulting from injudicious attempts to expedite delivery in the absence of fetal distress or maternal exhaustion. The incidence of neonatal jaundice may be increased in association with epidurals administered to the mother (Wood et al., 1979) but the reason for this, if it exists, is not understood, and is under further review.

CESAREAN SECTION

The advocated technique of administering a lumbar epidural for elective cesarean section has now been reasonably well systematized (Thorburn and Moir, 1980; Crawford, 1980). A profound sensory block should extend from T6 to S5, the drug of choice in the United Kingdom being 0.5% bupivacaine plain. In North American practice, 0.75% bupivacaine is favored although the advantages are not easily apparent (McGuiness et al., 1978; Datta et al., 1980). Three percent chloroprocaine is also used for this purpose in North America (Datta et al., 1980; James et al., 1980), but the recently reported neurotoxic effects of this agent makes it unlikely that it will be widely employed elsewhere (Covino et al., 1980). The satisfactory use of 1.0% etidocaine has been reported by Lund et al. (1977), but Datta et al. (1980) found the quality of analgesia provided by etidocaine to be poor compared with that afforded by bupivacaine (0.75%) or chloroprocaine.

The extensive vasomotor block which is an unavoidable characteristic of the technique involves the hazard of hypotension. This must be guarded against by preloading the mother with 2 liters of crystalloid solution intravenously before the block is established. The prospect of hypotension is further averted by administering the local anesthetic in incremental doses. The first dose, of 10 ml, is given while the mother reclines against a backrest (at about 45°). After 10 min are allowed for the drug to fix and spread to cease, the mother is helped into the full lateral horizontal position and a further dose of 10 ml is injected. Ten minutes later she is turned onto her other side and a third dose is given, the volume dependent on how high the sensory block has extended bilaterally. There is no good reason for trying to manage with the minimum possible dose of bupivacaine. A volume of less than 30 ml will infrequently provide good pain relief throughout the operation; we have, on many occasions, injected 40-50 ml or more. The advantages of the incremental technique are: it virtually eliminates suprapubic pain frequently experienced during suture of the uterine wound by patients who receive the full dose of drug as a single injection; it also permits a degree of autoregulation of maternal hemodynamics. Hypotension of a significant degree should very rarely occur when this technique is used. In our most recent series of almost 200 cases of elective section managed in this way, we have had to resort to the use of ephedrine to correct hypotension on only one occasion.

Contrary to when cesarean section is performed under general anesthesia, the direction of tilt required to avoid effects of aortocaval compression is critical when the operation is conducted under epidural analgesia (James et al., 1977). Most frequently, a tilt to the left is appropriate, but in possibly 10% of cases this will lead to maternal hypotension which is corrected by tilting her to the right.

The establishment of a satisfactory block undoubtedly takes a considerable length of time; 1 hr is not unusual in our department. This should occasion no distress or friction in a well-organized obstetric unit. Attempts to hurry what should be an orderly, planned procedure, can provoke the taking of ill-advised shortcuts with consequent distress to the mother.

There are no specific contraindications to the choice of an epidural for elective section beyond those enumerated for epidurals in obstetric practice generally. Some obstetricians dislike operating on an awake patient, and if this is likely to prove detrimental to the surgical procedure, the obstetric choice must be respected, if not fully comprehended. The majority of mothers, even in the United Kingdom, when offered the choice between general anesthesia and epidural analgesia, now opt for the latter, the dominant deciding factor being the prospect of seeing—and possibly of holding —the infant immediately after delivery.

Features which make the choice of an epidural inadvisable include distortion of intra-abdominal contents due to previous surgery, as for example, an ileostomy or a renal transplant. Under such circumstances the difficulty inherent in obtaining adequate access to the lower uterine segment can lead to pain or extreme discomfort for the mother.

The presence of a scar from a previous cesarean section certainly does not pose a contraindication. Indeed, this condition has been designated as providing a strong indication for the choice of epidural analgesia in preference to general anesthesia (Van Steenberg, 1980). The reason for such an opinion is that because the fetus is not being exposed to a progressively increasing quantity of centrally depressant drugs, the obstetrician does not feel compelled to hurry what might be a difficult procedure.

Placenta previa, or an anteriorly situated placenta, are not contraindications to the choice of an epidural. Hemorrhage at delivery can be as torrential in the absence of these features as in their presence, and the anesthetist should be well-equipped to cope with such an emergency. If these conditions are diagnosed prenatally, 4 u, instead of the customary 2 u of cross-matched blood should be made available for immediate infusion, whichever mode of anesthesia is to be used.

Ergometrine should not be given to a mother undergoing an "awake" cesarean section, unless there is an extremely powerful reason for so doing. This drug will almost invariably cause nausea and vomiting, and completely destroy the advantages attached to the choice of an epidural. If an oxytocic is required at the time of delivery—and this is unlikely in more than 10% of cases—oxytocin should be administered. The latter should be given as an infusion or injected in well-diluted form. If oxytocin is injected intravenously as a concentrated bolus, it will provoke maternal nausea, vomiting, and hypotension.

The epidural cannula may be used for administering postoperative pain relief. It should be remembered that at this stage the mother is no longer pregnant and so the capacity of her epidural space has increased. Thus, the dose of local anesthetic required to provide adequate analgesia will be somewhat larger than that needed for the operation.

There are no reported comparisons of general anesthesia with the recommended technique of epidural analgesia in respect to the condition of the neonate. However, it would be strange if the infants delivered under epidural block were found to be more depressed or acidotic. The potential of drug-induced depression is avoided when bupivacaine is used for the epidural, although it has been reported (Palahnuik et al., 1977) that infants tend to be "floppy but alert" when lignocaine is used. Provided that the mothers are appropriately positioned to avoid aortocaval compression (Datta et al., 1980) and do not become hypotensive (Downing et al., 1979) the neonatal acid-base status at delivery will be satisfactory, as will the infant's subsequent neurobehavioral condition (McGuiness et al., 1978; Hollmen et al., 1978; Fox et al., 1979). It is our practice to provide the mother with a supplementary supply of oxygen via a loosely applied mask from the time of establishment of the block to delivery of the infant. Although there is no reported evidence in support of this, it seems likely on the grounds of general principles that it is advantageous to the infant.

An epidural can be employed for emergency cesarean section, but the choice is limited by the degree of urgency involved. If an epidural is not already in progress, it is unlikely that there will be sufficient time to achieve a satisfactory block safely. If the mother has already received an epidural for labor, and the decision is made to deliver, the choice of technique of anesthesia will in part be dependent upon whether there is time to extend the level of the block to T6 (Milne et al., 1979). If such an extension is undertaken it must be accompanied—or preferably preceded—by the rapid intravenous infusion of 1 liter of crystalloid solution.

OTHER APPLICATIONS IN OBSTETRICS

A continuous epidural block is of value in situations additional to labor and cesarean section. We prefer to use it for patients who are having a Shirodkar suture inserted, because the discomfort and unpleasant sequelae of a general anesthetic are thereby avoided. Furthermore, top-up doses of bupivacaine (0.25%) can be administered during the subsequent 24 hr to relieve the post-operative pain that is an occasional feature of these cases.

Midtrimester abortion affords a strong indication for an epidural. Such labors are frequently very prolonged and there is no justification for failing to provide good analgesia without sensory disorientation in a situation which is inherently distressing. Such patients should also be given a tranquillizing drug (e.g., 5 mg diazepam every 6 hr) to reduce emotional distress.

There appears to be no defined limit to the length of time which an epidural cannula can be left in place, provided that access to its lumen is protected by a bacterial filter. Indeed, I have knowledge of one cannula having been maintained in situ for 42 days and of another which was in continuous placement for almost 2 years (both patients were "nonobstetric"). Thus it is quite acceptable to leave in place a cannula which has been in use during labor so that it can be utilized to provide analgesia for a post-partum sterilization. In such a situation it is advisable to inject a small volume of saline through the cannula at 6-8 hr intervals to avoid blockage of the lumen with coagulated protein.

ADMINISTRATION

The provision of a safe and efficient epidural service in a Department of Obstetrics requires that at least one competent anesthetist be available in the Department 24 hr a day throughout the year, with absolutely no clinical commitment elsewhere during the period of duty. It is generally agreed that only under the most unusual circumstance would an obstetric unit with a delivery rate less than 2000 (possibly less than 2500) annually be in a reasonable position to support the required anesthetic establishment. Certainly the practice of confining the services of one or two "occasional epiduralists" to high-risk patients and to those selected on a financial basis is an invitation to disaster. Fortunately, in the United Kingdom, the tendency of small maternity units to merge and the closure of isolated units is helping to remove difficulties of this kind.

In areas in which anesthetic assistance of an appropriate standard is unavailable and is unlikely to be gained, there is no valid reason why obstetricians should not give the epidurals provided that the following requirements are rigorously and consistently met: the obstetricians concerned must be capable of applying cardiorespiratory resuscitation (including endotracheal intubation) and must be responsible for maintaining the necessary associated equipment in a state of readiness; there must be assurance that competent anesthetic help is immediately available (within 5 min if required) should a complication arise; a brief annual refresher course on resuscitation—including intubation—should be undertaken by the obstetricians. We have instructed many obstetricians in the elements of epidural analgesia for labor and delivery and several of these now run their own very safe and efficient service (Taylor et al., 1977; Ghosh-Ray et al., 1980).

REFERENCES

Abouleish, E., Wadhwa, R. K., De La Vega, S., Tan, R. N., and Uy, N. T. L. (1975). Regional analgesia following epidural blood patch. *Curr. Res. Anesth. Analg. 54*:634.

Abouleish, E., Amortegui, A. J., and Taylor, F. H. (1977). Are bacterial filters needed in continuous epidural analgesia for obstetrics? *Anesthesiology 46*: 351.

Bleyaert, A., Sotens, M., Vaes, L., Van Steenberg, A., and Van der Donck, A. (1979). Bupivacaine 0.125 per cent in obstetric epidural analgesia. *Anesthesiology 51*:435.

Bray, M. C., and Carrie, L. E. S. (1978). Unblocked segments in obstetric epidural blocks. *Anaesthesia 33*:232.

Breeson, A. J., Kovacs, G. T., Pickles, B. G., and Hill, J. G. (1978). Extradural analgesia—the preferred method of analgesia for vaginal breech delivery. *Br. J. Anaesth. 50*:1227.

Bromage, P. R. (1967). Physiology and pharmacology of epidural analgesia. *Anesthesiology 28*:592.

Bromage, P. R. (1972). Unblocked segments in epidural analgesia for pain relief in labour. *Br. J. Anaesth. 44*:676.

Bromage, P. R. (1978). *Epidural Analgesia,* 2nd ed. Saunders, London.

Carlsson, C., Nybell-Lindahl, G., and Ingemarsson, I. (1980). Epidural block in patients who have previously undergone Caesarean section. *Br. J. Anaesth. 52*:827.

Carrie, L. E. S. (1971). The approach to the extradural space (Correspondence). *Anaesthesia 26*:252.

Covino, B. G., Marx, G. F., Finster, M., and Zsigmond, E. K. (1980). Prolonged sensory/motor deficits following inadvertent spinal anesthesia. *Curr. Res. Anesth. Analg. 58*:399.

Crawford, J. S. (1972). The prevention of headache consequent upon dural puncture. *Br. J. Anaesth. 44*:598.

Crawford, J. S. (1975). Pathology in the extradural space. *Br. J. Anaesth. 47*:412.

Crawford, J. S. (1976). The epidural sieve and MBC (minimum blocking concentration): An hypothesis. *Anaesthesia 31*:1277.

Crawford, J. S. (1978). *Principles and Practice of Obstetric Anaesthesia,* 4th ed. Blackwell, Oxford.

Crawford, J. S. (1980a). Experiences with epidural blood patch. *Anaesthesia 35*:513.

Crawford, J. S. (1980b). Experiences with lumbar extradural analgesia for Caesarean section. *Br. J. Anaesth. 52*:821.

Crawford, J. S., Williams, M. E., and Veales, S. (1975). Particulate matter in the extradural space. *Br. J. Anaesth. 47*:807.

Datta, S., Corke, B. C., Alper, M. H. Brown, W. U. Ostheimer, G. W., and Weiss, J. B. (1980). Epidural anesthesia for Cesarean section. *Anesthesiology 52*:48.

De Campo, T., Macias-Loza, M., Cohen, H., and Galindo, A. (1980). Lumbar epidural anaesthesia and sensory profiles in term pregnant patients. *Can. Anaesth. Soc. J. 27*:274.

De Crespigny, L. J. C., and Pepperell, R. J. (1979). Perinatal mortality in breech presentation. *Obstet. Gynecol. 53*:141.

Downing, J. W., Houlton, P. C., and Barclay, A. (1979). Extradural analgesia for Caesarean section: A comparison with general anaesthesia. *Br. J. Anaesth. 51*:367.

Ducrow, M. (1971). The occurrence of unblocked segments during continuous lumbar epidural analgesia. *Br. J. Anaesth. 43*:1172.

Enquist, A., Brandt, M. R., Fernandes, A., and Kehlet, N. (1977). Blocking effect of epidural analgesia on the adrenocortical and hyperglycaemic responses to surgery. *Acta Anaesthesiol. Scand. 21*:330.

Fox, G. S., Smith, J. B., Namba, Y., and Johnson, R. C. (1979). Anesthesia for Cesarean section: Further studies. *Am. J. Obstet. Gynecol. 133*:15.

Gal, D., Choudhry, R., Ung, K.-A., Abadir, A., and Tancer, M. L. (1979). Segmental epidural analgesia for labour and delivery. *Acta Obstet. Gynecol. Scand. 58*:429.

Gallery, E. D., Hunyor, S. N., and Gyory, A. Z. (1979). Plasma volume contraction. *Q. J. Med. 48*:593.

Ghosh-Ray, G., Taylor, A. B., and Alberts, F. (1980). An integrated pain relief service for labour: Cooperation between obstetricians, anaesthetists and midwives. *Anaesthesia 35*:510.

Gleicher, N., Midwall, J., Hochberger, D., and Jaffin, H. (1979). Eisenmenger's syndrome and pregnancy. *Obstet. Gynecol. Surv. 34*:721.

Glover, D. J. (1977). Continuous epidural analgesia in the obstetric patients: A feasibility study using a mechanical infusion pump. *Anaesthesia 32*:499.

Grundy, E. M., Zamora, A. M., and Winnie, A. P. (1978). Comparison of spread of epidural anesthesia in pregnant and nonpregnant women. *Curr. Res. Anesth. Analg. 57*:544.

Gullestad, S., and Sagan, N. (1977). Epidural block in twin labour and delivery. *Acta Anaesthesiol. Scand. 21*:504.

Hodgkinson, R., and Husain, F. J. (1980). Obesity and the cephalad spread of analgesia following epidural administration of bupivacaine for cesarian section. *Curr. Res. Anesth. Analg. 59*:89.

Hollmen, A., Jouppila, R., Pihlajiemi, R., Karvonen, P., and Sjostedt, E. (1977). Selective lumbar epidural block in labour. A clinical analysis. *Acta Anaesthesiol. Scand. 21*:174.

Hollmen, A. I., Jouppila, R., Koivisto, M., Maatta, L., Pilhajaniemi, R., Puukka, M., and Rantakyla, P. (1978). Neurological activity of infants following anesthesia for Cesarean section. *Anesthesiology 48*:350.

Hunton, J. (1979). The use of procaine hydrochloride as a continuous lumbar epidural epidural technique in labour. *Anaesthesia 34*:274.

Huovinen, K., Lehtovirta, P., Forss, M., Kivalo, I., and Teramo, K., (1979). Changes in placental intervillous blood flow measured by the ^{133}Xe method during lumbar epidural block for elective Caesarean section. *Acta Anaesthesiol. Scand. 23*:529.

Husemeyer, R. P., and White, D. C. (1980). Topography of the lumbar epidural space. *Anaesthesia 35*:7.

Husemeyer, R. P., and Crawley, J. C. W. (1979). Placental intervillous blood flow measured by inhaled ^{133}Xe clearance in relation to induction of epidural analgesia. *Br. J. Obstet. Gynaecol. 86*: 426.

James, F. M., George, R. H., Naiem, H., and White, G. J. (1976). Bacteriological aspects of epidural analgesia. *Curr. Res. Anesth. Analg. 55*:187.

James, F. M., Crawford, J. S., Hopkinson, R., Davies, P., and Naiem, H. (1977). Comparison of general anesthesia and lumbar epidural analgesia for elective Cesarean section. *Curr. Res. Anesth. Analg. 56*:228.

James, F. M., Dewan, D. M., Floyd, H. M., Wheeler, A. S., Grant, W. W., Rhyne, L., and Westmoreland, R. T. (1980). Chloroprocaine vs. bupivacaine for lumbar epidural analgesia for elective cesarian section. *Anesthesiology 52*:488.

Jaschevatzky, O. E., Shalit, A., Levy, Y., and Grunstein, S. (1977). Epidural analgesia during labour in twin pregnancy. *Br. J. Obstet. Gynaecol. 84*:327.

Jouppila, R., Hollmen, A., Jouppila, P., Kauppila, A., and Tuimala, R. (1976). Effect of segmental epidural analgesia on maternal ACTH, cortisol and TSH during labour. *Ann. Clin. Res. 8*:378.

Jouppila, P., Jouppila, R., Kaar, K., and Merila, M. (1977). Fetal heart rate patterns and uterine activity after segemental epidural analgesia. *Br. J. Obstet. Gynaecol. 84*:481.

Jouppila, R., Jouppila, P., Hollmen, A., and Kuikka, J. (1978). Effect of seg-mental extradural analgesia on placental blood flow during normal labour. *Br. J. Anaesth. 50*:563.

Jouppila, R., Jouppila, P., Hollmen, A., and Koivula, A. (1978). Epidural analgesia and placental blood flow during labour in pregnancies complicated by Hypertension. *Br. J. Obstet. Gynaecol. 86*:969.

Jouppila, R., Jouppila, P., Karinen, J. M., and Hollmen, A. (1979). Segmental epidural analgesia in labour: Related to the progress of labour, foetal malpositions and instrumental delivery. *Acta Obstet. Gynecol. Scand. 58*:135.

Jouppila, R., Louppila, P., Hollmen, A., and Koivula, A. (1980). Epidural analgesia and placental blood flow during labour in parturients with essential hypertension and EPH gestosis. *Excerpta Medica.*

Kaar, K., Jouppila, P., Kuikka, J., Luotola, H., Toivanen, J., and Rekonen, A. (1980). Intervillous blood flow in normal and complicated late pregnancy measured by means of an intravenous ^{133}Xe method. *Acta Obstet. Gynecol. Scand. 59*:7.

Lofstrom, B. (1980). Blocking characteristics of etidocaine (Duranest). *Acta Anaesthesiol. Scand. [Suppl.] 60*:21.

Lund, P. C., Cwik, J. C., Gannon, R. T., and Vassaool, H. G. (1977). Etidocaine for Caesarean section—effects on mother and baby. *Br. J. Anaesth. 49*:457.

Maltau, J. M., Eielsen, O. U., and Stokke, K. T. (1979). Effect of stress during labour on concentration of cortisol and estriol in maternal plasma. *Am. J. Obstet. Gynecol. 134*:681.

Maltau, J. M., and Egge, K. (1980). Epidural analgesia and perinatal retinal haemorrhages. *Acta Anaesthesiol. Scand. 24*:99.

Mather, L. E., and Thomas, J. (1978). Bupivacaine binding to plasma protein fractions. *J. Pharm. Pharmacol. 30*:653.

Matouskova, A. (1979). Epidural analgesia: continuous mini-infusion of bupivacaine into the epidural space during labour. *Acta Obstet. Gynecol. Scand. [Suppl.] 83.*

McGuiness, G. A., Merkow, A. J., Kennedy, R. L., and Erenberg, A. (1978). Epidural anesthesia with bupivacaine for Cesarean section. *Anesthesiology 49*:270.

Messih, M. N. A. (1981). Epidural space pressures in the lumbar region during pregnancy. *Anaesthesia 36*:775-782.

Milne, M. K., Dalrymple, D. C., Allison, R., and Lawson, J. I. M. (1979). Extension of labour epidural analgesia for Caesarean section. *Anaesthesia 34*: 992.

Modwig, J., Malmerg, P., and Karstrom, G. (1980). Effect of epidural versus general anaesthesia on calf blood flow. *Acta Anaesthesiol. Scand. 24*:305.

Moir, D. D., Slater, P. J., Thorburn, J., McLaren, R., and Moodie, J. (1976). Extradural analgesia in obstetrics: A controlled trial of carbonated lignocaine and bupivacaine hydrochloride with or without adrenaline. *Br. J. Anaesth. 48*:129.

Morishima, H. O., Pedersen, H., and Finster, M. (1978). Influence of maternal psychological stress on the fetus. *Am. J. Obstet. Gynecol. 131*:286.

Palahnuik, R. J., Scatliff, J., Biehl, D., Wieble, H., and Sankaran, K. (1977). Maternal and neonatal effects of methoxyflurane, nitrous oxide and lumbar epidural anaesthesia for Caesarean section. *Can. Anaesth. Soc. J. 24*:586.

Pearson, J. F., and Davies, P. (1973). Effect of continuous lumbar epidural analgesia on the acid-base status of maternal arterial blood during the first stage of labour. *J. Obstet. Gynaecol. Br. Commonw. 80*:218.

Pearson, J. F., and Davies, P. (1974). Effect of continuous lumbar epidural analgesia upon fetal acid-base status during the first stage of labour. *J. Obstet. Gynaecol. Br. Commonw. 81*:971.

Ravindran, R. S., Bond, U. K., Tasch, M. D., Gupta, C. D., and Luerssen, T. G. (1980). Prolonged neural blockade following regional anagesia with 2-chloroprocaine. *Curr. Res. Anesth. Analg. 59*:447.

Reisner, L. S., Hochman, B. N., and Plumer, M. H. (1980). Persistent neurologic deficit and adhesive arachnoiditis following intrathecal 2-chloroprocaine injection. *Curr. Res. Anesth. Analg. 59*:452.

Scott, D. B., McClure, J. H., Giasi, R. M., Seo, J., and Covino, B. G., (1980). Effects of concentration of local anaesthetic drugs in extradural block. *Br. J. Anaesth. 52*:1033.

Seltzer, J. L., Porretta, J. C., and Jackson, B. G. (1977). Plastic particulate contaminants in the medicine cups of disposable non-spinal regional anesthesia sets. *Anesthesiology 47*:378.

Stainthorpe, S. F., Bradshaw, E. G., Challen, P. D., and Tobias, M. A. (1978). 0.125% bupivacaine for obstetric analgesia? *Anaesthesia 33*:3.

Studd, J. W. W., Crawford, J. S., Duigan, N. M., Rowbotham, C. J. F., and Hughes, A. D. (1980). Effect of lumbar epidural analgesia on the rate of cervical dilatation and the outcome of labour of spontaneous onset. *Br. J. Obstet. Gynaecol. 87*:1015.

Talledo, O. E., Chesley, L. C., and Zuspan, F. P. (1968). Renin-angiotension system in normal and toxemic pregnancies. II Differential sensitivity to angiotension II and norepinephrine in toxemia of pregnancy. *Am. J. Obstet. Gynecol. 100*:218.

Taylor, A. B. W., Abuknalil, S. H., El-Guindi, M. M., and Watkins, J. A. (1977). Lumbar epidural analgesia in labour: A 24 hour service provided by obstetricians. *Br. Med. J.* 2:370.

Thorburn, J., and Moir, D. D. (1980). Epidural analgesia for elective Caesarean section. *Anaesthesia 35*:3.

Van Steenberg, R. (1980). Continuous epidural anaesthesia for Caesarean section. In *Epidural Analgesia in Obstetrics.* A. Doughty (Ed.), Lloyd-Luke, London, p. 159.

Weekes, A. R. L., Cheridjian, V. E., and Mwanje, D. K. (1977). Lumbar epidural analgesia in labour in twin pregnancy. *Br. Med. J.* 2:730.

Willdeck-Lund, G., Lindmark, G., and Nilsson, B. A. (1979a). Effect of segmental epidural block on the course of labour and on the condition of the infant during the neonatal period. *Acta Anaesthesiol. Scand. 23*:301.

Willdeck-Lund, G., Lindmark, G., and Nilsson, B. A. (1979b). Effect of segmental epidural analgesia upon uterine activity with special reference to the use of different local anaesthetic agents. *Acta Anaesthesiol. Scand. 23*: 519.

Wood, B., Culley, P., Roginski, C., Powell, J., and Waterhouse, J. (1979). Factors affecting neonatal jaundice. *Arch. Dis. Child. 54*:111.

Zador, G., and Nilsson, B. A. (1974). Continuous drip lumbar epidural anaesthesia with lidocaine for vaginal delivery. II Influence on labour and foetal acid-base balance. *Acta Obstet. Gynecol. Scand. [Suppl.] 34*:17.

Zuspan, F. P., Cibils, L. A., and Pose, S. V. (1962). Myometrial and cardiovascular responses to alterations in plasma epinephrine and norepinephrine. *Am. J. Obstet. Gynecol. 84*:841.

16

Obstetrical Anesthesia: Local Anesthetics and Regional Anesthetic Techniques for Labor and Delivery

JOSEPH J. KRYC / The Ohio State University, Columbus, Ohio

The relief of pain during labor and delivery has been of interest to many for centuries. Throughout time many varieties of medicinal concoctions have been used with varying degrees of success. Approximately 100 years ago, a new era began with the discovery of the first local anesthetic, cocaine. The ancient Incas used cocaine for centuries and considered it a divine gift from the gods. In 1860, this compound was isolated from the coca shrub by Albert Niemann (Koller, 1941). Its potential use in clinical situations however, was not realized for another 25 years. Studies concerning the clinical usefulness of cocaine in ophthalmology were presented to the Congress of the German Society of Ophthalmologists by Carl Koller in 1884. Shortly thereafter cocaine became a widely used local anesthetic. Although its benefits were great, so were its toxic properties. The quest for an "ideal" local anesthetic had now begun. This led to the synthesis of procaine in 1904 by Einhort (de Jong, 1977), which became the mainstay of local anesthetics for approximately 50 years. Modifications of the parent compound, an ester, resulted in the discovery of two other clinically useful agents, tetracaine and chloroprocaine. In 1948, lidocaine, the first amide local anesthetic was discovered by Lofgren, a Swedish chemist. A variety of amide agents have since been synthesized and introduced to clinical medicine. As a group, they are extremely stable and potent, and exhibit good tissue penetration and low systemic toxicity.

In anesthesiology, the classification of the effects of drugs and techniques can be described as producing either anesthesia or analgesia. Anesthesia implies

351

a loss of consciousness whereas analgesia does not. Local anesthetic agents produce a loss of sensation similar to general anesthetic agents. The similarity, however, ends there. Local anesthetics are selective in anesthetizing only those areas required, without the loss of consciousness. This single feature, combined with its safety, has resulted in their widespread use for the relief of pain during labor and delivery.

Functionally, labor has been divided into three distinct stages. The first stage is the active and progressive dilation and effacement of the cervix. The second stage is the expulsion and delivery of the fetus, and the third stage is the delivery of the placenta (Friedman, 1971). Although the pain of labor originates from multiple pain sensitive fibers in the uterus, parauterine, and perineal structures, the transmission of painful stimuli to the central nervous systems occurs by only two relatively distinct pathways.

Pain during the first stage of labor arises largely from the uterus, cervix, and upper vagina. Impulses originating in these areas travel through the paracervical (Frankenhauser's) ganglion to the pelvic plexus, and then to the middle and superior hypogastric plexuses. From there the impulses enter the spinal cord via the sympathetic rami communicantes between T_{10} and L_1 (Fig. 1).

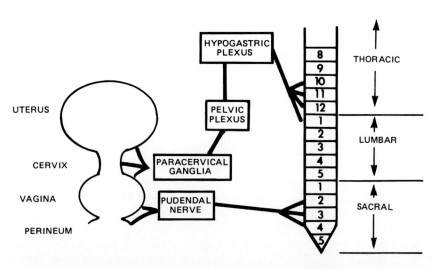

Figure 1. Diagrammatic representation of the neural pathways involved in the transmission of pain during labor and delivery (see text). (From Cleland, J. G. P., (1949). Continuous peridural and cotyl analgesia in obstetrics, *Anesth. Analg. 28*:61.

Table 1. Regional Anesthetic Techniques for Labor and Delivery

Labor	Technique	Area of anesthesia
	Paracervical	T_{10}-L_1
1st stage	Lumbar epidural	T_{10}-S_5
	Caudal	T_{10}-S_5
	Dual-catheter technique	
	epidural segmental	T_{10}-L_1
	caudal segmental	S_2-S_4
	Local infiltration	Portions of pudendal
	Pudendal	S_2-S_4
2nd stage	Lumbar epidural	T_{10}-S_5
	Caudal	T_{10}-S_5
	Dual-catheter technique	
	epidural segmental	T_{10}-L_1
	caudal segmental	S_2-S_5
	Subarachnoid (spinal)	
	saddle	S_1-S_5
	standard	T_{10}-S_5

Source: Shnider, Levinson, and Ralston, 1979. ©1979, The Williams & Wilkins Co., Baltimore.

Although uterine contractions continue during the second stage of labor, much of the pain during this portion of labor originates from the lower vagina, perineum, anus, and medial and inferior portion of the vulva and clitoris. Impulses originating in this area are transmitted along the pudendal nerve which travels across the sacrospinous ligament and enters the parasympathetic system via the sacral nerves S_2-S_4 (Fig. 1). Numerous regional anesthetic techniques are available for the relief of pain during labor and delivery. The most common forms are listed in Table 1 and include local infiltration, minor regional, and major conduction techniques (Shnider et al., 1973). Each of these is unique with respect to its effects on the fetus, mother, and the maternal-fetal unit. The selection of an appropriate local anesthetic and regional technique must therefore be considered in terms of the effects on the expulsive forces of labor, the muscle tone of the pelvis required for rotation of the presenting part, and the safety to the fetus and mother (Bromage, 1979).

PHYSIOLOGY OF NEURAL TRANSMISSION AND MECHANISM OF ACTION OF LOCAL ANESTHETICS

Neural structures are specialized tissues capable of transmitting electrical potentials, called impulses, from one part of the body to another. The cell membrane consists of a fluid matrix wherein a phospholipid bilayer is organized in such a way that the hydrophilic (water-soluble) polar groups are directed outward and the hydrophobic (water-insoluble) groups are directed inward. Floating in this lipid matrix are cholesterol and protein molecules. The protein molecules are orientated in a manner similar to the phospholipids, with the hydrophilic portion directed outward, and hydrophobic portion directed inward. It has been suggested that these protein structures penetrate the bilayered phospholipids and create pores or channels that connect the intracellular and extracellular spaces (Singer and Nicholsen, 1972). These channels vary in size and are selective for either sodium or potassium ions. Small gate-like structures are located on the internal portion of these channels and control the flow of ions into and out of the cell (Fig. 2a). During the resting state the cell membrane is more permeable to potassium than sodium ions. This selective permeability generates an electrochemical gradient of approximately −70 mv which is known as the resting membrane potential. If a stimulus of sufficient intensity is applied to the membrane, an electrical field is generated. Depolarization occurs when the sodium and potassium gates open and allow their respective ions to equilibrate with the intracellular and extracellular fluid. This gives rise to an action potential which is self-propagating (Fig. 2b). Following depolarization the gates then close and sodium is actively "pumped" out of the cell while potassium is actively "pumped" into the cell in an effort to re-establish the resting membrane potential. Local anesthetics appear to interfere with the process of depolarization by obstructing the influx of sodium ions (Fig. 2b). The mechanism for impulse blockade is unknown. It is known, however, that local anesthetics bond with a receptor on the internal portion of the cell membrane. This bonding may then alter the size of the sodium channel by "membrane expansion" and prevent sodium from entering the cell when a stimulus is applied. Physiologically this results in an obstruction to the transmission of a nerve impulse that is clinically interpreted as anesthesia.

PHARMACOLOGY OF LOCAL ANESTHETICS

To be efficient, a local anesthetic must penetrate the cell membrane, bind with a receptor for an appropriate period of time and inactivate the membrane, and, finally, it must disengage, leaving the cell membrane completely functional. It is not surprising then that there are a large number of local anesthetics

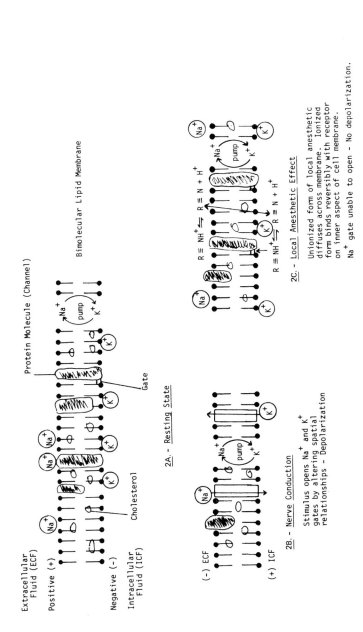

Figure 2. Diagrammatic representation of the biomolecular lipid membrane. A. Resting state membrane. Sodium and potassium ions are pumped out of and into the cell. Ion channels are closed. B. Nerve conduction. Sodium and potassium channels are open allowing the respective ions to pass through the membrane and equilibrate with the intracellular and extracellular fluid. C. Local anesthetic effect. Nonionized compound diffuses through the phospholipid matrix. In the intracellular space ionization of the molecule and bonding with the gate occur. Membrane expansion may prevent the channel from opening.

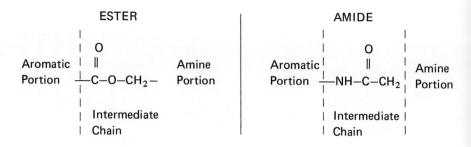

Figure 3. Classification of local anesthetics (see text).

available capable of fulfilling some but not all of these requirements. The clinically available local anesthetics are categorized by the type of linkage between the aromatic portion and the intermediate chain. The ester compounds have an ester linking the aromatic portion and the intermediate chain. The amide compounds have an amide linking these two portions (Fig. 3). In addition, local anesthetics may be classified according to their potency and duration of action. Three groups can be identified: a low potency and short duration group (procaine, chloroprocaine), an intermediate potency and duration group (lidocaine, mepivacaine) and a high potency and long duration group (bupivacaine, tetracaine, etidocaine) (Table 2). Although the pharmacologic properties of the local anesthetics are strongly influenced by their structure, lipid solubility, protein binding, and the dissociation constant (pK_a), they are nevertheless quite homogeneous as a group. Structurally, a local anesthetic consists of three parts: a hydrophilic component (amino portion), which is usually a derivative of a tertiary amine; an intermediate chain; and a lipophilic component (aromatic portion), usually a derivative of benzoic acid or aniline (Fig. 4).

The hydrophilic portion contains a tertiary amine group which is a trivalent uncharged nitrogen molecule with organic groups replacing the three hydrogen groups.

$$
\begin{array}{cc}
\text{H} & \text{R}_2 \\
| & | \\
\text{H-N} & \text{R}_1\text{-N} \\
| & | \\
\text{H} & \text{R}_3
\end{array}
$$

Tertiary Amine

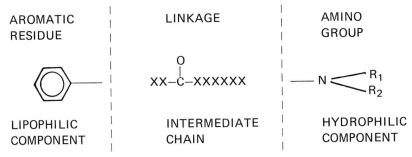

| AROMATIC RESIDUE | | LINKAGE | | AMINO GROUP |
| LIPOPHILIC COMPONENT | | INTERMEDIATE CHAIN | | HYDROPHILIC COMPONENT |

Figure 4. The three parts of a local anesthetic. R_1 and R_2 represent hydrogen atoms that have been replaced by organic groups.

Depending on the pH of the environment this uncharged nitrogen molecule is capable of changing to a "dissociated" electrically active form, which is important to the clinical properties exhibited by local anesthetics (Bromage, 1978).

$$R_1 - N \begin{array}{c} R_2 \\ R_3 \end{array}$$

The uncharged molecule is lipid-soluble, whereas the charged molecule is not. The receptor site is on the inside of the cell membrane and can accept only the charged form of the molecule. It can be easily appreciated that the uncharged form must pass through the lipid matrix of the cell membrane and once again become charged in order to bond with the receptor and inactivate the sodium channel.

The intermediate chain is crucial to the actual bonding of the molecule to the receptor site. It contains a carbonyl group which is important in electron transfer along the molecule, in the bonding characteristics, as well as the clinical qualities exhibited by the compound.

$$\overset{O}{\underset{\|}{-C-}}$$

Additions or alterations to this chain may alter the physiochemical and clinical properties dramatically. In addition, important spatial relationships between the polar groups are determined by the intermediate chain. For a local anesthetic to be effective clinically, a distance of 5-9 Å seems to be critical (Bromage, 1978).

Table 2. Classification of Local Anesthetics According to Potency and Duration

Agent	Structure	Trade name	Molecular weight	pK_a	Plasma protein % binding	Solution concentration (%)	Relative potency	Onset of action	Duration (min)
Group 1: Low potency, short duration									
Procaine	Ester	Novocaine	272	8.9		1	1	Slow	60-90
2-Chloroprocaine	Ester	Novocaine	307	8.7		2,3	1	Fast	30-45
Group 2: Intermediate potency and duration									
Lidocaine	Amide	Xylocaine	234	7.9	55	1, 1.5, 2.0	2	Fast	60-90
Mepivacaine	Amide	Carbocaine	246	7.6	65	1, 2	2	Fast	90-120
Group 3: High potency, long duration									
Tetracaine	Ester	Pontocaine	300	8.5		1	8	Slow	90-120
Bupivacaine	Amide	Marcaine	288	8.1	84	0.25, 0.5, 0.75	8	Slow	240-360
Etidocaine	Amide	Duranest	276	7.7	94	0.25, 0.5, 1.0, 1.5	6	Fast	300-1100

The lipophilic portion determines the duration of action and the protein-binding characteristics of the molecule. Substitutions and additions of hydrocarbon groups alter these characteristics markedly.

The local anesthetics are weak bases and as such are insoluble and unstable in aqueous solutions. To overcome this difficulty they are prepared commercially as acid salts which are much more stable and soluble in an aqueous solution. When the salt is placed in an aqueous solution, it ionizes almost completely to yield a positively charged cation and a negatively charged anion.

$$\text{Local anesthetic } -NH^+Cl^- + H_2O - \text{local anesthetic} - NH^+ + Cl^-$$

| (salt) | (cation) | (anion) |

The cation then further dissociates and equilibrates with the nonionized base form. The extent of dissociation is dependent upon the dissociation constant (pK_a) of the molecule and the pH (concentration of hydrogen ions) of the solution.

$$\text{Local anesthetic} - NH^+ \xrightarrow{pK_a} \text{local anesthetic} - NH + H^+$$

| (cation) | (base) |
| (lipid insoluble) | (lipid soluble) |

When a local anesthetic is deposited about a nerve, it exists in two forms: the cation, a charged molecule that is water-soluble and lipid-insoluble; and the base form, an uncharged molecule that is lipid-soluble and water-insoluble. The uncharged portion, being lipid-soluble, easily diffuses through the cell membrane. Inside the cell it must change back to the cation to maintain its activity (Fig. 2c).

The larger the dissociation constant (pK_a), the smaller the amount of nonionized base at any given pH (Fig. 5). By manipulating the acid-base environment, it is possible to direct the "flow" of local anesthetics into or out of a body cavity. This is called ion trapping and can become very important in clinical obstetric anesthesia when an acidotic infant is present.

Systemic uptake and distribution of local anesthetics is dependent on a number of variables which include: site of injection, dosage, vascularity of the injection site, use of vasopressors, rate of metabolism and excretion, and the physiochemical characteristics of the individual agents (Covino, 1980; Endler, 1980; Giasi et al., 1979; Pedersen et al., 1978). Absorption of local anesthetics is most rapid from areas that are highly vascular. In reference to the obstetrical patient, absorption is greatest with injection into the caudal canal followed by the lumbar epidural space, subarachnoid space, and subcutaneous tissue.

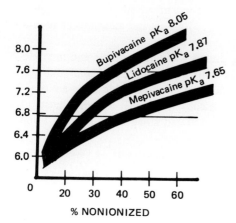

Figure 5. Effects of pH on local anesthetics with different dissociation constants (pK$_a$) with respect to the nonionized form available. (From Bromage, 1978.)

Paracervical block can result in an extremely rapid absorption of local anesthetic because of the proximity to the uterine vasculature.

The blood level of a local anesthetic achieved is most closely related to the total amount of drug injected rather than the volume or concentration used. The greater the amount of drug injected, the higher the maternal blood levels. This occurs in a linear manner. The addition of vasoconstrictors such as epinephrine or phenylephrine to local anesthetic solutions will decrease the rate of absorption as well as the peak level attained in the serum. In addition, the use of vasoconstrictors will prolong the duration and intensify the block. Although this is generally true of peripheral nerve blocks, the use of these agents seems to have little effect on the newer, long-acting, local anesthetics (such as bupivacaine and etidocaine) when used in the lumbar epidural space (Lund et al., 1975).

Vascular absorption of local anesthetics is also dependent on the agent utilized. Lidocaine and mepivacaine tend to be rapidly absorbed. This is probably due to the local vasodilation caused by these agents. Although bupivacaine is minimally absorbed compared with lidocaine and mepivacaine, it is much more rapidly absorbed than etidocaine. This is most likely due to etidocaine's greater lipid-solubility which enables it to be stored in the peripheral fat tissues.

Following the absorption of a local anesthetic from the injection site, distribution throughout the body occurs in two phases. The first, or alpha, phase of distribution is due to the uptake of the local anesthetic by its

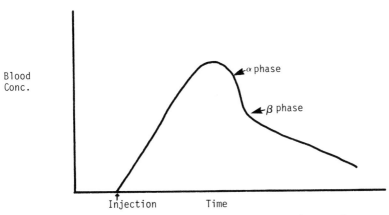

Figure 6. Uptake and distribution of local anesthetics (see text).

equilibration with the tissues. This is a relatively short and rapid occurrence. The second, or beta, phase of distribution is due to redistribution to poorly perfused tissues and to the metabolism and excretion of the compound. This process is slower and longer than the alpha phase and is dependent on the local anesthetic (Fig. 6).

Biotransformation of local anesthetics is determined by the linkage between the aromatic portion and the intermediate chain of the molecule. The esters are rapidly inactivated by plasma pseudocholinesterase to para-aminobenzoic acid and excreted in the urine. The half-life of these agents is very short. The amides are inactivated primarily in the liver by hydrolysis or dealkyation. This is a much slower process, therefore these agents tend to persist unchanged for longer periods of time than the ester agents. This prolonged elimination may result in cumulative effects if large doses are administered at frequent intervals.

SYSTEMIC TOXICITY OF LOCAL ANESTHETICS

When used in obstetrical patients, the systemic toxicity of local anesthetics can involve the mother, the fetus, or both. In addition, the effects on the maternal-fetal unit may be either direct or indirect.

Systemic toxicity in the mother is generally due to an intravascular injection resulting in high peak serum blood levels. The major organ systems involved are the cardiovascular and central nervous systems. The direct cardiovascular effects include myocardial depression and vasodilation. Lidocaine levels of 10 μg/ml have been associated with a decrease in myocardial contractility, a decreased intraventricular pressure, and a decrease in cardiac output. These changes are due to a prolongation of conduction through the heart, and a change in the threshold and automaticity of the sinus node. Sinus bradycardia with prolongation of the PR interval and the QRS interval are the elctro-cardiographic alterations that occur secondary to these changes. Concentrations of lidocaine above 10 μg/ml have been associated with asystole. The peripheral vasodilation is due to relaxation of the vascular smooth muscle. The decreased myocardial contractility and decreased peripheral vascular resistance can result in circulatory collapse and hypotension. Interesting, however, is the effect of local anesthetics on the uterine vasculature. When applied to the uterine artery, vasospasm occurs instead of vasodilation (Cibils, 1976).

The indirect cardiovascular changes are related more to the regional anesthesic technique than to any specific effect of the local anesthetic. Caudal, lumbar epidural, and spinal techniques may be complicated by total spinal anesthesia. This will result in a massive sympathetic blockade with a decrease in peripheral vascular resistance and hypotension. It may also cause a blockade of the cardio-accelerator area resulting in a decrease in heart rate and contractility.

In the central nervous system (CNS), local anesthetics easily cross the blood brain barrier producing CNS depression. Clinically this is seen as CNS excitation followed by marked CNS depression. CNS-inhibitory fibers are more sensitive to local anesthetics than are excitatory fibers. As a result, low levels of local anesthetics inhibit the inhibitory pathways, first causing an uncontrolled excitatory state. Clinically, this is evidenced by lightheadedness, dizziness, and auditory and visual disturbances. Higher levels can result in slurred speech, shivering, tremor of the face and extremities, which may all be precursors to seizure activity. Increasing levels eventually inhibit the excitatory pathways also and generalized central nervous system depression occur (Table 3).

Systemic toxicity may also result from an allergic reaction to the local anesthetic. This is rare and, when it occurs, is almost always due to the ester compounds. Para-aminobenzoic acid is a metabolite of these compounds and is a suspected allergen. Allergic reactions to the amide agents are extremely rare.

As recently as 20 years ago placental transfer of local anesthetics was not appreciated. In 1961, Bromage and Robson identified lidocaine in the cord blood of infants whose mothers had received this drug. Since then, local anesthetics have also been noted to produce effects in the fetus in a manner similar to the mother. Indirect fetal effects are due to alterations of the maternal hemodynamic state, which interferes with maternal-fetal exchange. The direct fetal effects include cardiovascular and CNS depression. The mech-anisms and clinical manifestations are identical to those produced by systemic toxicity in the mother. The placental transfer of local anesthetics is influenced by a variety of factors. The most important of these appears to be the physio-chemical properties of the local anesthetic and the status of the maternal-fetal unit (Ralston and Shnider, 1978). High maternal blood levels of local

Table 3. Cardiovascular and Central Nervous System Signs and Symptoms of
Local Anesthetic Toxicity

Cardiovascular Effects	Central Nervous System Effects
Mild	
↑ PR interval	Lightheadedness
↑ QRS duration	Dizziness
↓ Cardiac output	Tinnitus
↓ Blood pressure	Drowsiness
	Disorientation
Severe	
↑ PR interval	Muscle twitching
↑ QRS duration	Tremors of face and extremities
sinus bradycardia	Unconsciousness
AV block	Generalized convulsions
↓ Cardiac output	Respiratory arrest
Hypotension	
asystole	

Source: B. Covino, Pharmacology of local anesthetics, ASA Annual Refresher Course,
Park Ridge, Illinois: American Society of Anesthesiologists, 1980, by permission.

anesthetics, as may occur with intravascular injections and paracervical
anesthesia, can also enhance the transfer of these agents from mother to fetus.

The rate of transfer of a local anesthetic across the placenta is dependent on:
lipid solubility, molecular weight, degree of ionization, fetal hemodynamic state,
and uteroplacental blood flow. The placenta is a lipid membrane that easily
allows the transfer of lipid-soluble agents. Nonionized compounds are generally
highly lipid-soluble whereas ionized compounds are not. As discussed previously,
local anesthetics are salts of strong acids. As such they are capable of existing in
a nonionized and ionized state simultaneously. The fraction of nonionized
molecules present is dependent on the dissociation constant (pK_a) of that particular drug. The pK_as of the commonly employed local anesthetics range from 7.7
to 9.0 (Pedersen et al., 1978). The higher the pK_a the smaller the fraction of
nonionized molecules present at physiologic pH. In acidotic environments, that
is, distressed infants, the fraction of ionized molecules increases. Ionized molecules are unable to transfer across the placenta and therefore become "trapped"
in the fetus.

In addition to lipid solubility and ionization, the molecular weight of an
agent will also influence the rate of placental transfer. Pharmacologic agents
with molecular weights of 500 or less cross the placenta with relative ease. Those
agents with molecular weights of more than 1000 do not cross easily. This,
however, is not an all-or-none phenomenon. There seems to be a mechanism for

$$\frac{Q}{t} = \frac{(K)(A)(C_m - C_f)}{D}$$

where:

$\frac{Q}{t}$ = The rate of diffusion

A = The surface area available for diffusion

C_m = The maternal concentration

C_f = The fetal concentration

D = The thickness of the membrane

K = The diffusion constant

Figure 7. Fick's Diffusion Law.

placental discretion since maternal proteins with large molecular weights are easily transferable to the fetus (Mirkin, 1975). The molecular weights of all local anesthetics are less than 500. Placental transfer of these agents is by simple diffusion and depends on the concentration gradient across the membrane, the surface area available for transfer, and the thickness of the membrane. Mathematically, this has been described by Fick's Diffusion Law (Fig. 7).

The fetal circulation and hemodynamic state influences the distribution, metabolism, and "trapping" of drugs within the fetal unit. In utero, the fetal circulation contains a number of shunts that enable oxygenated blood access to important vital organs such as the myocardium and brain. Oxygenated blood flows from the placenta to the fetus via the umbilical vein. Upon entering the umbilicus a variable amount is shunted past the liver via the ductus venosus to the inferior vena cava to mix with the shunted portion. From here it travels to the right atrium where some mixing occurs with blood returning via the superior vena cava. The majority of right atrial blood is shunted through the foramen ovale to the left atrium. It then enters the left ventricle and is subsequently distributed throughout the fetus. The remaining portion of right atrial blood enters the right ventricle and then the pulmonary artery. In utero, the fetal pulmonary vascular resistance is extremely high and less than 10% of the blood in the pulmonary artery enters the pulmonary circulation. The majority is shunted to the aorta by means of the ductus arteriosus (Fig. 8). Because of this unique circulatory pattern, any drug entering the fetus will pass through the liver and be metabolized and inactivated to some degree. Prior to distribution to the rest of the fetus, the concentration of a drug is also decreased by progressive dilution at each stage. Fetal stress resulting in hypoxia and

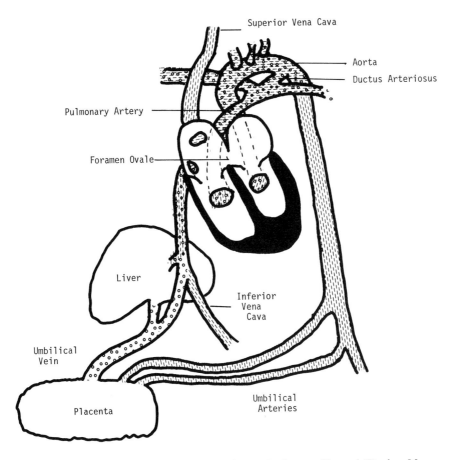

Superior Vena Cava

Aorta

Ductus Arteriosus

Pulmonary Artery

Foramen Ovale

Liver

Inferior
Vena
Cava

Umbilical
Vein

Umbilical
Arteries

Placenta

Figure 8. Fetal circulation (see text). (From Pedersen, H., and Finsler, M. (1977). Pharmacodynamics of analgesics and anesthetics. *Drug Therapy* 44-52).

acidosis alters the distribution of blood dramatically in an effort to maintain oxygenation to vital organs. There is an increase of flow through the ductus venosus, foramen ovale, and ductus arteriosus which in effect increases the flow to the brain, myocardium, placenta, and adrenals and decreases flow to the lungs and kidneys. The distribution of any drugs as well as the amount of active drug is also significantly altered with these changes. Since blood flow bypasses the fetal liver, more drug will enter the coronary and cerebral circulation and may further depress an already compromised fetus.

CHOICE OF REGIONAL ANESTHETIC TECHNIQUE

The appropriate choice of a regional anesthetic technique must be individualized to obtain the best risk-benefit ratio possible to both mother and fetus.
Although general anesthesia continues to be the most common form of
anesthesia administered in the United States, larger facilities and university
hospitals are utilizing regional techniques more frequently (Hicks et al., 1976).
In obstetrical patients, the use of regional anesthesia is associated with a
reduced risk of maternal aspiration syndromes. The mother is alert and cooperative and actively involved in the birthing process, and the neonate is less
influenced than if born to a mother who received narcotics or some form of
general anesthesia (Bonica, 1975). Although regional anesthesia is generally
safer for both the mother and fetus, it can be associated with major maternal
and fetal complications depending on the technique used.

Local Infiltration:

Technique
Local infiltration or field block of the perineum has been used extensively in
obstetrics. It is not only simple and effective but it is virtually devoid of
complications to the mother and fetus. This technique is effective in relieving
episiotomy pain. It cannot, however, eliminate the pain from perineal distention, nor is it capable of producing muscular relaxation. Field block of
the perineum is outlined in Figures 9 and 10. To prevent toxic doses of local
anesthetics from being administered to the mother, weak solutions of these
agents are indicated.

Field block of the perineum is performed under sterile conditions by in-
filtrating a small area of skin with local anesthetic at a point medial and
slightly posterior to the ischial tuberosity. This can be most easily accomplished
with a small 25-gauge needle. Infiltration of the soft tissues is carried out as
indicated in the diagrams. It is advisable to insert a finger into the rectum to
prevent accidental puncture of the rectum.

A local block of the perineum can be easily performed at any time during
delivery as illustrated in Figure 11. When performing this block it is important
to produce several fanwise injections to assure adequate anesthesia.

Paracervical/Pudendal Anesthesia

Paracervical and pudendal anesthesia have been used by obstetricians for
approximately 50 years (Petrie et al., 1974). During the past few years
paracervical anesthesia has been associated with some controversy regarding
its safety. Of particular concern are the frequent reports of perinatal
morbidity and mortality and the phenomena of fetal bradycardia following
the institution of a block. Postinjection fetal bradycardia generally appears

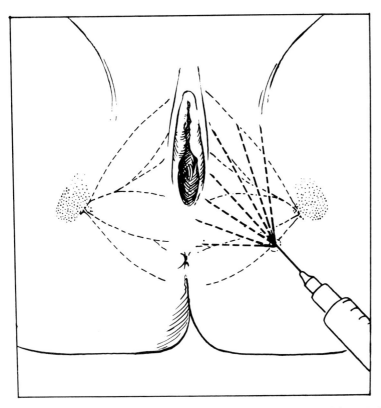

Figure 9. Technique of perineal infiltration: heavy dashed lines indicate areas of injection, light dashed lines indicate nerves. (From Bonica, 1969.)

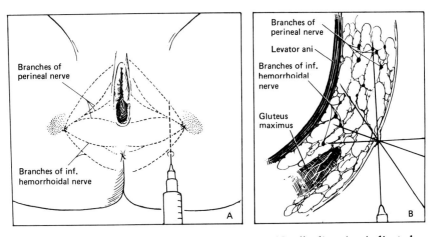

Figure 10. Technique of perineal infiltration. A. Needle direction indicated by heavy dashed lines. B. Sagittal view indicating fanwise infiltration technique. (From Bonica, 1969.)

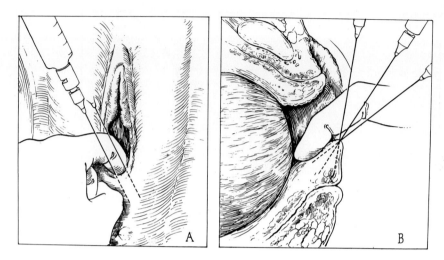

Figure 11. Technique of local infiltration for episiotomy. A. Anterior view: heavy dashed lines indicate direction of needle. B. Sagittal view shows fanwise injection pattern. (From Bonica, 1969.)

within 2-10 min of injection, may last for as long as 30 min, and is usually associated with fetal acidosis and an increased likelihood of fetal depression (Ralston and Shnider, 1978). The etiology of fetal bradycardia remains unknown, however, multiple factors acting directly and indirectly on the fetus may be involved.

In 1974, Petrie et al. investigated 10 normal patients in labor receiving paracervical blocks with 1% xylocaine. Postinjection fetal bradycardia coincided with the mean maximum maternal and fetal concentrations approximately 9-10 min after injection. However, it was also shown that postinjection fetal bradycardia occurred when very low concentrations of Xylocaine were obtained from the fetus. This implies that other mechanisms may be involved. When local anesthetics are injected in the paracervical space, a relatively high concentration of drug is available for rapid uptake and distribution to the fetus. In addition, local anesthetics cause uterine artery spasm and an increase in myometrical contractions, in a dose-dependent manner (Greiss et al., 1976). The combination of increased intrauterine pressure and arterial spasm result in a decreased uteroplacental perfusion which may interfere with fetal oxygenation.

Regardless of the cause, bradycardia is associated with an increased frequency of fetal acidosis, morbidity, and mortality (Ralston and Shnider, 1978; Shnider et al., 1970). The incidence of fetal bradycardia following paracervical block is approximately 22%. The range, however, varies between

3 and 70% depending on the local anesthetic used and the status of the fetus prior to institution of the block (Baskett and Carson, 1974; Cib's and Stantonja-Lucas, 1978; Ralston and Shnider, 1978; Shnider and Gildea, 1963). When paracervical anesthesia is used in patients with no prior fetal distress, post-injection bradycardia varies between 10 and 20%. If fetal distress is present prior to injection, the frequency of bradycardia more than doubles and in some series approaches 60-70%. Of equal concern are the reports of fetal mortality and long-term neurological complications that may occur following para-cervical anesthesia (Nyirjersy et al., 1963; Rosefoky and Petersiel, 1968). It is therefore recommended that this form of anesthesia be avoided in high-risk patients, especially those exhibiting uteroplacental insufficiency (Terrano and Widholm, 1967).

Pudendal anesthesia is frequently used during the second stage of labor. It is frequently employed just prior to delivery and provides excellent anesthesia of the perineum and lower vagina. It has not been associated with any direct fetal complications. Maternal systemic toxicity due to intra-arterial injection in the pudendal artery has, however, been reported. Simple surgical obstetrical procedures may be easily performed under pudendal anesthesia, however, relax-ation of the levator muscles and perineum is lacking. Because of this, more complicated obstetrical maneuvers requiring relaxation require other forms of anesthesia.

Technique

Paracervical anesthesia can be performed in the patient's labor room. It can be easily accomplished when the cervix is approximately 4-5-cm dilated. The technique becomes much more difficult, if not impossible, as the cervix becomes completely effaced and dilated. Injections of local anesthetic are made into the lateral fornices of the vagina at the 3 and 4 o'clock positions and at the 8 and 9 o'clock positions. This effectively interupts the painful stimuli transmitted by these nerves to the spinal cord (Fig. 12).

The procedure is performed under sterile conditions by inserting a hollow needle guide over the examining hand into the lateral fornix of the vagina (Fig. 13). The needle with a syringe attached is passed through the guide and advanced approximately 0.5 cm into the vaginal mucosa. Aspiration prior to injection will identify arterial placement of the needle (Fig. 14). If blood is aspirated, a change in needle position is indicated. If blood is aspirated on subsequent attempts it is best to abandon the procedure completely.

It is extremely important that a minimal amount of local anesthetic (2-3 cc) be used at each injection site. The fetal heart tones must be monitored closely before, during, and after the injection. Approximately 3-5 min should elapse before the procedure is performed on the opposite side. The duration of pain relief will range from 45 to 90 min depending on the local anesthetic used.

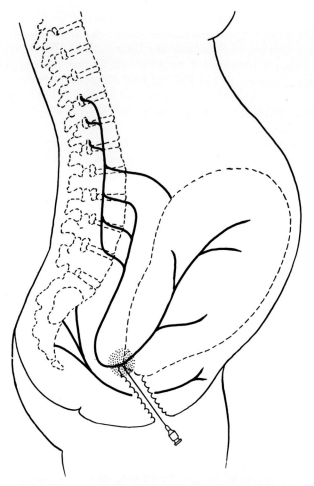

Figure 12. Schematic diagram showing sensory (pain) pathways interrupted when using a paracervical block. These pathways do not contain fibers from the vagina or perineum. (From Bonica, 1969.)

Because of the potential hazards of this technique, extreme care should be utilized at all times. It should not be used in patients with fetal distress or uteroplacental insufficiency.

Pudendal anesthesia is also relatively simple and easy to do. It is generally used prior to delivery when the patient has received systemic medication and paracervical blocks for labor. This nerve block can be approached by either the transvaginal or transperineal apprach (the former being most common). Both techniques are most easily performed with the patient in the dorsal

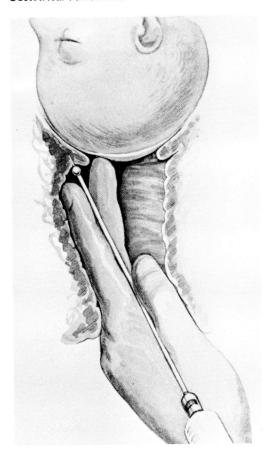

Figure 13. Technique of paracervical block. Gloved examining hand directs the needle guide to the lateral fornix. Care is taken not to inject into the uterine artery or fetal head. (From Bonica, 1969.)

lithotomy position. The pudendal nerve passes under the ischial spine and sacrospinous ligament on the lateral pelvic wall (Fig. 15).

When the transvaginal approach is used, the examining hand is inserted into the vagina and the location of the ischial spine is determined. A hollow needle guide is then directed to this area (Fig. 16). A needle with a syringe attached is introduced into the needle guide and into the vaginal mucosa (Fig. 17). A small skin wheal is created in the vaginal mucosa and injection is carried out at this point. The needle is then advanced 0.5-1 cm beyond the sacrospinous ligament. Aspiration is now performed and if negative then the local anesthetic (approximately 10 cc per side) is injected. The procedure is then performed on the opposite side.

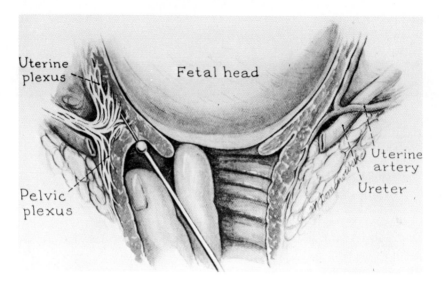

Figure 14. Technique of paracervical block. Enlarged view showing the cervix and upper portion of the vagina. Relationship of the needle to the uterine artery, ureter, and paracervical nerves is illustrated. (From Bonica, 1969.)

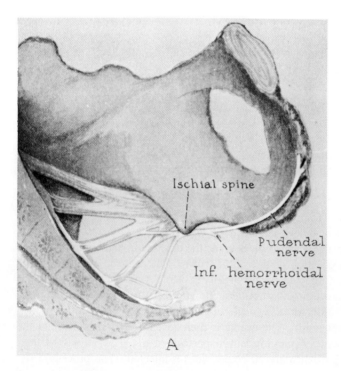

Figure 15. Origin and course of the pudendal nerve and its relationship to the bones of the pelvis. (From Bonica, 1969.)

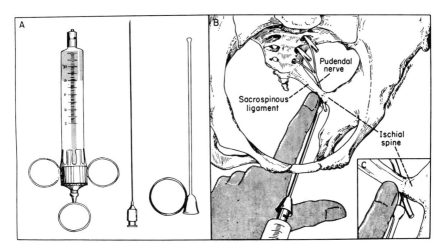

Figure 16. A. Equipment for pudendal nerve block: 10-cc syringe with finger grips, 6-in. 20-gauge needle, needle guide "Iowa trumpet." B. View showing index finger used to guide "Iowa trumpet" and needle to appropriate location. C. Enlarged view: relationship between spine, ligament, nerve, and needle. (From Bonica, 1969.)

When the transperineal approach is to be used the technique is modified to some extent. A small skin wheal is made approximately 2.5 cm posterior and medial to the ischial tuberosity. A long pudendal needle is now inserted and advanced slightly toward the ischiorectal fossa. The index finger of either the right or left hand is now introduced into the rectum to guide the needle to sacrospinous ligament (Fig. 18). As the needle approaches the ligament near the ischial spine the examining finger directs the tip of the needle posterior to the ligament and into the pudendal canal (Figs. 19 and 20). The patient may experience paresthesia at this time, if so then advancement of the needle should cease. Aspiration for blood is performed and if negative 10 cc of a local anesthetic solution is injected. It is best to inject 4-5 cc and then advance the needle forward 2-3 cm (if a paresthesia was not elicited). At this point an additional 4-5 cc of solution is injected. This is done in an attempt to block the inferior hemorrhoidal nerve which may arise as a separate trunk in some patients. The physician may now identify the ischial spine on the opposite side with the same examining finger and repeat the procedure. If the operator elects to change hands before repeating the procedure on the opposite side, a change of gloves is required to maintain sterility.

The procedure may also be performed with the examining finger located in the vagina as illustrated in Fig. 21.

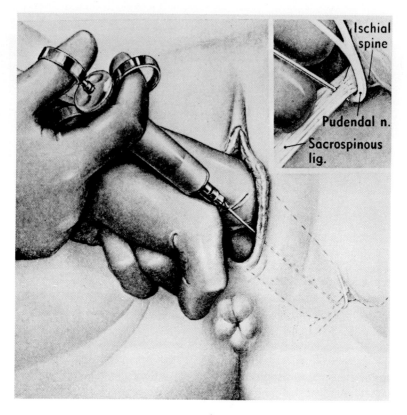

Figure 17. Technique of paracervical block, transvaginal approach.
Examining finger identifies the ischial spine laterally. Medial to the spine
is the bandlike sacrospinous ligament. Inset: enlargement of injection site.
Pudendal nerve passes posterior to the junction of the ischial spine and
sacrospinous ligament. The needle must pass through the ligament prior to
injection. (From Bonica, 1969.)

Conduction Anesthesia

The most frequently employed conduction techniques in obstetrics include
lumbar epidural, caudal, and subarachnoid blocks. Caudal anesthesia, once
the preferred technique in obstetrical units, has decreased in popularity for a
variety of reasons. This includes the large amounts of anesthetic agents required to achieve pain relief during the first stage of labor, and the loss of
pelvic sensation and motor tone essential to the successful expulsion of the
fetus during the second stage.

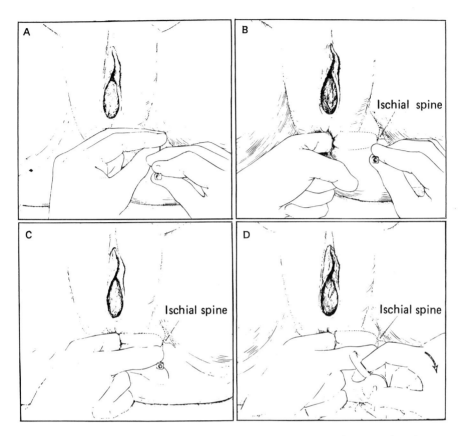

Figure 18. Technique of pudendal nerve block, transperineal approach. A. Introduction of needle through the skin. Shaft is protected by the left hand to prevent buckling. B. Index finger is inserted into rectum and used to guide needle to appropriate location. C. Technique of holding hub for attachment of syringe. D. Adaptation of syringe to hub. Arrow indicates clockwise rotation of syringe. (From Bonica, 1969.)

In major teaching universities lumbar epidural anesthesia has become the technique of choice (Hicks et al., 1976). It may be used alone or in combination with a caudal block as a segmental technique. Although the use of lumbar epidural anesthesia during labor is increasing in frequency, controversy continues to exist concerning its effect on the course of labor and the incidence of forceps deliveries. It is difficult to evaluate and compare the effects of epidural anesthesia on the course of labor because different local anesthetics and concentrations are used in each study. This situation is further

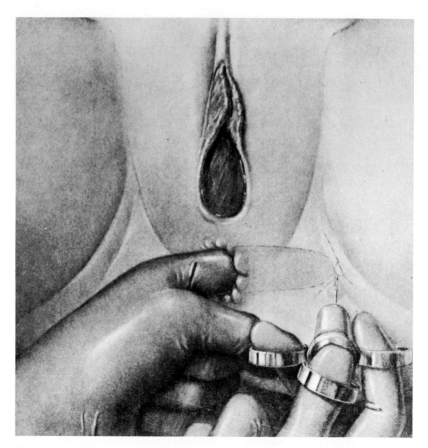

Figure 19. Enlarged view of pudendal nerve block, transperineal approach. Index finger locates spine and ligament and directs the needle. (From Bonica, 1969.)

clouded by use of vasoconstrictors such as epinephrine, which can interfere with uterine activity and alter the progress of labor (Gunther et al., 1969, 1972, Rosenfeld et al., 1974).

Lowenson et al., in 1974, reported on the effects of lumbar epidural anesthesia on uterine activity. Uterine activity was measured in two groups of patients. The control group contained patients who received no medication or anesthesia before the study period. The regional anesthesia group contained patients who received an epidural block with 1% Xylocaine and epinephrine. The authors demonstrated that in the control group, uterine activity increased

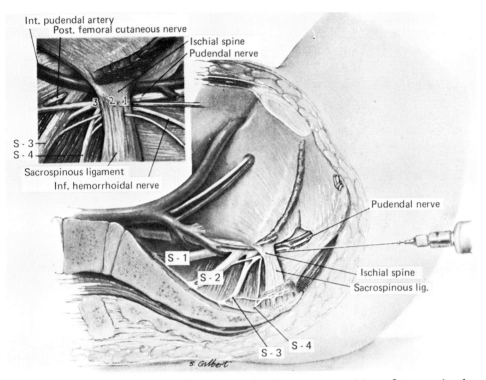

Figure 20. Sagittal section of perineum showing correct position of transperineal pudendal needle. Inset: area of ischial spine. Numbers indicate injection points. (From Bonica, 1969.)

progressively during the time period studied. In the regional anesthesia group however, uterine activity decreased for 10-30 min after institution of anesthesia. In all of these cases, uterine activity returned to preblock levels within 30 min. Whether or not the total course of labor was affected was not studied. Subsequently Phillips et al. (1977) reported on the use of 0.125% bupivacaine with epinephrine in 875 women in labor with term, vertex, singleton infant. The labor curves of three categories of patients were studied: spontaneous labor, augmented labor, and induced labor. These were then compared to each other as well as to those generated by Freidman and Hendricks in patients who had not received epidural anesthesia. They reported no statistically significant differences between the labor curves of the three groups studied. Nor were there any statistical differences noted between these curves and those reported by Freidman and Hendricks. Although uterine activity may be affected transiently by epidural anesthesia, the duration of labor does not seem to be affected.

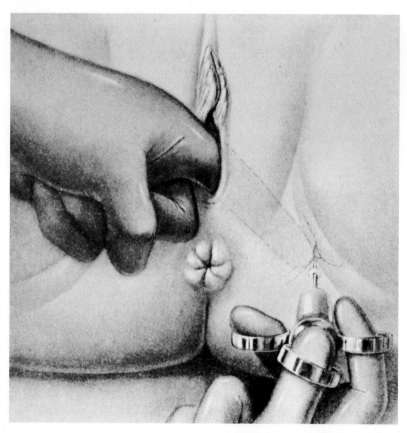

Figure 21. Technique for pudendal nerve block, transperineal approach. Examining finger in the vagina is used to direct the needle to its appropriate location. (From Bonica, 1969.)

The frequency of operative obstetrical procedures (forceps) can be greatly influenced by regional anesthetic techniques. As the concentration and volume of local anesthetic agent increases so does the relaxation of the levator muscles and loss of sensation in the rectal and perineal areas. This may result in a loss of the normal rotational mechanisms required for delivery as well as a loss of maternal expulsive efforts due to a lack of sensation. The use of appropriate local anesthetic concentrations and volumes, however, does not interfere with these mechanisms and does not increase the frequency of forceps. Philips et al. in their study (1977) reported an incidency of midforceps of 3% and an incidence of low forceps in approximately 14%.

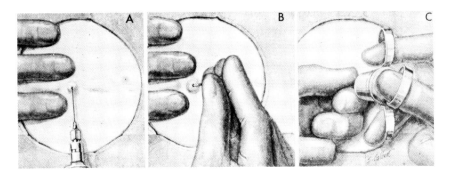

Figure 22. Technique of lumbar epidural, midline approach. A. Skin wheal
formed with local anesthetic and 25-gauge needle. B. Insertion of epidural
needle through the skin. C. Syringe attached to the needle hub. Dorsal aspect
of the left hand rests against the patient's back. Needle hub is grasped between
index finger and thumb. Right hand is used to exert pressure on the plunger
of syringe. (From Bonica, 1969.)

Although fetal deaths have not been reported in any study involving
epidural anesthesia, fetal bradycardia following the institution of the block
has been reported by several investigators (Brotanek et al., 1973; Maltare, 1975).
This occurs indirectly by an alteration of uterine blood flow due to a sympathetic
blockade and maternal hypotension rather than to any direct effect of the local
anesthetic agent on the fetus. Arterial hypotension is the most common complication of conduction anesthesia in pregnant patients. Mild to moderate decreases
in maternal blood pressure may not affect the mother, however, these changes
may result in fetal hypoxia and acidosis and subsequent fetal heart rate alterations. If maternal hypotension is prevented by preblock intravenous hydration,
left uterine displacement, and ephedrine, then fetal bradycardia does not occur.

Subarachnoid (spinal) anesthesia is not widely employed during labor because
of the rapid and profound motor and sensory block it occasions. Its duration is
also very short when compared with the time required for labor, making it an unacceptable form of anesthesia for labor. It is, however, an appropriate choice of
anesthesia when surgical intervention is anticipated. It can be performed
rapidly, simply, and easily with excellent results. Presently, two anesthetic
agents may be employed for subarachnoid anesthesia: 1% tetracaine (Pontocaine)
and 5% lidocaine (Xylocaine) in 7.5% dextrose. Tetracaine produces a block
of longer duration than Xylocaine, however, both result in excellent analgesia
and muscle relaxation. Until recently, it was thought that anesthetic agents
placed within the subarachnoid space resulted in very low blood levels. Giasi
et al. (1979) studied absorption of local anesthetics from the subarachnoid space

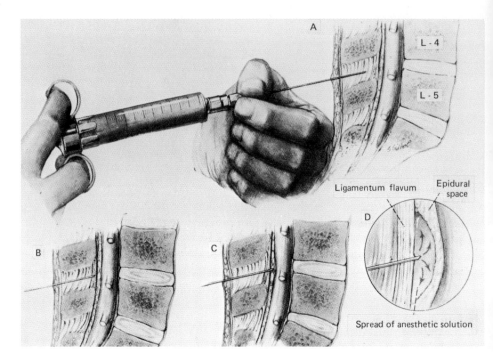

Figure 23. Technique of lumbar epidural, midline approach. A. Side view showing position of hands once needle point is properly located within the interspinous ligament. Injection of fluid will meet with increased resistance. B. Needle point in the ligamentum flavum. There is marked resistance and it is almost impossible to inject fluid. C. Entrance into the epidural space is indicated by sudden loss of resistance. D. Injected solution pushes dura away from needle point. (From Bonica, 1969.)

in a group of patients and compared the results obtained from patients receiving an epidural block with the same agents. The results showed that the peak plasma levels of Xylocaine from either technique were statistically insignificant. However, the rate of rise was greater following epidural injection than subarachnoid injection.

Lumbar Epidural
Lumbar epidural anesthesia can be performed with the patient in either the sitting or lateral position. In either situation, it is important to position the patient appropriately before starting the procedure. Adequate flexion of the spine is an important technical point because this simple maneuver increases the width of the interspace between the spinous processes and allows easier placement

of the epidural needle. Successful epidural anesthesia is also dependent on
accurate identification of the epidural space. A variety of techniques and
mechanical aids have been introduced in an effort to help identify this area.
The best technique however, involves a "loss of resistance" of either air or
fluid (normal saline).

Most lumbar epidural anesthetics are performed at either the L_2-L_3 or
L_3-L_4 interspace. Identification of the L_3-L_4 interspace is easily accomplished
by drawing an imaginary line connecting the posterior superior portion of the
iliac crest on each side of the pelvis. This line intersects the L_3-L_4 interspace.
Once the appropriate interspace is identified a sterile field is created using an
appropriate antiseptic solution. The epidural space may now be entered utilizing either the midline or paramedian approach.

When the midline approach is used a gloved finger is placed on the L_3-L_4
interspace. Local anesthesia is administered using a small 25-gauge needle
directed between the spinous processes (Fig. 22). An epidural needle is now
advanced through the skin. Once it has entered the skin, it is directed toward
the patient's umbilicus. This gives the approximate angle between the spinous
processes of L_3-L_4. The needle will meet some resistance as it passes through
the supraspinous and interspinous ligaments. When it enters the ligamentum
flava, however, a noticeable increase in resistance usually occurs. The stylet
is now removed and a 10-cc syringe filled with either air or normal saline is
attached. If the operator is right-handed, the back of the left hand is placed
on the patient's back and the hub of the needle is grasped between the index
finger and thumb. The syringe is then operated with the right hand and
constant pressure is placed on the plunger (Fig. 23). If the needle has been
appropriately placed in the ligamentum flava there will be considerable
resistance to the flow of fluid or air. If the plunger advances easily, then
the needle is advanced slightly until resistance to the flow of fluid occurs.
When the needle has been placed in the ligamentum flava, the needle is advanced *slowly* with constant pressure on the syringe and plunger. As soon as
the bevel of the needle enters the epidural space there is a "loss of resistance"
and free flow of air or saline occurs. The needle is advanced no further.
The syringe is removed and the hub is checked for a free return of fluid
(either blood or cerebral spinal fluid).

If a single "shot" epidural is to be performed, a test dose of 2-3 cc anesthetic
is given. If after 5 min no adverse reactions have occurred then the remainder
of the anesthetic solution is injected through the needle and the needle withdrawn. If a catheter is to be placed this is done before any anesthetic is injected. After the catheter has been appropriately placed the needle is removed
and the catheter inspected for blood or cerebral spinal fluid. This is performed
by holding the end of the catheter below the patient's back or by gentle aspiration with a syringe. If there is no return of fluid then a 2-3-cc test dose is

given. If after 5 min there have been no adverse reactions, the remainder of the anesthetic is injected through the catheter.

When the paramedian approach is used, the identification and preparation of the L_3-L_4 interspace is performed in the same manner. With this technique the middle finger of the left hand is placed in the L_3-L_4 interspace and the index finger of the same hand is placed in the L_4-L_5 interspace. This identifies the spinous process of L_4. Approximately 1 cm caudad and 1 cm lateral to the middle finger a skin wheal is created with a local anesthetic using a 25-gauge needle. The needle is advanced deep into and perpendicular to the skin. The lamina of the vertebras will now be encountered (approximately 2-4 cm below the skin). The periosteum is injected with a small amount of anesthetic agent to prevent any discomfort and the needle is withdrawn. The almina is an important landmark. The ligamentum flava attaches to the dorsal aspect of adjoining vertebral lamina, therefore, identification of the lamina indicates the approximate depth of the ligamentum flava. The epidural needle is now placed perpendicularly through the skin at the area of the skin wheal and is advanced until the lamina is encountered. The needle is now backed off the lamina slightly (approximately 1 cm), angled medially and cephadly, and advanced approximately 1 cm. If bone is encountered the needle is again backed off slightly and redirected. In this manner the needle can be made to "walk off" the lamina into the ligamentum flava (Fig. 24). When the ligament is appropriately identified the stylet is removed and a 10-cc syringe of either air or normal saline is attached. Identification of the epidural space is now accomplished in the manner previously described.

For obstetrical anesthesia, the epidural needle can be placed at any interspace from the second to the fifth lumbar verterbrae. In a small number of people (5-10%), however, the spinal cord ends at the level of the second lumbar vertebra. Attempts at this level should therefore be undertaken very cautiously since there is a danger of trauma to the spinal cord.

Subarachnoid (Spinal) Anesthesia

Subarachnoid anesthesia is accomplished by injecting a local anesthetic into the subarachnoid space. The landmarks, techniques, and approaches are identical to those described previously for lumbar epidural anesthesia. The end-point is the return of spinal fluid rather than the loss of resistance. The technique is therefore modified as shown in Figures 25-27 and outlined below.

The midline approach is performed by introducing a small (25-gauge) spinal needle through the skin between the appropriate spinous processes. The needle is advanced slowly through the ligament until a slight change in resistance is experienced. The stylet is then removed and the hub of the needle examined for the return of spinal fluid. If there is no return of fluid, the needle is rotated slowly through 360°. If, after this maneuver, there is

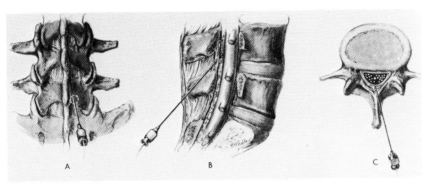

Figure 24. Technique of lumbar epidural, paramedian appraoch. A. Dorsal view: relationship of spinous process, lamina, site of puncture, and direction of epidural needle. B. Side view showing same relationships. Lamina and pedicles have been removed. C. Superior view: relationship of needle point to midsagittal plane and position of needle point in epidural space. (From Bonica, 1969.)

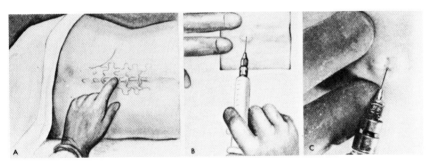

Figure 25. Technique of subarachnoid (spinal) puncture, midline approach. A. Appropriate interspace identified (see text). Note: an imaginary line connecting the two iliac crests intersects the L_3-L_4 interspace. B. Formation of skin wheal with local anesthesia and 25-gauge needle. C. Enlarged view: fingers straddle interspace in an effort to identify the appropriate area for injection and to immobilize the skin. (From Bonica, 1969.)

still no return of spinal fluid, the stylet is replaced and the needle is advanced 1-2 mm. The stylet is again removed and the hub of the needle examined for spinal fluid. This is repeated until spinal fluid is obtained, which indicates successful placement of the needle.

When the subarachnoid space has been accurately identified the syringe containing the anesthetic solution is attached to the hub of the needle. This

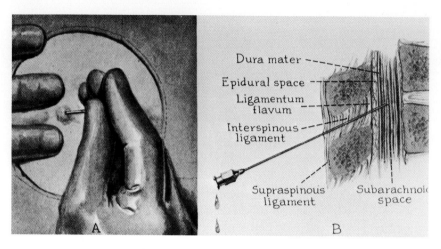

Figure 26. Technique of subarachnoid (spinal) puncture, midline approach. A. Introduction of spinal needle: needle is held like a dart. Index finger is held over the stylet to prevent displacement. The bevel of the needle should be facing laterally so that when it pierces the dura it will spread the longitudinal fibers in a wedgelike manner. B. Advancement of the needle through the ligamentum flavum produces marked resistance. As the needle enters the epidural space a loss of resistance is felt. The needle is now advanced 5-6 mm. Generally a distinctive "pop" is felt indicating penetration through the dura. The stylet is removed and the hub examined for spinal fluid. (From Bonica, 1969.)

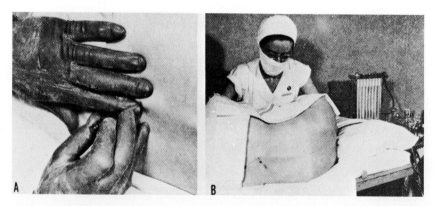

Figure 27. Technique of subarachnoid (spinal) puncture, midline approach. A. Approach with fingers of left hand straddling the midline and right hand introducing the spinal needle. B. Correct placement of spinal needle. Assistant holds patient gently in a "tuck" position. (From Bonica, 1969.)

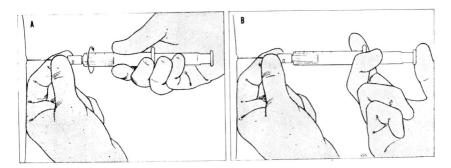

Figure 28. Technique of adapting syringe to the spinal needle. A. Dorsum of left hand rests against patient's back. Hub of needle is grasped between index finger and thumb, the syringe is gently adapted to the needle hub and rotated clockwise to assure good attachment. B. Technique of injection. Left hand continues to hold spinal needle while rotating against patient's back. This prevents inadvertant needle movement. (From Bonica, 1969.)

is best performed by placing the back of the left hand on the patient's back and grasping the hub of the needle with the index finger and thumb. The syringe is attached by gently touching it to the needle hub and rotating it clockwise with the right hand (Fig. 28). This prevents inadvertent advancement of the needle. A small amount of spinal fluid (0.1 cc) is now aspirated to ascertain proper needle placement before injection of local anesthetic. Injection is carried out slowly and, at the end, a second small aspiration is performed to be certain that the needle did not move during the injection period. The needle and syringe are then withdrawn.

CHOICE OF LOCAL ANESTHETIC AGENT

Selection of a regional anesthetic technique must be made intelligently if alterations to the maternal-fetal unit are to be minimal. Of equal importance is the local anesthetic agent itself. Table 2 lists the commonly employed agents and their physical characteristics. Criteria for utilization in the parturient includes safety first and foremost, for both mother and fetus. The agent must also provide adequate analgesia for the mother without interfering with her muscle tone or the expulsive forces required for the second stage of labor.

The local anesthetics include the two categories discussed previously: the ester and amide agents. The esters include procaine (Novocaine), 2-chloroprocaine (Nesacaine) and tetracaine (Pontocaine). These agents are rapidly metabolized by plasma pseudocholinesterase and fetal effects are therefore negligible. Procaine (Novocaine) is an excellent agent when used for local anesthesia, however, it has relatively poor permeability and diffusion qualities when used for epidural anesthesia. This frequently results in spotty and poor quality blockade (Lund et al., 1975). In addition it has a prolonged time of onset (latency) and a short duration of action which limits its usefulness. Chloroprocaine (Nescaine) is an excellent agent for use in obstetrical patients. It has a short latency period, good quality of sensory blockade, and short duration. The plasma half-life of this agent is extremely short due to the rapid rate of hydrolysis in both mother and fetus. Unfortunately it has recently been associated with prolonged and possibly permanent neurologic damage, thus limiting its popularity (Covino et al., 1980; Reisner et al., 1980). Tetracaine (pontocaine) is a popular agent for subarachnoid (spinal) anesthesia. It is extremely potent and long-acting resulting in excellent analgesia and relaxation in a short period of time. When used for epidural anesthetic procedures, it produces a profound motor block with a weak sensory blockade, which is undesirable in obstetrics. Its usefulness is therefore limited to subarachnoid techniques.

The amides include Xylocaine (lidocaine), mepivacaine (Carbocaine), bupivacaine (Marcaine), and etidocaine (Duranest). This group includes agents that are very potent and have an extremely long duration of action. These agents are metabolized by the liver and their half-life, compared with the esters, is extremely long (hours versus seconds). Xylocaine and mepivacaine are very similar in nature. Both agents have short latency periods and produce excellent anesthesia. They both exhibit a duration of action longer than chloroprocaine and shorter than bupivacaine. Unfortunately, the pK_as of these agents are relatively low. This results in a larger proportion of nonionized drug available for placental transfer in the range of physiologic pH. Clinically this produces a transient motor retardation in the infant. In addition, fetal metabolism of mepivacaine is extremely long and removal from the neonate may require partial exchange transfusions. The use of these agents in obstetrical patients has therefore decreased.

Bupivacaine (Marcaine) and etidocaine (Duranest) are relatively new local anesthetic agents. Each has a long duration of action. Here, however, the similarity ends. Bupivacaine produces excellent anesthesia with a greater sensory blockade than motor blockade with extremely low concentrations. The pK_a is quite high, and therefore, very little of this agent exists in the nonionized form at any given pH when compared with Xylocaine and mepivacaine. This agent is also highly bound to maternal proteins. These two characteristics result in decreased placental transfer and make it an ideal agent for use in obstetrics. Etidocaine also produces excellent anesthetic conditions; however, in contrast with bupivacaine, it produces a profound motor block that tends to outlast sensory analgesia (Moore et al., 1974, 1975). This characteristic limits its usefulness in obstetrics where good motor tone needs to be preserved. The pK_a of etidocaine is similar to that of Xylocaine, however, it is highly lipid-soluble and has a large volume of distribution within the mother. Therefore, transfer to the fetus is limited.

CONCLUSION

When properly administered, local anesthetics and regional anesthesia are safe for both mother and fetus. When narcotics and tranquilizers are avoided, the mother is awake, alert, and cooperative and can participate actively in the birthing process. Local anesthetic agents that are appropriately chosen will result in minimal fetal effects when the appropriate regional technique is utilized.

REFERENCES

Baskett, T. R., and Carson, R. M. (1974). Paracervical block with bupivacaine. *Can. Med. Assoc. J. 110*:1363.

Bonica, J. J. (1969). *Principles and Practice of Obstetric Analgesia and Anesthesia.* Davis, Philadelphia.

Bonica, J. J. (1975). Basic considerations. *Clin. Obstet. Gynecol. 2:* 469.

Bromage, P. R. (1978). Pharmacology. In *Epidural Analgesia.* P. R. Bromage (Ed.), Saunders, Philadelphia, London, Toronto, p. 77.

Bromage, P. (1979). Choice of local anesthetics in obstetrics. In *Anesthesia for Obstetrics.* S. M. Shnider and Levinson (Eds.), Williams & Wilkins, Baltimore/London, p. 109.

Bromage, P. R., and Robson, J. G. (1961). Concentrations of lignocaine in the blood after intravenous, intramuscular, epidural and endotracheal administration. *Anaesthesia 16*:461.

Brotanek, V., Vasicka, A., et al. (1973). The influence of epidural anesthesia on uterine blood flow. *Obstet. Gynecol. 42*:276.

Cibils, L. A. (1976). Response of human uterine arteries to local anesthetics. *Am. J. Obstet. Gynecol. 126*:202.

Cibils, L. A., and Santonja-Lucas, J. J. (1978). Clinical significance of fetal heart rate patterns during labor III. Effect of paracervical block anesthesia. *Am. J. Obstet. Gynecol. 130*:73.

Covino, B. (1980). Pharmacology of local anesthetics. ASA Annual Refresher Course Lecture #224.

Covino, B. G., Marx, G. R., Finster, M., et al. (1980). Prolonged sensory/motor deficits following inadvertant spinal anesthesia. *Anesth. Analg. 59*:399.

deJong, R. H. (1977). A centennial in local anesthetics. In *Local Anesthetics,* 2nd ed. Chas. C Thomas, Springfield, Illinois, p. 6.

Endler, G. (1980). Conduction anesthesia in obstetrics and its effects upon the fetus and newborn. *J. Reprod. Med. 24*:83.

Friedman, E. (1971). The functional divisions of labor. *Am. J. Obstet. Gynecol. 120*:274.

Giasi, R. M., D'Agostino, E., and Covino, B. (1979). Absorption of Lidocaine following subarachnoid and epidural administration. *Anesth. Analg. 58*:360.

Greiss, F. C., Stills, J. G., Anderson, S. G. (1976). Effects of local anesthetic agents on the uterine vasculatures and myometrium. *Am. J. Obstet. Gynecol. 124*:889.

Gunther, R. E., and Bauman, J. (1969). Obstetrical caudal anesthesia I. A randomized study comparing 1 percent lidocaine plus epinephrine. *Anesthesiology 37*:5.

Gunther, R. E. Belville, J. W. (1972). Obstetrical caudal anesthesia II. A randomized study comparing 1 percent Mepivacaine with 1 percent mepivacaine and epinephrine. *Anesthesiology 37*:288.

Hicks, J. S., Levinson, G., and Shnider, S. M. (1976). Obstetric training centers in the U.S.A., 1975. *Anesth. Analg. 55*:839.

Koller, C. (1941). History of cocaine as a local anesthetic. *JAMA 117*:1284.

Lowenson, R. I., Paul, R. H., Fales, S., Yeh, S., and Hon, E. H., (1974). Intrapartum epidural anesthesia: Evaluation of effects on uterine activity. *Obstet. Gynecol. 44*:388.

Lund, P. C., Bush, D. F., and Covino, B. G. (1975). Determinants of etidocaine concentration in the blood. *Anesthesiology 42*:497.

Lund, P. C. Wik, J. C., and Gannon, R. T. (1975). Extradural anaesthesia: Choice of local anesthetic agents. *Br. J. Anaesth. 47*:313.

Maltare, J. M. (1975). The frequency of fetal bradycardia during selective epidural anaesthesia. *Acta Obstet. Gynecol. Scand. 54*:357.

Mirkin, B. L. (1975). Perinatal pharmacology. Placental transfer, fetal localization and neonatal disposition of drugs. *Anesthesiology 43*:156.

Moore, D. C., Bridenbaugh, B., et al. (1979). A double blind study of bupivacaine and etidocaine for epidural (peridural) block. *Anesth. Analg. 53*:690.

Moore, D. C., Bridenbaugh, P., et al. (1975). Bupivacaine compared with etidocaine for vaginal delivery. *Anesth. Analg. 54*:250.

Nyirjersy, I., Hawks, B. L., Hebert, J. E., et al. (1963). Hazards of the use of paracervical block anesthesia in obstetrics. *Am. J. Obstet. Gynecol. 87*:235.

Pedersen, H., Morishima, H. O., and Mieczyslaw, F. (1978). Uptake and effects of local anesthetics in mother and fetus. *Int. Anesthesiol. Clin. 16*:(4)73.

Pederson, H., and Finsler, M. (1977). Pharmacodynamics of analgesies and anesthesia. *Drug Therapy,* April:44-52.

Petrie, R., Paul, W. L., Miller, F. C. et al. (1974). Placental transfer of lidocaine following paracervical block. *Am. J. Obstet. Gynecol. 120*:791.

Phillips, J. C., Hochberg, C. J., Petakis, J. K., and Van Winkle, J. (1977). Epidural analgesia and its effects on "normal" progress of labor. *Am. J. Obstet. Gynecol. 129*:316.

Ralston, D. H., and Shnider, S. M. (1978). The fetal and neonatal effects of regional anesthesia in obstetrics. *Anesthesiology 48*:34.

Reisner, L. S., Hochman, B. N., and Plumer, M. H. (1980). Persistent neurologic deficit and adhesive arachnoiditis following intrathecal 2-chloroprocaine injection. *Anesth. Analg. 59*:452.

Rosefoky, J. B., and Petersiel, M. E. (1968). Perinatal deaths associated with mepivacaine-paracervical block anesthesia in labor. *N. Engl. J. Med. 278*:530.

Rosenfeld, C. M., Barton, D., and Meschia, G. (1974). Effects of epinephrine on distribution of blood flow in the pregnant ewe. *Am. J. Obstet. Gynecol. 124*:156.

Shnider, S. M., and Gildea, J. (1963). Paracervical block anesthesia in obstetrics. III. Choice of drug: Fetal bradycardia following administration of lidocaine, mepivacaine and prolicaine. *Am. J. Obstet. Gynecol. 87*:235.

Shnider, S. M., Asling, J. H., Holl, J. W., et al. (1970). Paracervical block anesthesia in obstetrics I. Fetal complications and neonatal morbidity. *Am. J. Obstet. Gynecol. 107*:619.

Shnider, S. M., Levinson, G., Ralston, D. (1979). Regional anesthesia for obstetrics. In *Anesthesia for Obstetrics.* S. M. Shnider and Levinson (Eds.), Williams & Wilkins, Baltimore/London, p. 93.

Singer, S. J., and Nicholson, G. L. (1972). The fluid mosaic model of the structure of cell membrane. *Science 175*:720.

Terrano, K., and Widholm, O. (1967). Studies of the effects of anaesthetics on fetus. Part I. The effect of paracervical block with mepivacaine upon fetal acid-base values. *Acta Obstet. Gynecol. Scand. [Suppl.] 46*: 339.

17

Episiotomy and Perineal Repair

DAVID R. MILLAR / Jessop Hospital for Women, Sheffield, England

The art of obstetrics is a balance between expert observation of the normal process and the timely use of medical or surgical aid in the interests of either mother or baby. This balance is well-illustrated by the use of episiotomy at delivery. Errors can occur by being too passive or too active. At one extreme, in an attempt to achieve an intact perineum, the baby's head may be left distending the introitus until the mother is exhausted and the child hypoxic, or the baby may be born at the expense of an uncontrolled perineal tear. On the other hand, an early or overenthusiastic episiotomy may lead to unnecessary hemorrhage and pain for the mother.

DEFINITION

An episiotomy is an incision of the vulva, usually into the fourchette and perineal body, to aid delivery.

DERIVATION

Episiotomy is derived from the Greek words *Episeion* (external genitalia) and *temnein* (to cut).

INDICATIONS

1. To make delivery easier for a mother who cannot or should not bear down
2. To accelerate a slow second stage of labor if the delay is due to tight soft parts
3. To prevent maternal soft-tissue damage from tearing
4. To make delivery easier for a compromised baby

Maternal

Medical Condition of the Mother
When the mother has a condition as a result of which bearing down is unwise or impossible, an episiotomy is usually a planned procedure. This is most commonly the case when she has cardiorespiratory disease which is already causing dyspnea before or during labor. The effort of bearing down can increase maternal hypoxia and cardiac output to a dangerous degree so an assisted delivery, using an episiotomy, and often an epidural anesthetic, is the rule.

The Valsalva maneuver is also potentially dangerous in such diverse medical conditions as cerebral angioma and prolapsed intervertebral disc.

A mother with paralysis or weakness of the voluntary abdominal and pelvic muscles, due to paraplegia or other neurological or muscular disease, will often require an episiotomy because of her inability to bear down.

Relief of Soft-Tissue Obstruction
This is the most likely cause of delay in the second stage of labor in primigravidae. It is more common when the baby is large or when the larger diameters of the head present, as in the occipitoposterior position and facial presentation. It may be a limiting factor preventing delivery when the mother is tired or when the scar of an earlier perineal repair is rigid. The tissues are less elastic in older women.

In addition, when the bony outlet is reduced by a narrow subpubic arch, an episiotomy will allow the baby to pass more easily through the posterior part of the pelvis.

Prevention of Soft-Tissue Damage
Tearing of the introitus can usually be predicted as the presenting part distends the perineum at the height of an expulsive contraction, but any fresh bleeding during the second stage may be from a vaginal tear and is also an indication for an episiotomy. When a vaginal delivery is permitted in a mother who has a history of pelvic floor repair for prolapse, or of surgery to correct urinary incontinence due to bladder-neck weakness, or a fistula, it is wise to perform an elective episiotomy. However, many such cases are best delivered abdominally. Vaginal delivery following previous cesarean section may also be aided by

episiotomy, and it is usual to perform one prior to all assisted deliveries. However, whereas it is mandatory when using forceps, episiotomy may not be so essential with ventouse extractions (Chalmers, 1971).

Fetal

Potential Hypoxia
An episiotomy will reduce birth trauma and hypoxia for any baby already at particular risk from these hazards. Those presenting by the breech or experiencing preterm delivery or suffering from growth retardation are in this category. It is an old maxim in obstetrics that the smaller the baby, the bigger the episiotomy.

Fetal Distress
Episiotomy is preferable whenever vaginal delivery is possible in such cases, but particularly when the fetal heart rate shows decelerations that persist after contractions. Small decelerations synchronous with contractions are sometimes ignored, and even regarded as physiological and due to head compression, but any episode of bradycardia leads to hypoxia, poor tissue perfusion, and acidosis, and rapidly recurring episodes of bradycardia have a cumulative effect (Tipton and Finch, 1972).

INCIDENCE

In some modern obstetric units the births of almost all first babies are aided by episiotomy and the incidence is increasing (Alberman, 1977). The active management of labor may lead to a chain reaction of intervention ending in assisted delivery. However, the increased use of epidural or caudal analgesia does not necessarily result in the need for episiotomy and forceps delivery. An anxious mother, particularly if she has had a previous delivery, may be more likely to deliver *without* perineal trauma if her pelvic floor (and her mind) are relaxed by good pain relief.

ANALGESIA

Cutting the perineal skin without analgesia, as the presenting part distends it almost to the point of tearing at the height of a contraction, should have no place in modern obstetrics. There should always be a 20-ml syringe full of local anesthetic (e.g., 0.5% lidocaine [lignocaine, B.P.]) on the delivery trolley. The fourchette should be widely infiltrated as far as the anal sphincter in any case where episiotomy is anticipated. The only exception should be those cases where spinal, epidural, caudal, pudendal, or general anesthesia is already provided.

PROCEDURE

During the second stage of labor the rigidity and elasticity of the perineum is assessed digitally. When there is good analgesia the whole hand may be inserted along the posterior vaginal wall, and a gentle massage of the soft tissues may reduce the need for, or the size of, the subsequent cut. This maneuver also helps to disperse the analgesic agent. In spontaneous delivery the cut is made as the presenting part distends the tissues and when it is anticipated that delivery will be possible with the next contraction (Fig. 1).

In breech presentations, the timing is more critical and delivery may take rather longer, but the episiotomy should not be made until the trunk can be delivered to the level of the umbilicus immediately after the incision.

In forceps delivery, especially for the application of Kielland's blades, it may be preferable to make an episiotomy as the first step in the procedure. The length of the incision will depend on the size of the baby, and other factors, but a median cut should stop when the fibers of the superficial and sphincter are seen. It is important to ensure that the incision in the vaginal skin is adequate, otherwise, despite an apparently generous external cut, vaginal lacerations will still occur.

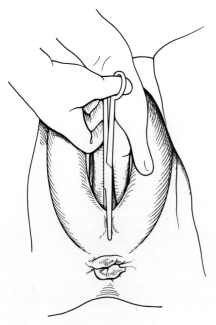

Figure 1. Midline incision.

As the presenting part is born, it may become apparent that the episiotomy is too small. An extension with scissors is preferable to uncontrolled extension by tearing.

Median or Mediolateral Incision?

An episiotomy should always start at the midpoint of the fourchette. A lateral incision gives poor exposure and is very awkward to suture. It is not recommended.

An incision in the median perineal raphe has many advantages. Firstly, because blood vessels and nerves supply the area from each pelvic side wall, the midline cut is less vascular, and less painful as it heals. Secondly, the muscles retract symmetrically and are easier to suture correctly, allowing both better healing and earlier resumption of coitus, with less dyspareunia (Beischer, 1967; Coats et al., 1960). Finally, the midline incision gives the maximum increase in pelvic space for a given length of cut. These advantages have been best expressed in the American literature (Eastman, 1948, Harris, 1970).

A mediolateral incision is generally favored in the United Kingdom and this method was advocated in 1967 when the Central Midwives Board recommended that their members carry out episiotomy (Burnett, 1967).

Midwives and less experienced doctors fear an extension of a median episiotomy into the anal sphincter causing a third- or fourth-degree tear. Such damage should not occur with skillful delivery and minor injury to the sphincter is amenable to simple repair resulting in no serious complications (O'Leary and O'Leary, 1965). Although the rectum may be involved after about 5% of midline episiotomies, the overall occurrence of rectovaginal fistula is only around 0.1% (Benyon, 1974). However, because of the risk of anal involvement, a mediolateral cut into the ischiorectal pad of fat is regarded as a reasonable compromise, especially for more difficult deliveries. The incision may be made at 5 or 7 o'clock directed towards a point no more than 2-3 cm lateral to the anus, or else a J-shaped cut may be made starting in the midline and, if necessary, then deviating to either side of the anus (Flew, 1944; Donald, 1979). Right-handed surgeons usually find a right-sided episiotomy easier.

Hemostasis

Although the episiotomy is made into vascular perineal tissues, the blood loss before delivery should be slight if the timing is correct because the descending presenting part acts as a hemostat. However, local pressure on the wound may be necessary between contractions, and sometimes brisk bleeding requires the application of a small pair of artery forceps. Varicosities in the perineum may sometimes cause anxiety but, in practice, if the incision avoids major varices, the bleeding can be controlled temporarily by pressure.

As soon as the baby is born a large sterile swab or pad is placed on the perineal wound and pressure applied with the hand, or the mother's legs are allowed to come together, until the placenta is delivered.

Bleeding from an episiotomy during and after the third stage of labor is the commonest cause of postpartum hemorrhage in modern obstetric practice. One of the advantages of the active management of the third stage is that the time between delivery and perineal repair is reduced.

It is never wise to embark on the repair before the placenta is delivered because, if its manual removal becomes necessary, the sutures will be disrupted. However, as soon as the third stage is complete sutures should be inserted in the episiotomy as soon as possible. If the birth attendant has no assistance, resuscitation of the newborn will take priority over delivery of the placenta and repair of the episiotomy, but in well-staffed maternity units pediatric care is not usually the responsibility of the obstetrician or midwife.

REPAIR

If this is done immediately, as suggested above, the analgesia used for making the episiotomy should remain adequate, but, if not, an additional infiltration of local anesthetic is required. A good operating light, shining into the wound over the surgeon's shoulder, is essential.

The first step is to palpate and inspect the vaginal walls to ensure that the incision has not extended and to exclude other vaginal lacerations. These are often easier to feel than to see. Small cervical tears are commonplace, but they seldom bleed significantly and rarely require sutures. Two pairs of sponge-holders attached to the anterior and posterior lips of the cervix allow it to be brought into view. If traumatic bleeding from the cervix is apparent, a more extensive tear up into the lower uterine segment should be suspected, and exploration and repair by the most senior surgeon available is recommended.

Fine sutures of 0 or 00 catgut or polyglycolic acid are used. Catgut is less inclined to cut through the tissues, but leads to more tissue reaction and discharge. Polyglycolic acid takes much longer to be absorbed, but this may prevent the breakdown of slowly healing wounds. It also gives a very clean surgical result when the wound is inspected several days later.

It is essential to use a needle stout enough not to break since it can be extremely difficult to trace the broken tip of a needle in the perineum. Most atraumatic sutures have needles which are unsuitable, especially for the beginner.

Before embarking on the repair it is usual to insert a small gauze pack, with a tape attached, high in the vagina to prevent the flow of blood from the uterus from obscuring the field (Fig. 2).

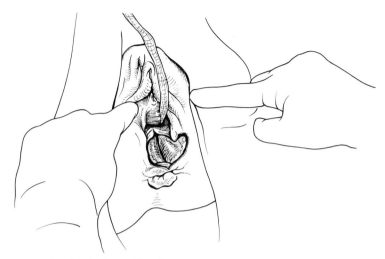

Figure 2. Swab inserted and exposure.

The first suture must be placed at the apex of the incision in the posterior vaginal wall (Fig. 3). The short end is cut, and a continuous running stitch is taken down the vagina as far as the hymenal remnants (carunculae myrtiformes) which are used as a guide to symmetry. It is important not to take this suture as far as the skin of the fourchette (Fig. 4) because as the last bite of tissue will tend to cause a bridge of skin at the introitus which may cause dyspareunia. A useful variation is to finish this vaginal skin suture in the subcuticular tissues of the fourchette, thus burying the knot.

The next step is to close the deepest part of the wound, bringing together the superficial perineal muscles with a series of interrupted sutures. These stitches are inserted parallel to the vagina and it is useful to place a finger along the posterior vaginal wall to help to keep the needle in the correct plane (Fig. 5). If this is done the rectum is unlikely to be included, but the sutures must pass deep enough to close the dead space. If the superficial anal sphincter is torn it should be repaired; remember that the ends of the muscle may have retracted. The repair of more extensive lacerations involving the anal canal is dealt with in Chapter 18.

Finally, the skin is closed by a series of interrupted subcuticular sutures (Fig. 6). With this technique no sutures have to be removed and the absence of skin sutures in the perineum increases the comfort of the patient. If skin stitches are preferred, nonabsorbable sutures are recommended. Less experienced surgeons pay particular attention to the skin closure, but the better the approximation of the skin edges seems to be at this stage, the

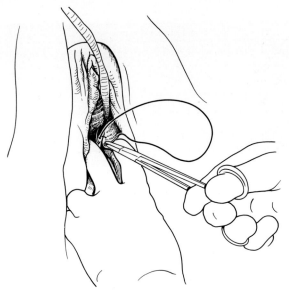

Figure 3. Continuous suture of posterior vaginal wall.

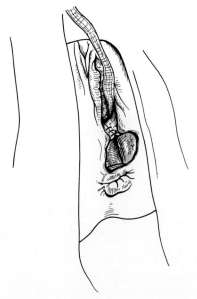

Figure 4. Completion of continuous suture at hymenal ring.

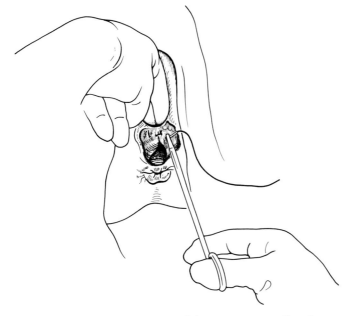

Figure 5. Interrupted sutures of deep structures of perineum.

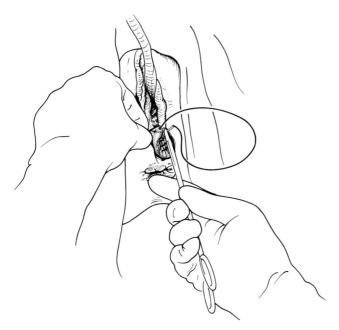

Figure 6. Final layer of subcuticular sutures.

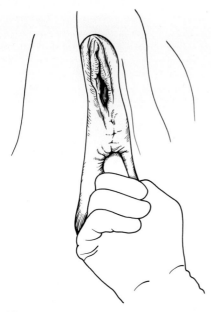

Figure 7. Insertion of finger into rectum at completion to check suturing.

more uncomfortable the patient will be the next day. There is always some edema after the repair and if skin sutures are used at all they should be tied quite loosely. Moir has described a method of repair involving one continuous suture throughout (Myerscough, 1977).

At the end of the repair the swab is removed from the vagina, any blood is expelled from the uterus by gentle suprapubic pressure, hemostasis is checked, and a finger is inserted in the rectum to ensure that no stitch has penetrated the mucosa (Fig. 7). A sterile pad is placed on the perineum.

AFTERCARE

When epidural analgesia has been used the patient may remain free from pain for several hours, but after more extensive repairs a "top-up" may be given before removing the epidural catheter. This will allow the mother a longer period of undisturbed rest. Later, oral analgesics are often required for 1 or 2 days, but acetaminophen (paracetamol B.P.) tablets are usually adequate. Further relief may be obtained by sitting in a hot bath, applying ice packs to the perineum, or sitting on a rubber ring.

The first bowel movement after delivery may be quite painful unless it is soft. A stool demulcent by mouth or a lubricant suppository will help.

The wound is inspected daily for bruising and healing. Sepsis is surprisingly rare if there is no hematoma. If skin sutures have been used they are removed in 5 days. Coitus should be discouraged for about a month.

COMPLICATIONS

Hematoma and Hemorrhage

This is the commonest problem within a few hours of delivery and usually arises from one of three errors of technique (1) failure to reach the apex of the vaginal cut, (2) failure to close the dead space between the vagina and rectum, or (3) failure to suture other vaginal lacerations.

Extravasation should always be suspected when the patient has unusual pain, or when there is clinical evidence of hypovolemic shock without external bleeding. When superficial bruising is seen a gentle digital examination is essential to exclude a large paravaginal hematoma. Any hematoma causing symptoms is best evacuated early. The bleeding point should be sought and ligated and a small drain left in the resutured cavity.

Failure to reoperate leads to a chronically swollen, painful, and sometimes infected, perineum from which the organized blood clot cannot be removed. It is fruitless to try to drain a hematoma which has been neglected for more than 2 days. These cases require a long convalescence. Emergency transfusion or subsequent iron therapy for anemia may be required.

A special watch is kept for bleeding when there has been a coagulation problem during delivery, or when anticoagulants have been prescribed.

Retention of Urine

Perineal pain may cause reflex spasm of the external voluntary urethral sphincter muscle and catheterization may be required.

If epidural analgesia is prolonged, the lack of bladder sensation may also result in urinary retention, in this case due to atony.

Breakdown of the Wound

This is uncommon if the suturing technique is correct and is usually due to infection of smaller hematomas. The slough on the wound edges may take several days to clear with the help of baths and antiseptic dressings. Small areas of dehiscence may be left to granulate, but when the wound is clean more major defects are best closed by secondary suture.

Rectovaginal Fistula

This is a very rare complication even after third-degree tears. Elective surgical repair of a persistent fistula is usually left for at least 3 months until infection has subsided and because some may close spontaneously.

POSTNATAL EXAMINATION

When the patient is seen 6 weeks after her delivery the episiotomy has usually healed soundly, but if a history of dyspareunia is noted, a particular check must be made for fibrous scarring in the vagina, or a tight skin bridge at the introitus. Occasionally scar tissue needs excision or the fourchette may require simple excision and resuturing transversely. More often, dyspareunia at this time is due to atrophic changes in the vaginal epithelium which accompany the ovarian suppression of lactation. The tender vagina recovers spontaneously when menstruation returns.

ACKNOWLEDGMENT

The author is grateful for help with the line drawings in this chapter from Mr. P. M. Elliott of the Department of Medical Illustration, Royal Hallamshire Hospital, Sheffield, England.

REFERENCES

Alberman, E. (1977). Facts and figures. In *Benefits and Hazards of the New Obstetrics*. T. Chard and M. Richards (Eds.), Heinemann, London, p. 15.

Beischer, N. A. (1967). The anatomical and functional results of mediolateral episiotomy. *Med. J. Aust. 2*:189-195.

Benyon, C. L. (1974). Midline episiotomy as a routine procedure. *J. Obstet. Gynaecol. Br. Commonw. 81*:126-130.

Burnett, C. W. F. (1967). *Midwives Chron. Nursing Notes 80*:388.

Chalmers, J. A. (1971). The effects of vacuum extraction upon the mother. In *The Ventouse: The Obstetric Vacuum Extractor*. Lloyd-Luke, Ondon, p. 70.

Coats, P. M., Chan, K. K., Wilkins, M., and Beard, R. J. (1980). A comparison between midline and mediolateral episiotomies. *Br. J. Obstet. Gynaecol. 87*: 408-412.

Donald, I. (1979). Maternal injuries. In *Practical Obstetric Problems*, 5th Ed. Lloyd-Luke, London, pp. 817-820.

Eastman, N. J. (1948). Editorial. *Obstet. Gynecol. Surv. 3*:828.

Flew, J. D. S. (1944). Episiotomy. *Br. Med. J. 2*:620.

Harris, R. E. (1970). An evaluation of the median episiotomy. *Am. J. Obstet. Gynecol. 106*:660-665.

Myerscough, P. R. (1977). Injuries to mother. In *Munro Kerr's Operative Obstetrics*, 9th Ed. Balliere-Tindall, London, pp. 794-798.

O'Leary, J. L., and O'Leary, J. A. (1965). The complete episiotomy. *Obstet. Gynecol. 25*:235-240.

Tipton, R., and Finch, A. K. (1972). The measurement and significance of transient fetal bradycardia during labour. *J. Obstet. Gynaecol. Br. Commonw. 79*:133.

18

Repair of Lacerations and Incisions of the Perineum

ZEPH J. R. HOLLENBECK / The Ohio State University College of Medicine, Columbus, Ohio

The true incidence of obstetric laceration of the rectal sphincter, anal canal, and lower rectum varies greatly from institution to institution (3-7%). It is dependent on the skill of the obstetrician and undoubtedly on the prevalence of the use of median rather than the mediolateral episiotomy. Complete laceration of the perineum does occur with the mediolateral episiotomy, however, and is much more difficult to repair than when it complicates the median incision. Third- and fourth-degree lacerations of the perineum comprise a very common maternal complication of vaginal delivery.

The term third-degree laceration has come, in recent years, to be identified with laceration of the rectal sphincter only, while the term fourth-degree laceration is used to indicate a tear involving the rectal sphincter, anal canal, and lower rectum. Laceration of the rectum also occurs without disruption of the sphincter muscle. On occasion the rectal wall may be forced to evaginate into the birth canal by the advancing fetal parts and may then be accidentally cut while making the episiotomy incision. It is very important to recognize and repair this type of "buttonhole" incision. If it is not recognized fecal material may be forced through this wound and the resulting abscess will usually cause a breakdown of the episiotomy repair or an episiotomy wound abscess that requires incision and drainage. A rectovaginal fistula may result. This troublesome complication probably occurs more often than is realized and may be thought to be caused by a suture being placed too deeply and through the rectal mucosa during the episiotomy repair whereas a small buttonhole incision or laceration of the rectum has gone unrecognized.

REPAIR OF THE COMPLETE PERINEAL LACERATION

After the delivery of the placenta the birth canal must be inspected. Lacerations of the vaginal wall, cervix, and lower uterine segment, and actual rupture of the corpus uteri demand immediate attention. Any or all may occur during the simplest of deliveries. Early and definitive management is necessary.

With the above problems, if any, under proper control, attention is directed to the repair of the rectum. Successful repair depends on adherence to two major principles of surgical technique. First, the sutures must not penetrate the rectal mucosa but must appose this layer by bringing together the rectal submucosa. Second, there must be no excessive tension on this line, only enough to appose the submucosal layers and no more.

Number 4-0 absorbable suture material (chromic gut or synthetic polyglactin type), with or without swedged-on needles, is used for this entire repair. The first suture is placed in the fascia just above the apex of the rectal laceration and tied (Fig. 1). A continuous suture is more desirable. In running the suture the needle should enter the rectal submucosa 3 mm from the edge of the laceration and, traveling in a horizontal plane, should emerge through the severed layer

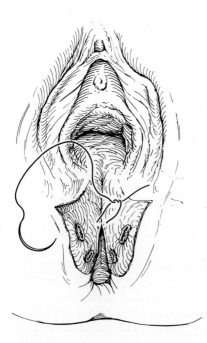

Figure 1. The first suture in the repair of a complete laceration of the perineum should be placed above the apex of the rectal defect.

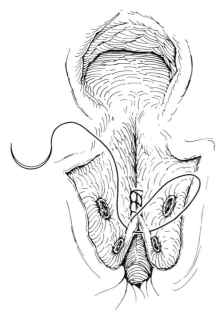

Figure 2. The running suture is placed so the rectal submucosa is brought together without tension.

of the submucosa. It then enters the submucosa of the opposite side and emerges
about 3 mm from the edge of the disrupted submucosa (Fig. 2). The stitches are
placed approximately 5 mm apart and the suture is run until it includes the subcuticulum of the skin of the anal canal posterior to the sphincter and is tied there.
As the suture line passes the sphincter muscle it includes the posterior portion of
this muscle and the posterior and inferior fascial support of the sphincter which
lies almost directly against the rectal submucosa (Fig. 3). It must be emphasized
again that only enough tension is placed on this line to bring the tissues into
approximation and no more.

A second layer of continuous suture, using 4-0, is begun in the fascia propria
of the rectum. The initial stitch is placed 4 or 5 mm above the first loop of the
submucosal closure. This is continued down to the sphincter, with the same
amount of tissue (3 mm) again included on either side and the sutures placed
the same distance apart (5 mm). When the sphincter is reached the line is
brought anteriorly to include a small bit of the perineal fascia, then through
the anterior portion of the tubular fascial support of the sphincter, coming to
the midline through a portion of the sphincter muscle itself (Fig. 4). The needle
then enters the sphincter muscle on the opposite side and again includes the

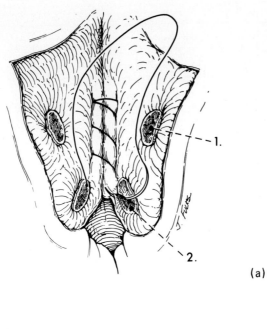

(a)

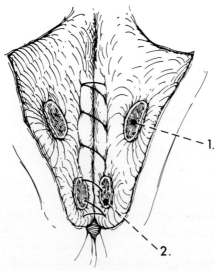

(b)

Figure 3. (a) The suture needle should enter the muscle substance of the anal sphincter (2) and emerge through the anal subepithelial layer. (b) The completed suturing of the rectal defect including the deep portion of the fascial support of the anal sphincter (2).

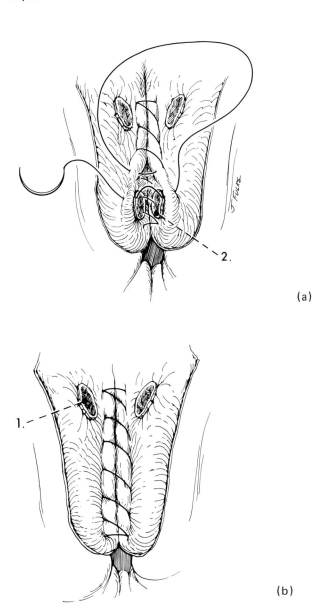

(a)

(b)

Figure 4. (a) The second or facial support layer of the rectal defect closure involves the more superficial support of the anal sphincter (2) and thus brings into apposition the cut or lacerated ends of this muscle. (b) The completed repair of the rectum, anal sphincter and the anal canal. This repair does not usually incorporate the posterior or deep fascial support of the transverse perineal muscle (1), although it may in a patient with a thin perineal body.

anterior tubular fascial sphincter support and a small bit of the perineal fascia. As the suture line continues toward the perineal skin, one or two more stitches include the sphincter and its support as just described. The suture line ends in the subcuticulum of the perineal skin. As this suture line closes the fascia propria of the rectum is usually approaches the posterior aspect of the tubular fascial support of the transverse perineal muscle. This layer and the muscle itself may be incorporated in this continuous suture line. In some patients the perineal body is much heavier than average and the transverse perineal muscle may lie too superficial to be included in the second (fascial) layer of closure of the rectum.

As the suture line approaches the lower end of the wound, bear in mind that it is not necessary to attempt to bring the ends of the sphincter together with separate sutures. Complete approximation is impossible unless the fascial support of this muscle is included in the sture. By following the steps just outlined, the fascia completely surrounding the sphincter has been apposed. This brings the ends of the disrupted sphincter together.

A word of caution must be given here. After the repair of the rectum or the subsequent repair of the episiotomy there seems to be a great desire by some operators to "test" the suture line by doing a digital rectal examination. This should *never* be done. Even in what appears grossly to be a clean field, it is possible to force a small bit of fecal material through the suture line into the submucosal space. This can easily result in a grossly infected perineum with resultant abscess and possible fistula formation.

REPAIR OF THE THIRD-DEGREE LACERATION

Disruption or laceration of the rectal sphincter without laceration of the rectum is not common but can occur. There is usually some separation of the anal canal for a short distance, however. If this is the case, the repair is the same as has been described for the "fourth-degree" laceration. Again, using two layers of continuous fine (4-0) absorbable suture, the subcuticulum of the anal canal and the beginning of perineal skin are brought together, the first layer also catching the posterior portion of the tubular sphincter fascia and a portion of the muscle itself. The second layer is begun in the fascia of the perineum above the torn sphincter and, as it is run toward the perineal skin, it incorporates the anterior and the more superficial portions of the tubular fascial support of the sphincter and finally ends bringing together the subcuticulum of the skin of the perineum.

REPAIR OF RECTAL LACERATION WITHOUT DISRUPTION OF THE ANAL SPHINCTER

If an incidental laceration of the rectal mucosa is found, it is repaired in the same manner as the rectum as described in Repair of the Complete Perineal Laceration, with one possible exception. These so-called "buttonhole" openings in the rectal wall are seen more frequently in the lower portion of the rectum and this places the inferior pole of the laceration behind or deep to the intact sphincter. If the repair is begun from the upper pole of the laceration as this suture line approaches the lower end of the traumatic opening, it becomes technically more and more difficult to place the sutures properly. It is better, therefore, to begin the repair at the lower end of the rectal tear and suture it upward. The sphincter can easily be retracted downward with a small curved retractor, such as a vein retractor, to give good exposure (Fig. 5).

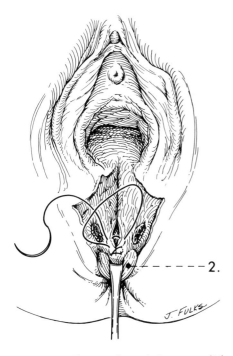

Figure 5. The rectal repair is accomplished in two layers using continuous suture, but beginning below the inferior end of the rectal defect and running the suture anteriorly. Frequently this part of the defect can be better visualized if the intact sphincter (2) is retracted downward with a small retractor.

Two layers of continuous fine (4-0) absorbable suture material are placed as described previously.

No special orders are necessary for patients who have had these rectal mucosa or sphincter reconstructions. Enemas may be used after 48 hr. It is important that constipation, and especially fecal impaction, does not occur. There is no more discomfort experienced by the patient following third- or fourth-degree laceration repair than that following episiotomy repair. Warm sitz baths may be used if desirable. Antibiotics are not routinely prescribed for the patient unless otherwise indicated.

MEDIAN EPISIOTOMY: PRO AND CON

Historically, an episiotomy, as performed in early obstetrics, meant a cutting of the vulva. These were lateral or bilateral incisions through the midvulvar tissues and are now obsolete. In modern usage the word episiotomy means a surgical incision of the perineum (perineotomy). There are two types: median and mediolateral.

The benefits of episiotomy are well-recognized and this surgical incision is used in most obstetric centers. Some controversy still exists as to the choice of the median or mediolateral operation. There are several advantages to the median episiotomy. The incision does not cross the belly of the levator ani muscle and there is much less bleeding, consequently there is better healing with less scar. The lateral pull of the separated muscles is even and equal. Repair is then easier and the anatomic approximation of the tissues can be accomplished with the minimal amount of suture material. Healing is usually perfect and much less painful. There is consequently less resultant scar tissue and dyspareunia is rare.

None of the foregoing attributes is characteristic of the mediolateral incision. It has, however, one advantage over the median. Complete laceration of the perineum through the sphincter and into the rectum is less common. If this type of laceration does occur with the mediolateral episiotomy, the repair of this triangular defect involving the rectal mucosa, anal sphincter, levator ani muscle, and the transverse perineal muscle (all three of these muscles pulling in a different direction) is by no means a simple procedure. On the other hand, a much simpler problem to handle technically exists when a complete perineal laceration follows a median episiotomy. The repair in this instance is easy and only requires the adherence to a few simple, standard, but important principles of surgical technique which have been described.

The episiotomy may be made with a scissors or a scalpel. Scissors should be straight, with blunt points and sharp cutting edges. Many obstetricians use a bandage scissor or a design modification of one because there is less danger of injury to the infant's scalp, and because the noncutting tip of the intravaginal blade will push a buldging rectocele away, should one be present. If a scalpel is used, a sterile wood tongue depressor is inserted between the infant's scalp and the perineal body. The incision is then made over the tongue depressor with a single firm, deft stroke from just anterior to the anal sphincter through the vaginal introitus and through the full thickness of the perineal body. If it becomes obvious, because of the size of the presenting part or the configuration of the maternal pelvis, that the episiotomy will extend to a third- or fourth-degree laceration, it may be better to extend the incision into the rectum rather than allowing the sphincter and the rectal wall to lacerate.

REPAIR OF THE EPISIOTOMY

This is simply a reapproximation of the tissues previously divided. It includes the repair of the vaginal epithelium, the subepithelial fascia support, the levator ani muscle and its fascia, the transverse perineal muscle and fascia, and the subcuticulum and skin.

The technique of the repair is shown in Fig. 6. The first of a series of interrupted, buried-knot sutures, using 4-0 absorbable material, is placed in the subepithelial layer of the vagina slightly above the apex of the incision. A second similar suture is placed between the apex of the wound and the hymenal ring but includes the fascia of the perineal body as well as the vaginal subepithelium. Insertion of the needle is begun at the deepest portion of the defect, directing the needle toward the vaginal subepithelium. The needle is then inserted on the opposite side into the subepithelium and directed toward the deepest portion of the incision in the body of the perineum. The needle emerges opposite the spot where it was first introduced. The suture is tied. Before tying the suture traction is made on both ends to pull the tissue together gently and at the same time tissue forceps are used to pull the more superficial portion of the wound together. The third suture is placed in a similar manner, but the needle is directed downward (toward the skin of the perineum) so that it will emerge through the subcuticulum about 0.5-1 cm from the lower angle of the skin incision. The needle is then inserted opposite its emergent point in the subcutis and directed upward through the fascia of the perineal body toward the deepest portion of the wound so that it emerges opposite the point of its original insertion. The suture is tied and, again, as tension is put on the suture, the skin edges are brought together with the tissue forceps.

The next suture is directed upward from the deepest point of the episiotomy wound toward the vaginal subepithelium, as was the second suture, so that the needle emerges just inside the hymenal ring. The opposite side is treated as before, with care taken to insert the needle exactly opposite where it emerges in relation to the hymenal ring. If the hymen is reapproximated in this manner so that the normal anatomic relationship of the cut hymeneal ring is re-established, mild but bothersome dyspareunia is eliminated.

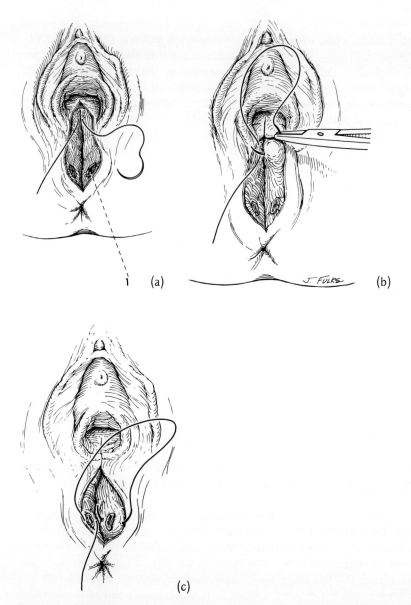

(a)

(b)

(c)

Figure 6. (a) In the episiotomy repair the first interrupted suture is placed at the apex of the defect in the vagina. The suture catches the subepithelial layer of the vaginal epithelium as well as the fascia beneath it. The suture is placed so the knot is buried. (b) At the hymenal ring, care is taken to approximate this structure in its normal anatomic relationship. (c) As the transverse perineal muscle is brought together, the suture passes through the fascial support of this muscle as well as through the muscle itself.

The next suture is directed downward (posteriorly) toward the perineal skin. This suture will usually pass through the belly of the transected transverse perineal muscle, catching its supporting fascia deep and superficial as it passes toward the subcutis, where it emerges about 1 cm closer to the vaginal orifice than the previously placed stitch.

It is important to bring the lower ends of the bulbocavernosus muscle together properly in the midline again so that there will be no gaping of the vulva following the repair of the episiotomy. This is accomplished by inserting the suture needle rather deeply into the belly of the muscle, pointing the needle toward the labium majus upward (as the patient lies on the delivery table). The curve of the needle makes it appear as though the point would penetrate the inner surface of the labium if it were allowed to continue in its course. Instead, downward pressure is made on the needle holder and at the same time the point of the needle is turned sharply downward and the skin of the inner surface of the labium majus is pushed upward with the tissue forceps so that the point of the needle emerges just beneath it in the edge of the episiotomy wound (Fig. 7). When the needle point is inserted on the opposite side, it is directed just a little beneath the skin (0.5 cm) but almost parallel with it and with the needle pointing upward (anteriorly). When the needle has been inserted about 2 cm into the bulbocavernosus muscle, it is turned sharply downward and the point of the needle emerges in the deepest part of the episiotomy. When this suture is tied, it pulls both of the bulbocavernosus muscles downward and brings the fascial support of these muscles together in the midline. Occasionally it will be necessary to bring the perineal skin together with one or two subcuticular sutures to complete the repair.

In repairing the mediolateral episiotomy, the operator must be aware that the two sides of the wound are not pulled directly apart, but that the muscle traction on the lateral side of the wound is not only lateral but also upward (anterior) and that the pull of the muscle on the medial side is not only medial but also downward (posterior). The vaginal portion, down to the hymenal ring, is repaired in the same manner as the median episiotomy. That portion of the mediolateral episiotomy involving the levator ani muscle, it must be remembered, involves the pubococcygeus and bulbocavernosus portions. It also transects the transverse perineal muscle. Interrupted, buried-knot sutures also serve well in the repair of this type of episiotomy. The placement of the suture is somewhat different from that used in the repair of the median episiotomy, however. The lateral half of the stitch travels forward (anteriorly) at about 45° from the horizontal and the median half is placed about 20° downward (posterior) from the horizontal (Fig. 8). When traction is placed on the suture as it is tied it pulls the lateral flap backward and medially to meet the medial flap being pulled laterally and

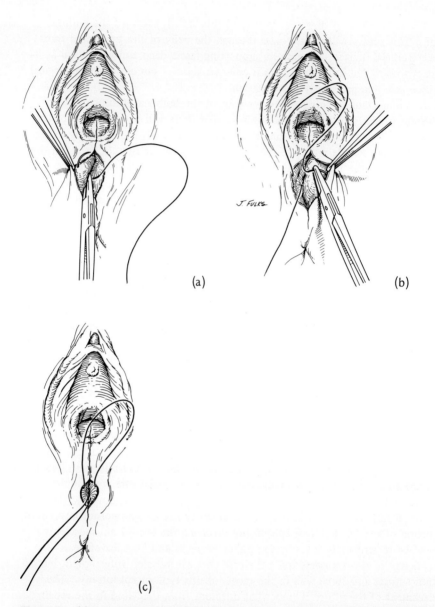

Figure 7. (a) Approximation of the fascial support of the muscle and the bulbo-cavernosus is begun by inserting the suture needle rather deeply into the belly of the muscle and bringing it out so that the point of the needle emerges close to the skin edge of the labium majus. (b) On the opposite side, the needle is inserted close to the skin edge of the labium majus. (c) The repair is completed with one or two subcuticular sutures if necessary. If the skin edges fall together with the patient in the dorsal lithotomy position no sutures are necessary.

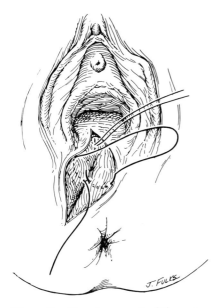

Figure 8. The placement of the sutures in the repair of a mediolateral episiotomy is different than that used in the repair of a median episiotomy. The lateral half travels foreward (anteriorly) about 45° from the horizontal and the medial half of the suture travels posteriorly (downward) about 20° from the horizontal.

somewhat forward. It is necessary to do this because of the parabolic arc of the pubococcygeus muscle and the forces resulting from cutting this muscle at an angle across its belly. Several sutures placed in this manner, and at the same time picking up the subcuticular layer of the perineal skin, will complete the repair as it does in suturing the median episiotomy.

19

Maternal Resuscitation

B. ALAN WALDRON / Nottingham City Hospital and University Hospital, Nottingham, England

Maternal collapse due to a variety of conditions that may occur during pregnancy and childbirth is a medical emergency of unique significance. The mother is often young and generally in good health. This patient has a particularly good chance of responding to resuscitation.

Unfortunately, the maternity unit medical staff, although they may be well-trained in resuscitation, are not usually called upon to carry it out frequently. Hence, the medical team should pay particular care to familiarizing themselves with resuscitation equipment and to keeping up with any advances in this area of medicine. There can be no doubt that for the maternity medical staff to practice and familiarize themselves with the techniques of resuscitation can have profound benefits in terms of successful resuscitation.

Maternal collapse may result from a variety of complications of childbirth, and resuscitation will therefore have to be relevant to the principal pathological processes, as well as appropriate to the restoration of basic functions such as respiration and heart beat.

PRINCIPLES OF RESUSCITATION PROCEDURES

Intravenous Infusion

All mothers who need to be resuscitated should have an intravenous cannula placed in as large a vein as possible. The cannula should preferably be 16-gauge or larger to facilitate the rapid infusion of fluids, should this be necessary.

Cannulas which have injection ports make it very easy to give extra drugs to the intravenous infusion, but the injection port may harbor bacteria if used for long periods and therefore probably should not be used for more than a few hours. The rapid infusion of fluids as would be required in cases of severe hemorrhage, such as abruption of the placenta or defibrination syndrome, will also lead to cooling of the tissues around the site of entry into the body. Once the tissues surrounding the vein delivering fluid rapidly to the heart have been cooled, the fluid will then be entering the heart directly at temperatures of not much more than 4°C in the case of blood, or 20°C (room temperature) for blood substitutes and electrolyte fluids. This cooling of the heart may lead to serious arrhythmias in a heart that is already severely stressed. The infusion of fluids rich in potassium, such as long-stored blood and plasma, will further increase the risks of arrhythmia. Stored blood has a low pH due to storage under hypoxic conditions, which leads to increasing hemolysis, and at the time of infusion the blood is inefficient in oxygen transportation. If all fluids to be infused rapidly are passed through a warming coil at 37°C, the heart is more likely to survive a multitude of insults without developing an arrhythmia. Storage of blood inevitably causes clumps of cells and debris to collect, and the longer it is stored, the more this process will develop. Most intravenous infusion sets have a filter for particles larger than 160 μ, but it is thought that particles should be filtered down to 20 μ. Such blood filters are available which can be placed between the fluid container and the intravenous set and will thus greatly reduce the debris that would otherwise lodge in the pulmonary circulation, possibly causing respiratory problems. These blood filters should be used whenever it is proposed to transfuse more than 500 ml of blood.

Intravenous infusions are best given into the arm because there is a considerable risk of thrombophlebitis if they are given into the lower limb. However, in dire emergency any vein that will accommodate a large cannula is appropriate. If no veins are readily visible, a cutdown onto a vein should be carried out.

In cases of severe hemorrhage, two infusions should always be used and, if possible, a central venous line set up to monitor the pressure in the right atrium. In addition, an accurate record should be kept of all fluids infused.

Fits due to eclampsia or epilepsy can be controlled by injecting intravenous boluses of thiopentone, phenytoin sodium, diazepam, or a continuous infusion of 0.8% chlormethiazole.

Artificial Ventilation

Severe respiratory depression or arrest is an emergency that requires immediate and efficient treatment. Respiratory arrest or dangerous depression of respiration can result from overdosage of analgesic drugs, accidental spinal injection during epidural anesthesia, and cardiac arrest.

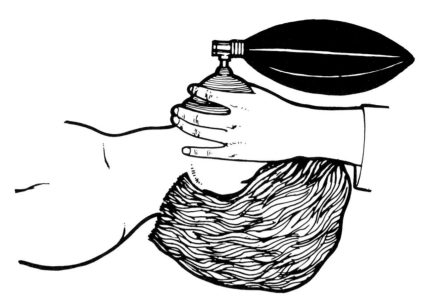

Figure 1. Application of anaesthetic mask to the face.

Successful and efficient ventilation of the lungs is entirely dependent on a gas-tight seal between an anesthetic mask and the patient's face or, in the event of mouth-to-mouth resuscitation, between the resuscitator's mouth and the patient's face. If an airway such as the Brooke airway is available, then it may not be necessary for the resucitator to come into direct contact with the patient's face. Holding an anesthetic mask onto the face needs considerable practice and requires pressure to be applied in two distinctly different directions. The mandible has to be elevated and the cervical spine extended in order to pull the tongue forwards in the mouth, thus helping to keep the airway patent (Fig. 1). In addition, the mask has to be pressed firmly onto the face in order to achieve a gas-tight seal. This technique seems simple, but often becomes very difficult in an emergency unless previously practiced. If an adequate airway cannot be achieved by this method, then the only alternative is endotracheal intubation, another difficult technique unless practiced regularly.

As soon as it has been recognized that artificial ventilation is required for a patient, the mouth must be cleared by sucking out any collected foreign material with a suction apparatus. Ideally, an oral airway should then be inserted before ventilation is begun, so that the tongue will not obstruct the posterior pharynx. The lungs should then be ventilated with air or oxygen from a self-inflating resuscitator bag. The only advantages of endotracheal intubation are that the airway is guaranteed, (especially important if the patient

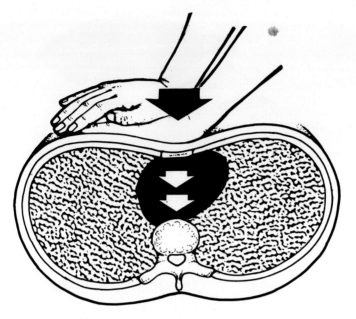

Figure 2. Efficient cardiac massage.

vomits) and all the ventilated gas enters the lungs. Ventilation with a mask pushes gas into the stomach as well as the lungs, and this might lead to the regurgitation of stomach contents, which will flood the pharynx and may enter the lungs.

Endotracheal intubation and the use of a mask in ventilation are skills that can be practiced on suitably constructed dummies. At the time of intubation, the cricoid cartilage of the larynx should be pressed back against the cervical vertebrae to occlude the esophagus and thus prevent stomach contents from passing up it to enter the pharynx.

Cardiac Massage

In the event of cardiac arrest, there will only be 3 min to restore an adequate cerebral circulation if brain damage is to be avoided. Time should not be wasted in trying to establish a diagnosis, but cardiac massage should be commenced immediately. For this to be sufficiently effective, the resuscitating person must strike a sharp blow on the lower end of the sternum, which may restart the heart. If this is unsuccessful, then repeated compressions of the lower chest must be made at about 60 times/min. Compression of the chest by pressing on the lower sternum must squeeze the heart between the anterior chest wall and the vertebrae behind (Fig. 2). It will only be possible to get adequate chest compression if the patient is placed on a firm surface such as a board or the floor. Between each five cardiac compressions the lungs should be ventilated once. If the cardiac massage is adequate, there should be good carotid and femoral pulses and, provided that ventilation is also adequate, the patient should become pink, with reacting pupils.

Cardiac Arrest Procedure

As soon as a cardiac arrest is discovered, medical aid should be sought; an arrest team is ideal if available. Emergency trolleys, defibrillator, suckers, and electrocardiograph should also be obtained quickly. An intravenous infusion of 100 ml 8.4% sodium bicarbonate should be run into a vein to correct the inevitable metabolic acidosis caused by tissue hypoxia. After this initial infusion 60 ml should be run in every 15 min while the arrest continues. When the defibrillator becomes available, the electrodes should be covered with a conductive jelly and one placed over the sternum and the other at the apex. Providing no one is touching the bed or the patient, a shock of 400 J DC should be sent through the patient.

To determine the next step, it will be necessary to attach the patient to an electrocardiograph monitor. The cardiac complexes can be observed on this monitor, but cardiac massage should only cease when there is a spontaneous cardiac output.

Normal Cardiac Complexes
Normal cardiac complexes may be associated with *sinus bradycardia* which can be treated by intravenous atropine 0.6 mg.

Heart Block
Heart block with a ventricular rate less than 40/min will require stimulation for the heart in the form of isoprenaline 2 mg/500 ml in 5% dextrose or dopamine 5-10 μg/kg body weight per min in 5% dextrose administered by infusion pump. Subsequent electrical pacing might also be required for a more prolonged effect.

Ventricular Fibrillation
If this persists after the initial stimulus of 400 J DC then this shock should be repeated. If ventricular fibrillation still persists then 100 mg lignocaine may be given as an intravenous bolus and the heart defibrillated again. Should there still be a failure to resume normal complexes, the following drugs can be given intravenously and further shocks given:

Lignocaine	200 mg
Oxyprenolol	2 mg
Procainamide	200 mg
Phenytoin sodium	100 mg

Efficient cardiac massage and ventilation must continue between shocks if cerebral damage is to be avoided.

Asystole

In the case of asystole, inject adrenaline 10 ml 1/10,000, isoprenaline 2 mg, or 10 ml calcium gluconate 10% intravenously or into the heart. This may cause either sinus rhythm or ventricular fibrillation. In the case of ventricular fibrillation, it will be necessary to defibrillate while, if asystole persists, the dose of adrenaline should be repeated every 3 min.

In the event of successful defibrillation, attacks of ventricular tachycardia or ventricular extrasystoles indicate an irritable focus in the myocardium. This can usually be abolished by 100 mg lignocaine intravenously followed by a lignocaine infusion of 1-4 mg/min. Later, this can be changed to procainamide 500 mg every 6 hr.

Long-term resuscitation will demand transfer of the mother to an intensive care unit which can offer more skilled monitoring and suitable environment for ventilation than a maternity unit. Renal blood flow can be encouraged immediately after cardiovascular collapse by giving doses of 40 mg frusemide intravenously.

Successful resuscitation in a maternity unit is most likely if the medical staff practice the resuscitation procedures. This may be carried out on life-like dummies. In the normal course of events in a maternity unit, staff do not have sufficient experience of maternal resuscitation to maintain a resuscitating team at a high standard of efficiency.

RESUSCITATION IN SPECIFIC CONDITIONS

Pre-Eclampsia and Eclampsia

This condition is a major cause of maternal morbidity and death and its management requires a variety of therapeutic approaches to restore an improved physiological state for both mother and fetus. Reduction of blood pressure is one of the first requirements and may be achieved by B-blockers, methyldopa, or hydralazine.

Prevention or control of convulsions will be effected by drugs such as chlormethiazole 0.8% intravenously or diazepam.

Pain relief is most efficiently provided by caudal or lumbar epidural anaesthesia. However, pethidine in combination with a phenothiazine such as chlorpromazine or promethazine can be effective.

Urine output and the maintenance of fluid and electrolyte balance is extremely important in these edematous, fluid-overloaded patients who, at the same time, have a low circulating blood volume. Some claim success with the intravenous administration of plasma leading to a diuresis and reduction of tissue fluid. In any event, strict detail should be paid to maintaining electrolyte levels near normal and at the same time ensuring there is adequate urine output with the help of diuretics and intravenous fluids, if necessary.

Early delivery of the fetus is the only guaranteed method of bringing this damaging pathological process to an end.

Sedation should only be sufficient to achieve the aims of lowering blood pressure and reducing the chance of convulsions. Oversedation will adversely affect the baby.

Acid Aspiration Syndrome

The only effective way of treating this syndrome is by preventing its occurrence. The administration of oral alkali and prevention of inhalation of vomitus by intubation during general anesthesia is the cornerstone of effective treatment. Ensuring that the stomach is empty before initiating general anesthesia has to be the most successful method of preventing this syndrome.

Pulmonary aspiration of the stomach contents is associated with a 70% mortality (Cameron and Zuidema, 1972) and may result from the inhalation of as little as 25 ml of gastric contents (Roberts and Shirley, 1974). Persistent cyanosis, tachycardia, and pulmonary edema will develop and these signs usually occur within 30-60 min. Bronchospasm is often present but not in every case. The acid in the respiratory tract causes tissue damage leading to an exudation of fluid into the alveoli which may lead to hypotension due to hypovolemia. Anoxia and tachycardia may progress to cardiac failure, thus causing even further congestion and edema within the lungs. Chest x-ray will demonstrate pulmonary edema and atelectasis. Infection of the lung tissue is a possible sequel to acid aspiration syndrome.

Treatment

Mild cases should be given oxygen by face mask and the cardiovascular and respiratory systems should be monitored closely over the next few hours. In those patients who develop serious symptoms and signs, the pharynx and trachea should be aspirated. A cuffed endotracheal tube is then placed in position and the patient's lungs ventilated with oxygen.

Corticosteroids are advocated by most, in spite of the fact that they are of slight (Lewinski, 1965) or even of no value (Awe et al., 1966). It has been suggested that these will relieve bronchospasm and reduce the inflammatory reaction in the respiratory tract. It has been suggested that if the inhaled fluid has a pH of less than 1.5, the mortality is almost 100% and therefore steroids do not help (Downs et al., 1974). If the pH is between 1.5 and 2.0, then the steroids may improve survival; when the pH is greater than 2.1, there is no progressive lung damage (Taylor and Prys-Davies, 1966).

Dexamethasone 10 mg followed by 5 mg every 6 hr for the first 72 hr is the treatment of choice since it does not cause sodium retention which would aggravate pulmonary edema, and at the same time it will prevent cerebral edema. Hydrocortisone 300 mg every 6 hr or methylprednisolone 30 mg/kg every 6 hr are alternative forms of steroid therapy advocated by some physicians.

Artificial ventilation is essential and should be carried out in an intensive care unit. If the patient with serious symptoms is to survive then she must be ventilated for 4-5 days. Some patients who survive may have permanent damage to their lung function.

Specific therapy for bronchospasm with bronchodilators and with digoxin and diuretics for cardiac failure may be required. Physiotherapy, intravenous fluids, monitoring of central venous pressure, and antibiotics may all be required to manage the patient through this very dangerous condition.

Amniotic Fluid Embolism

This is a rare condition occurring about once in every 80,000 pregnancies, but it has a very high mortality rate and therefore contributes as much as 5% of the maternal mortality rate.

When amniotic fluid enters the maternal circulation in significant quantity, it will cause intravascular coagulation. Coagulation affecting the pulmonary circulation is the principal lesion in amniotic fluid embolism. The patient will suddenly collapse with dyspnea, cyanosis, and hypotension usually occurring at delivery or towards the end of labor. The central venous pressure will rise rapidly due to obstruction of the pulmonary arterial circulation and there will consequently be a fall of arterial pressure. The normal gaseous exchange in the lungs will be severely impaired and this will be associated with a mottled chest x-ray appearance.

If the patient survives the initial symptoms, then a widespread coagulation defect will develop in response to thromboplastin release which will trigger the conversion of fibrinogen to fibrin and lead on to low fibrinogen levels, thrombocytopenia, and low factor V and VIII levels. In addition, fibrinolytic activity will be increased and uterine hemorrhage will nearly always occur.

In order to establish the exact diagnosis, the development of acid aspiration syndrome or emboli of air or blood clot must be excluded. Certain diagnosis can only be made at post mortem when amniotic fluid debris and fetal squamous epithelial cells are found in the pulmonary circulation.

Treatment requires oxygenation as a primary priority in a condition where there is impaired gaseous exchange in the lungs. This can be best achieved by ventilating the patient with a gas mixture rich in oxygen, usually for a number of days in an intensive care unit. Transfusion of large volumes of preferably fresh and warmed blood may be necessary to restore the circulating blood volume. The central venous pressure should be monitored in addition to the blood pressure to ensure that the right heart does not become overloaded. Isoprenaline 2 mg in 500 ml 5% dextrose or dopamine 5-10 μg/kg per min in 5% dextrose may be required to maintain pressure and cardiac output during the acute phase of the condition.

Uterine hemorrhage will require the use of an oxytocin infusion, bimanual compression of the uterus, or packing of the uterus. If there has been some major damage to the uterus during delivery, this will require surgical repair or even hysterectomy to stop the bleeding.

As soon as amniotic fluid embolism is considered the likely cause of collapse, heparin should be given as 10,000 U intravenously every 4 hr to prevent the intravascular coagulation. If there is a low fibrinogen level, then 6 G of fibrinogen should be given in 30 min or, alternatively, fresh frozen plasma containing 3 G fibrinogen liter can be used.

Fibrinolysis usually occurs but it is thought that hemorrhage and hypocoagulability should be treated by the transfusion of whole fresh blood as much as possible. If fibrinogen and drugs inhibiting fibrinolysis are to be used, then it should only be after consultation with a hematologist where this is practicable. Epsilon aminocapnoic acid and aprotinin inhibit plasminogen activation and plasmin activity which is the proteolytic enzyme that causes fibrinolysis. However, these drugs might exaggerate the accompanying thrombotic condition and should be used with caution. If they are used, epsilon aminocaproic acid is given as 5 G by slow intravenous infusion followed by 1 G/hr. Aprotinin is given as a dose of 50,000-150,000 kallikrein inactivator units (KIU) intravenously, followed by 300,000-500,000 KIU daily.

Abruption of the Placenta

The condition may occur without resuscitation being required, but should there be a large hemorrhage into the retroplacental space between the placenta and the uterus, there will be an urgent need to replace the lost blood, and massive transfusion might be needed. Coagulation failure develops in 20% of patients with abruption of the placenta (Hibbard and Jeffcoate, 1966). However, only one in four of these cases with a coagulation defect will have excessive postpartum or intrapartum bleeding, and, in this case, it is often uterine atony as well as the coagulation defect that causes bleeding.

Treatment must be based on early delivery of the infant vaginally or by cesarean section if it is alive and mature. It is difficult to estimate the amount of blood loss and therefore transfusion should be judged by the maternal blood pressure, with the additional help of the central venous pressure. The circulating volume should be maintained by blood rather than substitutes and, if this is fresh, it will also supply valuable clotting factors. An alternative is fresh frozen plasma and cryoprecipitate.

Intravascular coagulation, should it occur, may lead to renal failure due to the deposition of fibrin following the release of thromboplastins. Should oliguria develop, then this will be best checked by the initiation of diuresis by mannitol 20% solution or a large dose of frusemide.

Defibrination Syndrome

The treatment of this condition can be extremely complicated and it would be best to take the advice of a hematologist if one is available. This syndrome should be suspected when bleeding is excessive and associated with one of the usual accompanying obstetric conditions. Taking some blood and placing it in a glass bottle to time the development of a clot in the blood is the most rapid and convenient way of initially testing for the condition.

The syndrome may develop after a variety of pathological conditions in obstetrics. These will include eclampsia, hydatidiform mole, septic abortion, abruption of the placenta, and the presence of a dead fetus in the uterus for a prolonged period.

Disseminated intravascular coagulation is said to occur as a result of the release of thromboplastin into the blood. This usually occurs at the interface of the uterus and the placenta. This will lead to depletion of the stores of fibrinogen due to its deposition in retroplacental clot or throughout the vascular system. In addition, there will be activation of the fibrinolytic system at the placental site or in the blood stream. Increased blood levels of plasmin will lead to the breakdown of fibrin and fibrinogen and the resulting fibrin degradation products (FDPs) will act as a powerful anticoagulant.

If a low fibrinogen state develops, it is not necessary to give fibrinogen intravenously unless excessive bleeding develops. Only 1:4 patients with a low fibrinogen subsequently develops a severe hemorrhage (Leeton, 1974). However, should this occur, or if a cesarean section is planned, 6 G fibrinogen should be infused in 30 min. It is also not necessary to administer epsilon aminocaproic acid or aprotinin simply because fibrin degradation products are present in the blood.

Epidural and spinal anesthesia should not be used when there is a clotting deficiency, since this may lead to bleeding from the engorged epidural veins present in pregnancy. This could lead to the formation of a hematoma within the spinal canal and compression of the spinal cord or spinal nerves.

Cardiac Failure

This occurs most frequently immediately after delivery as a result of the sudden increase in blood volume which accompanies uterine retraction and placental separation. Intravenous ergometrine may precipitate heart failure by increasing the circulating blood volume and central venous pressure.

Naturally, any patient with congenital or acquired heart disease will be at risk during pregnancy, and particular care will have to be taken that failure is not precipitated during labor or delivery. Pulmonary edema may develop at any time during pregnancy if there is a tight mitral stenosis, and a tachycardia during labor is likely to lead to cardiac failure when there is associated heart disease.

Pulmonary Edema
If pulmonary edema develops, this should be treated with oxygen, intravenous frusemide 40 mg, 10 mg morphine, and 0.5 G aminophylline by slow intravenous injection. An alternative way of reducing circulating blood volume would be to apply sphygmomanometer cuffs to the limbs and keep them inflated above diastolic pressure for about 15 min and then release the cuffs slowly. Venesection of 250-500 ml blood would also be a rapid method of reducing the cardiac load. Aminophylline may relieve the bronchospasm that often accompanies pulmonary edema and may lead to an increase of cardiac output. Digitalis is not usually effective in pulmonary edema unless there is myocardial damage, and it is only by using diuretics and other methods of reducing the blood volume that treatment will be effective. Diazepam 5-10 mg should also be given to reduce anxiety. Epidural blockade of the pain of labor can reduce the likelihood of tachycardia with the associated inefficient heart function leading to failure. An epidural block might also relieve pulmonary edema by increasing the vascular space, leading to a reduction in the work load on the heart as well as heart rate.

Congestive Cardiac Failure
Congestive cardiac failure is less common, occurring mainly in patients with valvular incompetence and myocardial damage. Frusemide will again be required and also digitalis for any patient who has not already received this drug.

Oxygen therapy for dyspnea and the raising of the shoulders on pillows, along with good analgesia and the relief of anxiety, are very important principles of treatment. The second stage of labor should be shortened where possible by forceps delivery or vacuum extraction. Epidural analgesia is the ideal method of analgesia. Following delivery, it may be best to avoid all uterotonic drugs, but if one is required, then 10 u of intravenous oxytocin would be the best.

Pulmonary Embolism

This is particularly likely to follow cesarean section in patients with cardiac disease, obesity, enlarged varicose veins, and early postpartum sterilization.

It may be of variable severity, but in all cases the immediate treatment should consist of the administration of 10,000 u heparin, the use of oxygen to reduce hypoxia, and support for the circulation with drugs such as digitalis, isoprenaline, or dopamine.

Once the patient has survived the initial onset of the condition, an intravenous line should be set up to facilitate drug therapy. A failing myocardium may respond to drugs to stimulate cardiac output and cardiac efficiency. The primary problem is the chronic hypoxia caused by a large embolus. This might be helped by intubation and ventilation of the patient under sedation and the use of muscle relaxants. Unfortunately, ventilation will increase the intrathoracic pressure and this may further embarrass the already overstrained right heart.

If the pulmonary embolus is to be removed surgically, then it will be necessary to perform angiography before this can be carried out. Some emboli have been treated by the injection of streptokinase.

Respiratory Disease

Pateints with obstructive airways disease and asthma are usually little affected during pregnancy, but may become breathless during labor and delivery. Narcotic analgesics need not be given if epidural analgesia is employed, thus avoiding the respiratory depression of analgesic drugs. Tension pneumothorax may develop if an emphysematous bulla ruptures and would need relief by intercostal drainage of the air in the pleural space.

Septicemia

Once relatively common after self-procured abortion, this has now become much less common since many abortions are carried out in hospitals. Septic abortion and subsequent septicemia may result in cardiovascular collapse, acute renal failure, and septic thrombophlebitis.

Treatment will consist of maintaining adequate hydration, large doses of the appropriate antibiotics and, if the patient develops septic shock with low blood pressure and peripheral shut down, then a large dose of dexamethasone (56 mg in 24 hr) has been advocated (Weil et al., 1974). The latter is said to reduce peripheral resistance and increase cardiac output which will reverse the hemodynamic changes found in bacterial shock (Shubin and Weil, 1963).

Central venous pressure should be monitored and it may be necessary to ventilate very ill patients in an intensive care unit. Urine output should be monitored and, if not adequate, can be increased with large doses of frusemide.

REFERENCES

Awe, W. C., Fletcher, W. S., and Jacob, S. W. (1966). Pathophysiology of aspiration pneumonitis. *Surgery 60*:232.

Cameron, J. L., and Zuidema, G. D. (1972). Aspiration pneumonia: Magnitude and frequency of the problem. *JAMA 219*:1194.

Downs, J. B., Chapman, R. L. Jr., Modell, J. H., and Hood, I. (1974). An evaluation of steroid therapy in aspiration pneumonitis. *Anesthesiology 40*:129.

Hibbard, B. M., and Jeffcoate, T. N. A. (1966). Abruptio placentae. *Obstet. Gynecol. 27*:155.

Leeton, J. F. (1974). Emergency complications of the third stage of labour and early puerperium. In *Obstetric Therapeutics*. D. F. Hawkins (Ed.), Bailliere Tindall, London.

Lewinski, A. (1965). Evaluation of methods employed in the treatment of chemical pneumonitis of aspiration. *Anesthesiology 26*:37.

Roberts, R. B., and Shirley, M. A. (1974). Reducing the risk of acid-aspiration during Cesarean section. *Anesth. Analg. Curr. Res. 53*:859.

Shubin, H., and Weil, M. H. (1963). Bacterial shock. *JAMA 185*:850.

Taylor, G., and Prys-Davies, J. (1966). The prophylactic use of antacids in the prevention of the acid-pulmonary-aspiration syndrome (Mendelson's syndrome). *Lancet i*:288.

Weil, M. H., Shubin, H., and Nishijima, H. (1974). Corticosteroid therapy in circulatory shock. *Int. Surg. 59*:589.

20
Fetal Resuscitation

A. D. MILNER / University Hospital, Nottingham, England
H. VYAS / City Hospital, Nottingham, England

It may not always be possible to protect the unborn baby from death or permanent brain damage as a result of intrauterine asphyxia. It is totally unacceptable that the child should fail to reach his or her full potential as a result of hypoxia in the minutes after birth. There is no doubt that the first priority when setting up even the minimum of neonatal services is to ensure an adequate resuscitation service.

Neonatal resuscitation by intermittent positive pressure ventilation (IPPV) via an endotracheal tube was first popularized by Flagg in the United States (1928) and shortly after in Britain by Blaikley and Gibberd (1935). These methods were slow to gain general acceptance but have become widely used over the last 20 years. This chapter will discuss how, and in what situations, these established techniques should be used.

ONSET OF SPONTANEOUS RESPIRATIONS

We now have considerable knowledge of the changes occurring in the respiratory system during the period of adaptation at birth. We know from long-term fetal animal experiments and from ultrasound studies (Davies et al., 1972; Boddy and Robinson, 1971) that rapid shallow respiratory movements are certainly present intermittently from the end of the third trimester. These respiratory movements are very sensitive to hypoxia and are probably limited to periods of rapid eye movement sleep when the respiratory drive is controlled by the cortex.

There is good evidence that the central and peripheral chemoreceptor drive is, to a large extent, turned off until after delivery. Once born, the child is barraged with stimuli, of which cold and touch are probably the most important, normally leading to the first inspiration within 10 sec (Vyas et al., 1981). The factors activating the chemoreceptor drive are not known. A small group of babies, those with the central hypoventilation syndrome (Ondine's curse) (Severinghaus and Mitchell, 1962) fail to develop normal drive and tend to become apneic when sleeping. The apnea in preterm babies also probably represents a failure of maturation of the normal control mechanisms. The cerebral and chemoreceptor components of respiratory drive can obviously also be impaired by cerebral damage from trauma or hypoxia and suppressed by a variety of drugs, including the opiates and Valium.

We also know that in utero the fetal lung is not collapsed but has a fluid volume which is probably similar to the 30-35 ml/kg body weight of air in the neonatal period. This fluid is actively secreted during pregnancy and has a chemical composition strikingly different from that of amniotic fluid (Adams, 1966). The rate of flow in the fetal lamb is 3-5 ml/hr per kg (Normand et al., 1971) and is under hormonal control (Walters et al., 1978). The surge in catecholamines during labor and in the immediate neonatal period not only turns the secretion off but also results in a process of reabsorption, possibly creating a potential space for air to enter.

The process of vaginal delivery also prepares the lungs by squeezing the chest with pressures of up to 250 cmH$_2$O, which wrings fluid out (Fig. 1). The air remaining in the lung after the first spontaneous breath probably represents the combined effects of these two processes.

The baby, on average, generates a negative intrathoracic pressure of 30-40 cmH$_2$O (Saunders and Milner, 1978), lasting for approximately 300 msec (Milner and Vyas, 1982). This draws approximately 40 ml into the lung. The baby almost always then produces a high positive intrathoracic pressure of up to 110 cmH$_2$O which is maintained for up to 3 sec, this being the baby's first cry. At the end of this first breath, about 20 ml of air will typically remain in the lungs, known as the functional residual capacity. Babies born by elective section have neither the conditioning effects of the catecholamine nor the prolonged squeeze of the birth canal but are exposed to transitory squeeze as they are pulled out of the uterine incision (Vyas et al., 1981). These babies are much less likely to have a reservoir of air in their lungs at the end of the first breath and have considerably less air in their lungs than their vaginally delivered counterparts for the next 48 hr of life (Milner et al., 1978). This is the likely explanation for the increased incidence of respiratory problems in babies born by cesarean section.

Experiments carried out on higher animals have shown characteristic series of events occurring following total asphyxia (Dawes et al., 1960). Within

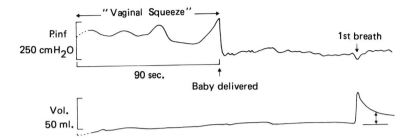

Figure 1. Longitudinal tracing of positive inflation pressure (P.inf) and volume with respect to time of a typical infant. The prolonged vaginal squeeze of 250 cmH$_2$O is shown. At the end of the first breath, the baby has formed a functional residual capacity.

30 sec of asphyxia, the animal starts making rhythmic respiratory efforts. During this phase the animal becomes cyanosed and then, within a few minutes, white as a result of vasoconstriction. The initial apneic episode, referred to as primary apnea, lasts for up to 1 min and is followed by gasping. The rate of gasping increases 4-5 min after total asphyxia; however, the gasps become weaker and eventually terminal or secondary apnea sets in. Without active resuscitation all animals in secondary apnea will die. Whether this pattern occurs in humans is not known.

INDICATIONS FOR RESUSCITATION

There is no doubt that the newborn is far more tolerant to asphyxia than the adult or older child (Brown, 1976). There are well-authenticated cases (Grossman and Williams, 1971) of babies surviving apparently neurologically intact despite not having commenced regular respiration for 10 or even 15 min after delivery (Bullough, 1958). This cannot be used as a guideline as it is impossible to know how much asphyxia the baby has suffered by the time of delivery. As a result the current guidelines generally accepted for resuscitation are:

1. Failure of regular respiration to occur by 2 min after delivery
2. Apnea and a heart rate of less than 80/min before the age of 2 min
3. Heart rate recorded within 20 min of delivery but absent at birth

Using these indications babies will be resuscitated who would have breathed spontaneously if left alone but will identify all those who are asphyxiated.

Table 1. Causes of Prolonged Time between Uterine Incision and Delivery

Transverse lie
Breech presentation
Multiple pregnancy, affecting the second or third baby
Anterior placenta previa
Head deeply impacted in the pelvis
Large baby
Uterine anomaly
Poor anesthesia and relaxation
Inadequate abdominal incision

Table 2. Babies (Vaginally Delivered) Particularly Likely to Require Resuscitation

Breech
Second of twins
Deep transverse arrest requiring Kielland's rotation
Heavy maternal sedation

The incidence of babies requiring intubation has changed over the years. In the 1960s rates as high as 10% were recorded. In 1978 the rate at the City Hospital, Nottingham, was 3.5% and had fallen to 2% in 1980. Babies most likely to fulfill the requirements for intubation are those born by cesarean section, particularly those who are difficult to extract and in whom there is a long period between incision of the uterus and delivery, for example, in cases of transverse arrest (Table 1). This incidence is also related to the anesthetic technique. More babies need resuscitation when the interval between induction and delivery is greater than 15 min or when halothane is used generously. Only 1.5 and 0.8% of full-term babies born after a normal pregnancy fulfilled the requirements in 1978 and 1980, respectively. Those particularly likely to require resuscitation were delivered after Kielland's rotation for deep transverse arrest, fetal asphyxia, breech delivery, and the second of twins (Table 2).

PROCEDURE

Someone skilled in resuscitation should be present at all high-risk deliveries (Table 3). Wherever possible, trained staff should be available to resuscitate other babies who are delivered after an uneventful pregnancy and labor but who are unexpectedly slow to establish respiration. Although the need for intubation is rare these represent more than 30% of those needing help.

Table 3. High-Risk Deliveries Requiring Presence of a Pediatric Resident

Cesarean section
Breech delivery
Multiple pregnancy
Preterm delivery
Meconium staining with fetal distress
Rh incompatibility in moderately to severely affected fetus (as judged
   by antibodies)
Instrumentation: All Kielland's deliveries
                 Neville Barnes or Wrigleys liftout when associated with
                    fetal distress
Prepartum hemorrhage if associated with fetal distress or bleeding

The first step after the delivery of any baby must be to get rid of excess surface fluid since a wet baby can drop its core temperature by 4°C within 10 min
due predominantly to evaporative water loss. A quick check should also be
made for major congenital abnormalities; occasionally babies with massive
myelomeningocoele are inappropriately resuscitated. If the baby has not
established regular respiration by 15-30 sec additional stimuli can be provided
by flicking the baby's feet. Nasopharyngeal aspiration is acceptable and
indeed mandatory if there is evidence of meconium aspiration but should be
carried out gently. Vigorous stimulation can undoubtedly delay the onset of
regular respiration and also lead to severe bradycardia (Cordero and Hon, 1971).
For this procedure, a manual disposable sucker is safe and most likely to clear
thick secretions.

If the baby is not breathing by 30 sec he or she should be transferred to a
resuscitation system consisting of a sloping table which can be fixed to a wall
or on wheels. An overhead radiant heater is essential to reduce heat loss
(Fig. 2). Other essential equipment includes a stop-clock and a system for
producing IPPV and suction (Table 4). The Apgar score should be assessed at
1 min (Apgar, 1953) (Table 5). If the baby has still not established regular
respiration by this time blow either pure oxygen or, preferably, 40% oxygen
over the baby's face using a funnel or mask. Not infrequently, the local cooling
effect of the gas on the face stimulates the onset of respiration. By now the
baby will be approximately 1½-min old, which is the time to commence the
process of intubation if he or she is still apneic. The laryngoscope, preferably
of the straight-bladed variety, must be held in the left hand. The tip of the
blade is inserted into the mouth and eased down into the pharynx until the
epiglottis is identified. The cords are best visualized if the tip is placed over
the epiglottis and the laryngoscope blade elevated. A suction catheter held
in the right hand can be used to clear excessive secretions and aid vision. If

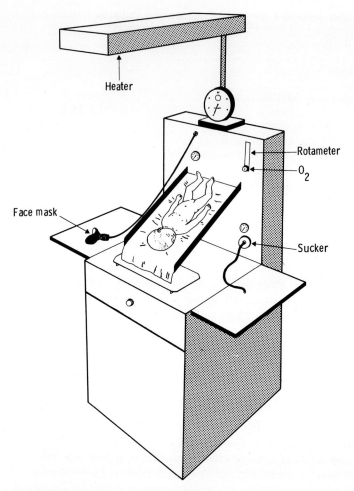

Heater

Rotameter

O$_2$

Face mask

Sucker

Figure 2. Standard resuscitaire with an overhead heater. Spring-loaded valve set at 30 cmH$_2$O in the inspiratory line has replaced the traditional water column.

the view is still not good, press the larynx downwards, with the little finger of the hand holding the laryngoscope. Sometimes the laryngoscope is inserted too far, passing down the esophagus behind the larynx. Under these circumstances withdraw the laryngoscope slowly; the entrance to the larynx will then fall into view.

If the cords are readily visible and the laryngoscope held in the midline there is usually little difficulty inserting an endotracheal (ET) tube. This may be either straight or tapered. The largest tube likely to fit comfortably should

Table 4. Essential Equipment for Resuscitation

Infant laryngoscope: straight-blade
Geudel airways
Nelaton catheter for suction
Infant resuscitation set
Mediswabs
Surgical blades
Syringes/needles
Umbilical catheters

Drugs: Sodium bicarbonate 8.4%
           Adrenaline 1 : 10,000
           Neonatal Narcan
           10% dextrose

Table 5. Apgar Score at 1 Minute

Sign	Score		
	2	1	0
Heart rate	More than 100	Less than 100	Absent
Respiration	Good	Poor	Absent
Color	Pink	Pink body Blue extremities	Blue/white
Tone	Well-flexed	Some flexion	Flaccid
Response (to catheter in nose)	Cough or sneeze	Grimace	Absent

Source: Adapted from data of Apgar, 1953.

be selected. Selection of too small a tube will often result in a large leak and may lead to selective intubation of the right main, or even the right middle, lobe bronchus. Resuscitation tubes incorporating "T-pieces" are undoubtedly least likely to create problems, and prevent the frantic search for a correct fitting T-piece at a time when the baby's heart rate has all but disappeared.

Pressure Limitation

Lung inflation is usually achieved by connecting the ET tube to a supply of gas across a T-piece and intermittently obstructing the egress of gas. Before this is begun, it is essential to ensure that there is a safety blow-off system in the line; inflow directly from a cylinder or wall supply will lead to almost certain death.

The traditional water column device is no longer acceptable on its own because, on occlusion of the T-piece, there will be an initial high pressure often exceeding 70 cmH$_2$O, due to the inertia of the system. This is of relatively short duration and may not be dangerous. A greater worry is the recent finding that the static pressure generated is related to the flow rate more than to the depth of the tube in the water column, presumably due to turbulence at the end so that pressures may be two or even three times higher than those the operator considers he or she is applying (Hey and Lenney, 1973). Most commercially available systems have been modified by incorporating a safety-spring or gravity-loaded valve set at 30 or 40 cmH$_2$O. Even these tend to be flow-dependent and can not be relied on to limit the pressure to safe limits under all conditions. Alternatively, one of the hand-operated resuscitation systems can be used. These, again, can generate high pressures if used overvigorously.

Gas Selection

The gas most commonly used for resuscitation is 100% oxygen since this is readily available. Some authorities (Davies et al., 1972) have recommended 40% oxygen because there is a fear that exposure of the very early preterm baby to high oxygen concentrations for even relatively short periods may lead to retrolental fibroplasia. There is currently no evidence to suggest this. The other anxiety that breathing 100% oxygen may lead to atelectasis is also probably not justified. A recent work measuring lung volume after the breathing of more than 80% oxygen for up to 20 min in the first 6 h of life showed that newborns are uniquely resistant to this effect (Boon et al., 1981), possibly due to foam formation within the lungs (Scarpelli, 1978). Conversely, there is little evidence that 100% oxygen has any advantages other than the easier availability of more than 40% oxygen.

Pattern of Resuscitation

An inflation pressure of 30 cmH$_2$O is generally selected. This has proved a reasonable compromise in clinical practice but is based on very little hard data. Blaikley and Gibberd (1935) found this pressure was sufficient to inflate the lungs of a small group of stillborn babies. More recently, workers have found that isolated newborn lungs tend to rupture when exposed to pressures above 50 cmH$_2$O (Gruenwold, 1963; Rosen and Laurence, 1965). This measurement is, however, of little relevance since in the normal situation the lungs, like a car's inner tube, are protected from overexpansion to some extent by the chest wall. Measurements of pressure generated during the onset of spontaneous respiration ranged widely from less than 10 to more than 80 cmH$_2$O, indicating that no one pressure will be ideal on all occasions. The 30-cm limit is, however, close to the mean spontaneous value (Karlberg et al., 1962; Milner and Saunders, 1977; Saunders and Milner, 1978). The mean amount of air entering the lung on the first inflation with a pressure of 30 cmH_2O maintained for 1 sec was 18.6 ml. in babies requiring resuscitation after delivery by cesarean section (Boon et al., 1979). On three occasions this pressure failed to produce any measurable lung-volume change, suggesting that we should be more flexible. On all these occasions adequate tidal volume was achieved within 15 sec. Our conclusions are that 30 cmH_2O is probably a reasonably safe compromise but that pressures of 40 cm or even higher may be needed for the first inflation. As already stated, the traditional pattern of ventilation has been to apply a square pressure wave to the airway. Some authorities consider, from the data available on spontaneously breathing babies, that 300 msec should not be exceeded and that longer inflations would increase the risk of pneumothorax. In practice, a 30-cm pressure applied for 1 sec is approximately half as effective as the same negative pressure generated for 200-300 msec by the spontaneously breathing baby. We also find that, unlike in the spontaneously breathing baby, air rarely remains in the lung after each inflation until the baby makes inspiratory respiratory efforts of his or her own. For some reason air enters the lung only slowly in response to a positive inflation pressure (Fig. 3). An initial inflation pressure maintained for 5 sec

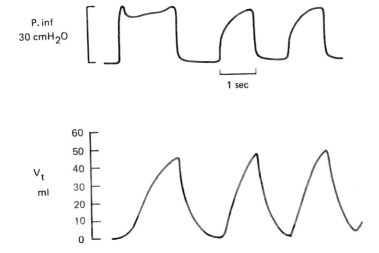

Figure 3. Longitudinal trace showing air entering slowly in response to a positive inflation pressure (P.inf). No air remained in the lungs at the end of the first inflation.

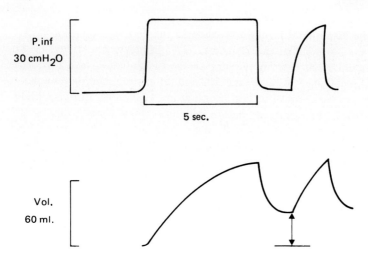

Figure 4. Formation of a functional residual capacity is seen at the end of a prolonged inflation of 5 sec.

will double the inflation volume and will lead to immediate formation of a functional residual capacity (Vyas et al., 1981) (Fig. 4). Whether this is entirely safe, or indeed advisable, is not yet known.

Reassessment

As soon as IPPV has commenced it is essential to check by auscultation that air is entering both lungs. It is also important to assess chest movement to assure equal movement on both sides. Failure to hear air entering either side strongly suggests that the tube is lying in the esophagus. Under these circumstances it is often possible to hear bubbling over the stomach. If this is suspected the tube should be withdrawn immediately and the baby reintubated.

Air entering only one lung, usually the right, is most frequently due to overgenerous insertion of too small an endotracheal tube so that the end is lying in the right main bronchus. In these situations place the bell of the stethoscope over the left lung, continue inflating at 20-30 breaths/min, and slowly withdraw the endotracheal tube by 1-2 cm. If the diagnosis is correct air entry will suddenly occur and the baby's condition will improve dramatically.

Failure of this to occur raises two further possibilities:

1. There is a pneumothorax
2. The baby has a large diaphragmatic hernia

If the baby's condition permits, an emergency x-ray should be taken while IPPV is maintained. Any pneumothorax will almost certainly be of the tension variety and will need draining. Initially a 21-gauge needle and a large syringe can be used to aspirate air but it will almost certainly be necessary to insert an intercostal drain and connect it to an underwater seal. The improvement on release of the air is again very dramatic.

A diaphragmatic hernia is more difficult to diagnose. The gut, which is almost always in the left chest, will not be aerated and will have the appearance of dense opacity. Appearance of a scaphoid abdomen is often the only physical sign. These children require urgent referral to a neonatal surgical unit but often do not have a good prognosis due to underlying lung hypoplasia.

A small group of babies will fail to respond to IPPV alone due to gross hypoxia and metabolic acidosis which have suppressed the cardiac output. The heart rate will almost always be low under these circumstances, less than 60/min. If air is undoubtedly entering the lung, commence external cardiac massage, pressing down on the sternum approximately 100 times/min with the index and middle finger while continuing IPPV. Meanwhile, an assistant can draw up 8.4% sodium bicarbonate into a syringe. It is possible to insert an umbilical vein catheter within a few seconds in this situation, taking care not to introduce air into the circulation. If the catheter is not immediately available inject into the umbilical vein in the cord using a 21-gauge needle. A large baby will require 5 ml, a small baby 2.5 ml. These volumes should be given over 2-3 min, preferably diluted in an equal volume of water. Five ml of 10% dextrose solution should also be infused at the same time. Adamson et al. (1964) found the combination of glucose and alkali speed the recovery of the heart rate but also shorten the time to the first gasp.

Babies not responding even to this require 1 ml of 1 : 10,000 adrenaline, either via the umbilical catheter or directly into the heart. Steiner and Neligan (1975) and Scott (1976) have shown that the outcome of infants who have not established their own respiratory efforts by 30 min is poor. This should be used as a clinical guideline for residents in the labor ward to discontinue further resuscitatory efforts.

SUBSEQUENT MANAGEMENT

The large majority of babies readily respond to IPPV with increase in heart rate, disappearance of cyanosis, and onset of respiration. Interestingly, the first respiratory efforts are usually positive and expiratory and appear to be generated by the abdominal muscles. They may be powerful enough to result in expiration during a period of inflation. These are soon followed by inspiratory gasps in response to the applied pressure, the so-called Head's paradoxical reflex. As already stated the initial lung volumes are relatively small. These tend to increase with repeated inflation, presumably representing changes in the mechanical characteristics of the respiratory system. The formation of the functional residual capacity does not usually occur until the baby's first effective inspiration, which is often a Head's paradoxical reflex.

Once the baby has made regular respirations for 30-60 sec the endotracheal tube can be withdrawn, the baby wrapped up, and, where appropriate, given to the mother. If the baby has responded rapidly there is no need for it to be admitted to a special-care baby unit provided there are no other indications. In our unit any baby requiring more than 10 min of IPPV is admitted for observation.

Some babies fail to make adequate respiratory efforts once their hypoxia and acidosis have been relieved. This is often due to transplacental passage of maternal drugs, particularly pethidine. If this is suspected, give naloxone, 2 ml, i.v. This will counteract the effects within 1-2 min. Babies still not responding may need IPPV for the next 24-48 hr. There is then a major worry that irreversible brain damage has occurred. A reasonable plan is to continue IPPV for 48 hr and then extubate the baby. (Using these criteria more than 85% of even those babies born with an absent heart beat and surviving for 2 days of life will subsequently have no evidence of brain damage.)

If facilities for intubation are not available, resuscitation can often be achieved using a hand-held resuscitator and face mask or even by mouth-to-mouth inflation. The positive pressure is likely to produce considerable gastric distention which will tend to splint the diaphragm and impede ventilation. Passage of a nasogastric tube would counteract this.

Using the techniques described above, intubation and resuscitation are safe procedures that rarely produce a pneumothorax or laryngeal edema. The main problem has been to ensure that junior staff receive sufficient training to become competent. For these reasons full use should be made of resuscitation models and the tragic, but occasional, fresh stillbirth.

REFERENCES

Adams, F. (1966). Functional development of the fetal lung. *J. Pediatr. 68*: 794.

Adamsons, K., Behman, R., Dawes, G. S., James, L. S., and Koford, C. (1964). Resuscitation by positive pressure ventilation and Tris-Hydroxymethyl-animomethane of rhesus monkeys asphyxiated at birth. *J. Pediatr. 65*:807.

Apgar (1953). *Curr. Res. Anesth. Analg. 32*:260.

Blaikeley, J. E., and Gibberd, G. F. (1935). Asphyxia neonatorum; its treatment by tracheal intubation. *Lancet 1*:736.

Boddy, K., and Robinson, J. S. (1971). External methods for detection of foetal breathing in utero. *Lancet 2*:1231.

Boon, A. W., Milner, A. D., and Hopkin, I. E. (1979). Lung expansion, tidal exchange and formation of the functional residual capacity during resuscitation of asphyxiated neonates. *J. Pediatr. 95*:1031-1036.

Boon, A. W., Ward-McQuaid, M., Milner, A. D., and Hopkin, I. E. (1981). Thoracic gas volume, helium functional residual capacity and airtrapping in the first six hours of life: The effect of oxygen administration. *Early Hum. Dev.*

Brown, J. K. (1976). Infants damaged during birth. In *Recent Advances in Paediatrics*, 5th Ed. D. Hull (Ed.).

Bullough, J. (1958). Protracted foetal and neonatal asphyxia. *Lancet 1*: 999-1000.

Cordero, L., and Hon, E. J. (1971). Neonatal bradycardia following nasopharyngeal stimulation. *J. Pediatr. 78*:441.

Davies et al. (1972). *Medical Case of the Newborn, Clinics in Developmental Medicine,* Spastics International Medical Publication, Heinemann Medical, London.

Dawes, G. S., Fox, H. E., et al. (1972). Respiratory movements and REM sleep in the foetal lamb. *J. Physiol. 220*:119.

Dawes, G. S., Jacobson, H. N., Mott, J. C., and Shelley, H. J. (1960). Some observations in fetal and newborn rhesus monkeys. *J. Physiol. 152*:271-278.

Flagg, P. J. (1928). The treatment of asphyxia in the newborn. *JAMA 91*: 788.

Grossman and Williams. Electrical activity and ultrastructure of cortical neurons and synapses in ischaemia. In *Brain Hypoxia, Clinics in Developmental Medicine.* J. B. Brierley, and B. S. Meldrum (Eds.), Heinemann, London, pp. 61-78.

Gruenwold, P. (1963). Normal and abnormal expansion of the lungs of newborn infants obtained at autopsy. II. Opening pressure, maximal volume and stability of expansion. *Lab. Invest. 12*:563.

Hey, E., and Lenney, W. (1973). Letter to the Editor. *Lancet 2*:103-104.

Karlberg, P., Cherry, R. B., Escardo, F. E., and Koch, G. (1962). Pulmonary ventilation and mechanics of breathing in the first minutes of life, including the onset of respirations. *Acta. Paediatr. 51*:121-136.

Milner, A. D., and Saunders, R. A. (1977). Pressure and volume changes during the first breath of human neonates. *Arch. Dis. Child 52*:918-924.

Milner, A. D., Saunders, R. A., and Hopkin, I. E. (1978). Effects of delivery by Caesarean section on lung mechanics and lung volume in the human neonate. *Arch. Dis. Child 53*:545-548.

Milner, A. D., and Vyas, H. (1982). Lung expansion at birth. *J. Pediatr. 101*: 879-886.

Normand, I. C. S., Olver, R. E., Reynolds, E. O. R., and Strang, L. B. (1971). Permeability of lung capillaries and alveoli to non-electrolytes in the foetal lamb. *J. Physiol. 219*:303-330.

Rosen, M. and Laurence, K. M. (1965). *Lancet 2*:721-722.

Saunders, R. A., and Milner, A. D. (1978). Pulmonary pressure/volume relationships during the last phase of delivery and the first postnatal breaths in humans subjects. *J. Pediatr. 93*:667-673.

Scarpelli, E. (1978). Intrapulmonary foam at birth. An adaptational phenomenon. *Pediatr. Res. 12*:1070-1076.

Scott, H. (1976). Outcome of very severe birth asphyxia. *Arch. Dis. Child 51*: 712-716.

Severinghaus, J. W., and Mitchell, R. A. (1962). Ondine's curse—Failure of respiratory centre automacity while awake. *Clin. Res. 10*:122.

Steiner, H., and Neligan, G. (1975). Perinatal cardiac arrest. Quality of survivors. *Arch. Dis. Child 50*:696-702.

Vyas, H., Milner, A. D., and Hopkin, I. E. Physiological responses to prolonged and slow rise inflation in the resuscitation of the asphyxiated newborn. For publication.

Vyas, H., Milner, A. D., and Hopkin, I. E. (1900). Comparison of the intrathoracic pressure and volume changes during the spontaneous onset of respiration in babies born by Cesarian section and by vaginal delivery. *J. Pediatr. 99*:787-791.

Walters, D. V., and Olver, R. E. (1978). The role of catecholamines in lung liquid absorption at birth. *Pediatr. Res. 12*:239-242.

Author Index

Numbers indicate the page on which an author's work is referred to; numbers in italic indicate page on which the complete reference is listed.

Abadir, A., 329, *346*
Abouleish, E., 324, 326, *344*
Abramovici, H., 257, *284*
Abuknalil, S. H., 344, *349*
Adam, A. H., 6, *20*
Adams, E. C., 9, *20*
Adams, D. W., 91, *97*
Adams, F., 432, *442*
Adamsons, K., 176, *190*, 299, 313, 315, *316*, *318*, 441, *442*
Adeleye, J. A., 141, *149*
Adrian, T. E., 257, *286*
Agress, R. L., 221, *230*
Agüero, O., 107, *126*
Alberman, E., 393, *402*
Alberts, F., 337, *346*
Allen, L. C., 90, *95*

Allison, R., 343, *348*
Alper, M. H., 340, 341, 343, *345*
Alter, B. P., 53, *76*
Althabe, O., 176, 185, *188*
Alvarez, H., 251, *252*
Amato, J. C., 174, 184, *190*, 248, *251*, *284*
Amortegui, A. J., 324, *344*
Anderson, A. B. M., 220, 221, *231*, *232*
Anderson, G. G., 52, *78*, 79, 85, *95*
Anderson, I., 265, *287*
Anderson, M. M., 222, *230*
Anderson, S. G., 368, *388*
Andresen, B. D., 86, *94*
Andros, G. J., 205, *211*
Apgar, 435, 437, *442*

Subject Index

about the book . . .

The first part of this unique two-volume reference set provides clinicians with a convenient, detailed single source of up-to-date information on day-to-day clinical obstetrical procedures—written by a distinguished panel of international contributors.

Part A: Obstetrics offers step-by-step guidelines on such subjects as techniques used for prenatal diagnosis, including fetoscopy . . . prenatal and postnatal fetal monitoring methods and their relevant merits . . . the use of ultrasound for checking fetal growth and placental localization . . . epidural anesthesia techniques and applications . . . and more!

Written especially for the practitioner, *Clinical and Diagnostic Procedures in Obstetrics and Gynecology, Part A: Obstetrics* serves as an excellent, easy-access, clinical companion for obstetricians/gynecologists; residents training in obstetrics, perinatal medicine, and family medicine; and nurses specializing in obstetrics.

about the editors . . .

E. MALCOLM SYMONDS is Foundation Professor of Obstetrics and Gynaecology at The University of Nottingham, England. His main research interests involve the maternal and fetal renin-angiotensin systems, and hypertension in pregnancy, and he has written extensively on these subjects. He is Corresponding Editor of the *American Journal of Obstetrics and Gynecology*, Coeditor of the journal *Clinical and Experimental Hypertension in Pregnancy* (Marcel Dekker, Inc.), as well as Coeditor of Marcel Dekker, Inc.'s *Reproductive Medicine Series* of books. Dr. Symonds is a Fellow of the High Blood Pressure Council of the American Heart Association.

FREDERICK P. ZUSPAN is Professor and Chairman of the Department of Obstetrics and Gynecology at The Ohio State University College of Medicine, and Obstetrician-Gynecologist-in-Chief, University Hospitals and Clinics, Columbus, Ohio. Dr. Zuspan serves on the editorial board of many medical journals including Editor of the *American Journal of Obstetrics and Gynecology*, Founding Editor of *The Journal of Reproductive Medicine*, Associate Editor of *Obstetrical and Gynecological Survey*, and Coeditor of *Clinical and Experimental Hypertension in Pregnancy* (Marcel Dekker, Inc.). He is the author/coauthor of over 180 scientific articles, coeditor of four books and seven monographs, coauthor of one book, contributing author to numerous book chapters, and Coeditor of Marcel Dekker, Inc.'s *Reproductive Medicine Series* of books. Dr. Zuspan is a member of many professional societies including the American Gynecologic and Obstetric Society, American College of Obstetricians and Gynecologists, American College of Surgeons, Society of Gynecologic Investigation, Perinatal Research Society, American Society of Clinical Pharmacology and Therapeutics, and the International Society for the Study of Hypertension in Pregnancy.